FOOD MATTERS

Alonso Quijano's Diet and the Discourse of Food
in Early Modern Spain

Food Matters

Alonso Quijano's Diet and the Discourse of Food in Early Modern Spain

CAROLYN A. NADEAU

86 Tannahill   90
268, 270, 272, 273, 277
244 _ Malaguzzi (270)
264 Long Solis
112 ✓ 114
264 - Ferguson
260 Castro Martinez
186 - via
170 177 180

UNIVERSITY OF TORONTO PRESS
Toronto Buffalo London

ISBN 978-1-4426-3730-6

Library and Archives Canada Cataloguing in Publication

Nadeau, Carolyn A., 1963–, author
Food matters : Alonso Quijano's diet and the discourse of food in early modern Spain / Carolyn A. Nadeau.

(Toronto Iberic)
Includes bibliographical references and index.
ISBN 978-1-4426-3730-6 (bound)

1. Food habits – Spain – History.   2. Food habits – Social aspects – Spain –
History.   3. Food – Spain – History.   4. Food – Social aspects – Spain –
History.   5. Diet – Spain – History.   6. Gastronomy – Spain – History.
7. Spain – Social life and customs.   8. Cooking – Spain – History.   9. Cookery,
Spanish – History.   I. Title.   II. Series: Toronto Iberic

GT2853.S7N34 2016   394.1'20946   C2015-906107-5

University of Toronto Press acknowledges the financial assistance to its
publishing program of the Canada Council for the Arts and the Ontario Arts
Council, an agency of the Government of Ontario.

Canada Council   Conseil des Arts
for the Arts   du Canada

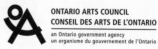

ONTARIO ARTS COUNCIL
CONSEIL DES ARTS DE L'ONTARIO
an Ontario government agency
un organisme du gouvernement de l'Ontario

Funded by the   Financé par le
Government   gouvernement
of Canada   du Canada

Canadä

To Mom and Dad

Contents

Illustrations

Preface

Why do we eat what we eat and what does it matter? These questions are at the root of this book on the role of food in the formation of identity in early modern Spain. Apart from the biological necessity that defines living beings' relationship with food, humans identify themselves both individually and collectively through the food they prepare and consume. Food events are constitutive moments that shape and are shaped by cultural, social, and even spiritual values. Used universally to celebrate rites of passage such as birth, marriage, and death, food is also one of the major defining elements of identity, whether it be national, regional, ethnic, or class based.

In addition to its resounding cultural significance, food carries enormous buying power and shifts economic policies of nations great and small. The medieval butchers' and bakers' guilds, the rise and fall of the Mesta (the powerful guild of sheep herders) during the Middle Ages and early modern period, or the legal ordinances and regulations that formed village policies on where and from whom people could buy foodstuffs are some of the ways that food shaped community identity in early modern Spain. Today we need only think of the million-dollar business deals that are brokered over lunch or the lobbying power of, for example, a certain multinational, agricultural biotechnology corporation to understand that food continues to dominate political and economic policy around the world.

Because of its tremendous role both historically and globally today, it is fitting to examine Spanish foodways as a cultural, social, and economic marker during the early modern period, a time when Spain's Hapsburg empire dominated the world landscape and then lost that position, a time when the country produced dozens of literary and visual artists that are still recognized for their creative genius, a time when the country, like others in Europe, experienced a gastronomic revolution with dramatic changes in the foodstuffs and methods of preparation.[1]

This study examines the representation of food in a multiplicity of discourses in early modern Spain. It considers cooking manuals as literary texts; brings to light the figurative significance of foodstuffs and food events in their literary, historic, and prescriptive contexts; and elucidates on food as an important historical cultural marker. Food merits study as a subject in and of itself because it is essential to life and creativity. It is also imperative to understand food representation because it reveals how and what individuals and society valued. These opinions are manifested in the voices of cooks, poets, villagers, lawmakers, and travellers who recorded their perceptions. I approach these texts primarily as a literary critic but I also draw from multiple disciplines including anthropology, sociology, economics, and history.

The legacy of structuralists Claude Lévi-Strauss and Mary Douglas, who have shown that food habits are culturally shaped and socially controlled, has opened the door to a wide variety of approaches to food practices in western society.[2] In Lévi-Strauss's seminal work, *The Raw and the Cooked*, he emphasizes binary oppositions, for example, between the raw and the cooked, arguing that "the raw/cooked axis is characteristic of culture ... since cooking brings about the cultural transformation of the raw" (142). Lévi-Strauss developed the now celebrated "triangle of recipes," in which he argues that types of cooking are representative of states of food (fig. 0.1).

Grilling and roasting are connected to the raw as these techniques directly expose food (and Lévi-Strauss focuses on meat) to the heat source. Smoking meat correlates with the cooked as smoking is a slower, more intentional process than grilling or roasting that involves a more thoughtful (cultural) transformational process. Boiling meat is directly associated with the rotten, a natural progression of both the raw and the cooked, as this technique requires a receptacle and even greater cultural input. His work on food is a result of his efforts to examine structures of human thought and an attempt to find universality encoded in the language and techniques of cooking.

Like Lévi-Strauss, Douglas looks at the complex web of foodways and social relations. However, she moves away from binary oppositions and the expectation of discovering a universal message in the way food is treated across cultures (62). In her study on British food she argues that food and eating encode social boundaries that are revealed

Figure 0.1. Lévi-Strauss's "Triangle of recipes."

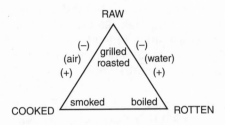

when one studies the daily, annual, and life-cycle patterns of eating. "Between breakfast and the last nightcap, the food of the day comes in an ordered pattern. Between Monday and Sunday, the food of the week is patterned again. Then there is the sequence of holidays and fast days through the year, to say nothing of life cycle feasts, birthdays, and weddings" (62). The structure of my investigation is thoroughly indebted to Douglas's notion of food patterns as I use the weekly meal of Alonso Quijano, Cervantes' humble hidalgo turned knight errant, to give meaning to food and the role it plays in understanding expressions of class hierarchy, cultural webs of inclusion and exclusion, and other forms of social identity.

Whether consciously or not, all work on food and identity has been influenced by the findings of both Lévi-Strauss and Douglas. The scholarship of structuralists, like Pierre Bourdieu, and developmentalists like Stephen Mennell, whose approaches heavily influence my own, are no exception. In developing his own theories of taste and social relations, Bourdieu took from Lévi-Strauss the idea that social systems reproduce themselves but, like Douglas, moved away from concepts of binary oppositions. He also drew from Karl Marx, Emile Durkheim, and Marcel Mauss, as he insisted that the taste for food needed to connect with taste for "high culture" in order to understand culture and organize social life.[3] In *Distinction: A Social Critique of the Judgement of Taste,* he looks at cultural preferences of different social classes and explains them as a combination of *habitus* and "fields." Bourdieu defines *habitus* as a complex set of social structures such as class, race, and gender that are reinforced through taste and culture. "Fields" consist of a set of social positions, i.e., a profession, and the power struggles that incur within that set. Finally, an individual's capital, whether it be economic, cultural, or symbolic, is another important variable in understanding both an individual's class position and that person's taste. Bourdieu's theory, which explains how preferences and subjectivities are produced both consciously as ideologies and unconsciously through daily practices such as cooking and eating, infuses my entire study of food and identity and is particularly relevant to issues of class in early modern Spain.

In Mennell's persuasive study *All Manners of Food*, he analyses changing food preferences and emerging cuisines as a reflection of the developments of the state in both England and France. Mennell notes that for sociologists concerned with the process of development, "modes of individual behaviour, cultural tastes, intellectual ideas, social stratification, political power and economic organization are all entangled with each other in complex ways" (15). Mennell seeks to understand how "changing structures of social interdependence and changing balances of power within society have been reflected in one particular cultural domain, that of food" (16). These complexities are very much present within the pages of my study on early modern food representations. In this book a dialogue of discourses that begins with cooking manuals and includes novels, plays, poems, travel logs, requisitions, lawsuits, and other legal proceedings brings to light how food is perceived from a multitude of perspectives. Together these representations uncover food's role as a cultural and social force that defines identity in terms of class, region, ethnicity, nutrition, and celebration in early modern Spain. These discourses also reveal patterns of interdependence as observed, for example, in how Muslim and Jewish aversion to pork played into Spain's passion for ham, how cities relied on towns' bread baking to feed its citizens, how foodstuffs imported from the New World entered into Old World kitchens, how scientific authorities rationalized that certain foodstuffs were appropriate for the elite and others for the working class, and how food and sexual urges so often came together, regardless of class, ethnicity, or gender at defining moments of communal celebration. Like Douglas's work on weekly food patterns that informs the entire structure of this study, so too does Mennell's strategy of examining food from various discourses to better understand the relationship between food and identity.

The methodology for this book is also informed by the work of cultural historians. In *The Culture of Food*, Massimo Montanari identifies the production, preparation, and consumption of food as cultural acts. The choices made on what to grow or raise; on how to prepare food; and how, when, where, and with whom to consume it are all decisive moments in the construction of individual and social identity. In particular his notion of how medical assertions of nutritional privilege affect class hierarchies shapes my research on food choices and social class in chapter 5. Several other historians in Spain, among them Manuela Marín, Joan Santanach i Suñol, Teresa de Castro Martínez, Juan Cruz Cruz, and María de los Ángeles Pérez Samper, are contextualizing gastronomic developments within the sociopolitical and historic trends of the day; their studies have been excellent resources for my own research.[4]

But I am, at heart, a literary critic and have read with fascination dozens of monographs and essays that have appeared in the last twenty or thirty years that have brought to light significant food practices in the works of European writers.[5] To understand what people ate at home in early modern Spain, we must turn to literature, to the fictional form that reflects human existence, daily life and struggles, and a search for, or perhaps a questioning of, taste and pleasure. In the early modern period, literature is also experiencing a revolution that peaks in the creation of the modern novel. Both the culinary and the literary arts foreground traditions of creating illusions. As Ronald Tobin so eloquently described in the opening to his study on food in Moliere, "The cook and the poet both work at *bricolage* – making something new out of something old – and through a process of selection, renovation, and imagination, they perform an archetypal, sacred, and creative act that produces original, complex products which change the consumer emotionally, intellectually, and physically" (4). Mennell, Montanari, and others deeply understood that cuisine is a product of a double orality: taste and language. The writer's role in the formation of food identity is almost as important as the food itself as an author's words can prove invaluable to understanding defining moments of culture.[6]

In literature, writers describe images of food that, in turn, define characters and regions, lend verisimilitude to the text, transform relationships, and offer a fixed social identity to readers. Food images create a culinary sense of materiality with which the readers can identify. For example, in Miguel de Cervantes' *Don Quixote* the essence of Alonso Quijano, the humble hidalgo who transforms into Don Quixote, is defined by the food he eats in the second sentence of the novel.

Una olla de algo más vaca que carnero, salpicón las más noches, duelos y quebrantos los sábados, lantejas los viernes, algún palomino de añadidura los domingos, consumían las tres partes de su hacienda. (69–70)[7]

[A stew made of more beef than mutton, cold salad on most nights, abstinence eggs on Saturdays, lentils on Fridays, and an additional squab on
Sundays consumed three quarters of his income.][8]

These dishes regularly consumed by Alonso Quijano give the readers
insight both into who he is and into the social values of Castile in the
early modern period. Cervantes summarizes the hidalgo's dietary habits as those consisting of one-pot meals and salads and guided by religious mores associated with abstinence and feasting. This single phrase,
together with the works of other early modern writers, confirms the
relationship between food and social inclusion and exclusion. It distinguishes midday meals from those taken at night. It accentuates the religious mores that guided a country's eating habits and sought to unify
Spain under one religion. His weekly food description recalls Spain's
history of multifaiths that, although it ended in the expulsion of both
Jews and Muslims, demonstrates the vestiges of both in Spain's culinary heritage. Through this single phrase, Cervantes alludes to food's
primacy in the early modern understanding of health and diet and also
references the role of food in celebrations, even those as simple as a
Sunday dinner. Undoubtedly, the early modern period is one of the biggest transformative moments for foodstuffs and food preparation in
Spain (as in other parts of Europe) due to Europe's contact with the
New World, but, as seen in the meals served in Alonso Quijano's home,
the basic food selections of the late sixteenth and early seventeenth centuries and how they are prepared come from long-established culinary
traditions that play a fundamental role in Spain's national and regional
gastronomy today.

Cervantes' introductory sentence, which sets the stage for understanding the novel's hero and is arguably the most discussed phrase
of food imagery in the early modern period, provides the structure for
this monograph. After an initial chapter on cooking manuals in Spain
before 1700, each subsequent chapter explores one of the five sections
that describe his diet – a stew made of more beef than mutton, cold
salad on most nights, abstinence eggs on Saturdays, lentils on Fridays,
and an additional squab on Sundays – in terms of identity construction.
Chapter 1, "El Ante: The Rise of Cooking Manuals in Spain," stands
apart from the other chapters as it focuses exclusively on cooking
manuals. It provides a much-needed and overdue examination of the
contributions of five medieval and four early modern cooking manuals to the development of Spanish cuisine. Cooking manuals are key

to understanding culinary history because, unlike any other discourse, they reveal what food was consumed and privileged and how dishes were prepared. Dietary treatises, regulations controlling the sale of prepared foods, etiquette manuals, novels, plays, and poems also contribute to our understanding of early modern foodways in Spain, but only cookbooks concentrate exclusively on food preparation from start to finish. Beginning with the notion that cookbooks conform to the characteristics of a "discourse colony," in other words, that their meaning is not derived from sequence and that the individual units do not form continual prose or depend on one another for meaning, this chapter explores notions of authorship and implied reader; the works' structures and shared culinary lexicon; strategies of imitation, from vague shared cultural tastes to cited sources; and diverse narrative voices that express pride, satisfaction, or even disappointment in describing different recipes.[9] In addition, it examines both the unique and repetitive features of each work that contribute to Spain's culinary history. A second reason for opening the monograph with a study of the most salient cookbooks of the day is that they define the cultural norms for food preparation and eating and, as such, are significant agents of cultural capital. To understand the culinary literature and history of Spain, one must return to these early manuscripts and books because they provide a foundation for subsequent culinary publications and offer insight into the cultural and social identity of the people of early modern Spain.

Chapter 2, "'Una olla de algo más vaca que carnero': Privileging Meat in the Early Modern Diet," examines food and identity in terms of class and draws primarily on the theories of Pierre Bourdieu, whose work in this area still dominates the field. In *Distinction* Bourdieu explains that individuals define themselves and are defined by larger force fields such as class or nation. Individual subjectivities are then produced in tension with others and practised, mostly unconsciously, in everyday habits like eating. In this chapter, meat's privileged position over vegetables and specifically, society's preference for mutton over beef, become signifiers for how class identity is tied to meat preferences. Through cookbooks, novels, plays, travellers' logs, and legal accounts we can understand how meat was regulated and consumed at different economic and regional levels of society and how it became a type of cultural capital which defined social status and played out even in the lives of fictional characters like Alonso Quijano. Other literary works by Mateo Alemán, Alonso de Contreras, Agustín de Rojas, Pedro Calderón de la Barca, Antonio Mira de Amescua, Antonio de Solís, and

Antonio de Guevara provide additional proof that meat is, without a doubt, a cultural marker of social status. However, upon careful study of who ate what meat and how often these texts reveal that meat preferences also present what Mennell terms "diminishing contrasts" between social classes. The chapter also addresses the other mainstay of any Spanish table, bread, and explains its place in the diet and social life of Spaniards living in the sixteenth and seventeenth centuries.

Chapter 3, "'Salpicón las más noches': Salads, Vegetables, and New World Contributions to Spanish Fare," turns away from meat to examine vegetables. This chapter explains how specific foodstuffs, for example, vinegar, lettuce, and four New World products that forever changed Spanish gastronomy – tomatoes, peppers, potatoes, and chocolate – impacted what was served at the early modern table and for which meal. Drawing from what Alonso Quijano eats for dinner, salpicon, this chapter seeks to answer the following series of questions. What do the ingredients of a traditional salpicon and its place on the table as an alternative to a salad dish tell us about dinner fare in the early modern period? What are the main ingredients in a salad in the early modern period and how do they differ from our understanding of a salad today? When do key ingredients of today's salpicon and salad, namely the tomato but, to a lesser extent, the pepper, and the potato, become part of the menu in Spain? And finally, how do writers across discourses describe and respond to Old World vegetables found in salpicon and salad, and New World products that are appearing in Spain for the first time. In the second part of the chapter Mary Louis Pratt's work on cultural contact points between the colonizer and the colonized proves useful in exploring the moment of confluence where traditions of the past blend with revolutionary discoveries from the New World. As food travelled into Spain we witness a key stage of transculturation through food that laid the groundwork for revolutionizing Spanish cuisine. Using the tomato, potato, pepper, and chocolate, and the literary works of Bernardino de Sahagún, Tirso de Molina, Sor Marcela de San Félix, Gabriel Lobo Lasso de la Vega, Cervantes, Agustín Moreto, and Mariana de Caravajal, whose works reveal a curiosity for New World products, this chapter shows how New World "peripheral" products transform "metropolitan" Western world food identity in unprecedented ways.

Shifting gears away from food revolutions, chapter 4, "'Duelos y quebrantos los sábados': Jewish and Muslim Influences on Early Modern Eating Habits," examines how longstanding Jewish and Muslim food traditions contributed to Spain's gastronomy. Both chapters 3 and 4 examine moments of transculturation but while the former looks at the introduction of new foodstuffs, the latter defines and deciphers different ethnic contributions to long-established culinary contact zones. This chapter explores how specific foodstuffs from pork to rosewater to eggs shaped culinary habits of the early modern period not only through food taboos and defining cultural otherness but also through repeated usage and cultural integration. It compares the cooking of Jews and Muslims stating both their commonalties and their unique features. Rather than drawing from many literary sources as seen in chapters 2 and 3, the latter part of chapter 4 focuses on one specific work, Francisco Delicado's picaresque novel *La lozana andaluza* to make connections between the food memories of the protagonist Aldonza and the elite cooking manuals of Al-Andalus, Aragon, and Castile. Aldonza's selective and seductive food memories do more than position the reader in her childhood kitchen. Using Stoler and Strassler's research on food and memory, we find that Francisco Delicado's fictional account of a *conversa*'s kitchen memories becomes key to understanding Spain's culinary history as it reveals similarities and differences between Jewish and Muslim kitchens and how these two ethnic groups shaped the Spanish cuisine of the early modern period. Aldonza's famous culinary passage, coupled with cooking manuals and other legal and prescriptive discourses, stands as the nexus between the food habits of Jewish, Muslim, and Christian ethnicities, between elite and underprivileged communities, and across centuries.

While chapters 3 and 4 examine how different foodstuffs and cuisines contributed to the shaping of Spain's early modern gastronomy, chapter 5 returns to issues of food consumption and the making of social identity explored in chapter 2 but here, focuses on food's role in the perception of nutrition and spirituality. "'Lantejas los viernes': Perceptions of Health and Christian Abstinence" examines the way in which writers, doctors, and cooks wrote about lentils and other legumes and how specific food items played into concepts of privilege, both nutritional and spiritual. In terms of nutrition the chapter summarizes important natural philosophical texts specifically related to the theory of humorism. In particular, the chapter draws on the work of the medieval doctor Ibn Zuhr, whose writing went on to influence Maimonides, Arnau de Vilanova, and other medical writers through the early modern era. Ibn Zuhr explained specific foodstuffs in terms of the theory of humorism and in turn, these accepted notions of nutrition formed part of a theory of nutritional privilege. Massimo Montanari's work on nutritional privilege informs the interpretation of literary responses to food's connection to privilege and health that follows. For Montanari, medical treatises on nutrition produced the type of social stratification that ruling classes embraced. This accepted principle was found not only in learned treatises on natural philosophy but also in the fictional pages of *Don Quixote* and works by other writers. Plays by Lope de Vega and Tirso de Molina, Quevedo's picaresque novel *El buscón*, the travel journals of Madame d'Aulnoy and Albert Jouvin, Sephardic poetry, and a treatise on Trinitarian Reform penned by San Juan Bautista de la Concepción all discuss lentils and other pulses as food for the poor or as a marker of spirituality. Cervantes and Juan Luis Vives, among others, also exemplify how eggs have restorative properties that, like lentils, were frequently associated with religious dietary restrictions. The latter part of the chapter looks at Spain's eating practices during periods of abstinence and shows how they differ from those of other European countries and how consuming lentils and other pulses demonstrated religious identity.

Food choices reflect not only dietary and nutritional values but also notions of community and celebration. In chapter 6, "'Algún palomino de añadidura los domingos': The Theatrics of Food and Celebration," these concepts are explored with particular focus on how acts of feasting and celebration are played out on the stage. The chapter begins with poultry, its place on the king's table, its significance as a social marker, and how writers used various fowl in their works. The chapter then explores celebratory meals more generally by examining both real banquets and imagined ones. Drawing from Ficino's banquet of senses, today's sociological theories on the banquet, and primary texts that record banquets both real and imagined, we can see how both real and fictional representations of banquets recognize and celebrate the established social order. Lévi-Strauss's early work on binary oppositions within food choices is effective for understanding food on the early modern stage. Literary artists such as Lope de Rueda, Ruiz de Alarcón, and Cervantes, whose characters create fictional banquets, delve into perceptions of desire and combine food fantasies with sexual ones. Writers take the biological need of eating as survival and convert it into a site of feasting, social pleasure, and social order. By comparing contemporary cookbooks, shopping lists, dietary manuals, and early modern representations of banquets we can understand more fully the meaning of celebratory foods in early modern Spain and their contribution to the cultural identity of Spain.

After chapter 7, "*La sobremesa*: Final Reflections on the Discourse of Food in Early Modern Spain," which offers some concluding remarks about the complexity of food discourse in early modern Spain, the appendix brings together a number of medieval and early modern recipes that are discussed throughout the book. My hope is that readers may try a couple of them, perhaps share with students in the classroom, and savour the tastes of the early modern era.

My intention in writing this book is to add to the rich conversation of Spain's gastronomic heritage. In the following chapters readers will learn about the history of specific foodstuffs, the way medieval and early modern writers described food events and infused them with meaning, and how food is intimately tied to notions of identity. I hope that readers will gain a deeper appreciation for how early modern foodways influenced and were influenced by the many cultural, social, and economic practices that inform Spain's history. Finally, it is also my aim to enrich our understanding of literature by highlighting how food shapes literature and to inspire further research on topics that are raised in this work but not fully developed such as the staging of food in the *comedia*, diet and hygiene, food and sex, and food and material culture, because ultimately, in life and in fiction, food matters.

Acknowledgments

Humble words of gratitude could never sufficiently express my heartfelt thanks to my family and many friends and colleagues who have listened patiently, read over sections of this book, and time and again offered their wise counsel. I am so fortunate to have such unconditional support from all of you. I begin then by acknowledging my partner, Chad Sanders, who knows this work better than anyone and who has discussed every aspect of it with me, morning, noon, and night. I'd like to think that while discussing food in the early modern era and trying out some of the recipes mentioned within these pages he has enjoyed our dialogues and culinary experiments as much as I have. Thank you, my friend. I would also like to acknowledge the support of our children, Miranda, Camille, Daniel, and Ethan who have grown up with the project, and probably now know more than they want to know about tomatoes, eggplant, and mutton stew! They have accepted my absences from home, sometimes with a grumble or two, and know how important conference presentations, research at libraries and archives, and time for writing are for my research and professional identity. I would also like to thank my siblings, who share my passion for food and have provided words of love and support and a healthy sense of humour at stressful times in the years during the writing of this book. And of course, I deeply appreciate my parents, to whom I dedicate this book, for instilling in me a sense of inquiry and a spirit of adventure, and for their unconditional love.

In addition to family, I am also grateful to my friends and role models, Carmela Ferradáns, Kathleen Montgomery, and Lynda Duke, with whom I have gathered on more than one occasion to share extraordinary meals and discuss our scholarly and artistic pursuits. Carmela's close readings of many sections of this book and her advice based on my countless food inquiries have inspired significant changes to the book. My friendship with all of them has deepened over the years and their encouragement has proved vital to both my work and general sanity. Also, I am grateful to Virginia Bell for her insights as she read over parts of the project. Her feedback, in particular regarding literary theory and New World-Old World food exchanges, enhanced both the introduction and chapter 3. Carlota Larrea and Cristina Sáenz de Tejada have also provided me with long-distance support for which I am deeply grateful, as well as Luis F. Hebrero, Concha Valderas, and Guille Fernández, who have fed me countless times while in Spain and taught Chad and me the secret to a perfect tortilla. And, I deeply appreciate the Sunday dinner group – Ken, Mary, Laura, Giovanni, Dave, and Amanda – all of whom have been incredibly supportive throughout the project.

I would also like to thank my distant mentor and friend, Charles Ganelin, who regularly shares excellent scholarship with me. Our years of email exchanges and, when possible, live conversations over taste, gastronomy, and food representations in literature have helped to keep me current and been an incredible source of validation for this project. I would also like to thank Howard Mancing, Steve Wagschal, Javier Irigoyen, Valeria Finucci, Kate Regan, Fr. Liddy, and Rita de Maeseneer who have invited me to speak on sections of these projects at their respective institutions. At these lectures and other conference presentations, I have found feedback from colleagues and students invaluable. Conference presentations in Spain have proved especially helpful as anecdotes from scholars familiar with different regions of Spain have helped to clarify uses of spices, ways of making bread, wine varieties, and other subtleties that complement information from primary written texts. I am especially indebted to Joan Santanach who patiently clarified many of my questions regarding the *Sent Soví*. I would also like to thank Fred de Armas who, as dissertation advisor began counselling me over twenty years ago, continues to serve as an outstanding role model.

I would also like to acknowledge the excellent work of the librarians and archivists at the National Library of Spain and the Regional Archives of the Community of Madrid. These nameless people have assisted in uncovering documents that may have gone unnoticed were it not for their help. The Rare Books librarian at the University of Illinois, Urbana-Champaign, Jane Somera, was also helpful in locating some of the earliest visual representations of tomatoes and other food stuffs.

Another large debt of gratitude is for Natalia Maillard who transcribed dozens of legal documents to provide me with regulations on, among other things, the weight of bread, the sale of prepared food at roadside establishments, and the census of household possessions in sixteenth-century Spanish villages.

Finally, I would like to acknowledge the institutions that offered financial support for this project. In its earliest stage, the Spanish Ministry of Culture supported this project with a Program for Cultural Cooperation Grant. Additionally, I have received substantial support from Illinois Wesleyan University which provided me with two Artistic and Scholarly Development grants and a sabbatical leave, and has contributed to the production costs of this publication. I have taught at Illinois Wesleyan for over twenty years and continued to feel incredibly privileged to work with such outstanding colleagues and gifted students. In particular, I have shared sections of this research with the students of the 2012 senior seminar, "*Don Quijote* y su legado cultural," and with students in the culture class, "Food as Social Signifier in Early Modern Spain," and in both cases students have raised insightful questions about food representation in literary texts.

Sections of this book have appeared in earlier publications and I thank the editors of the following journals for permission to incorporate sections of those publications into this book. In chapter 1, "Contributions of Medieval Food Manuals to Spain's Culinary Heritage," Monographic Issue of *Cincinnati Romance Review,* "Writing About Food: Culinary Literature in the Hispanic World," ed. María Paz Moreno (winter 2012) 59–77 and "Early Modern Spanish Cookbooks: The Curious Case of Diego Granado," *Food and Language: Proceedings of the Oxford Symposium on Food and Cookery 2009,* ed. Richard Hosking, Totnes, England: Prospect Books, 2010, 237–46. In chapter 2, "Critiquing the Elite in the Barataria and 'Ricote' Food Episodes in *Don Quijote II,*" *Hispanófila* 146 (Jan. 2006): 59–75, and "Spanish Culinary History in Cervantes' 'Bodas de Camacho,'" *Revista canadiense de estudios hispánicos* 29.2 (winter 2005): 347–61. In chapter 4, "'Duelos y quebrantos los sábados': la influencia judía y musulmana en la dieta del s. XVII," *Comentarios a Cervantes: Actas selectas del VIII Congreso international de la Asociación de Cervantistas,* ed. Emilio Martínez Mata and María Fernández Ferreiro (Oviedo: Fundación María Cristina Masaveu Peterson, 2014), 236–44. And, finally, in chapter 6, "Sweetmeats and Preserves: Food, Eroticism, and Society in Lope de Rueda's *Pasos,*" *Texto y espectáculo: Selected Proceedings of the Fifteenth International Golden Age Spanish Theater*

Symposium (March 8–11, 1995) at the University of Texas, El Paso, ed. José Luis Suárez García (York, SC: Spanish Literature Publications, 1996), 86–94. Finally, I would like to extend my heartfelt thanks to Suzanne Rancourt, executive editor at the University of Toronto Press, and to Barb Porter, associate managing editor, for their encouragement and patience throughout the process; to Miriam Skey, for her incomparable copy editing; and to the readers of my manuscript whose insightful comments significantly improved this work.

FOOD MATTERS

Alonso Quijano's Diet and the Discourse of Food
in Early Modern Spain

El Ante: The Rise of Cooking Manuals in Spain

todas son cosas mias, y ninguna escrita por relacion de nadie

[All of these (recipes) are mine, and none are written by the hand of another]
Martínez Montiño, on the originality of his cookbook

Cooking manuals hold a preeminent position in understanding culinary history because, unlike dietary treatises, regulations controlling the sale of prepared foods, etiquette manuals, novels, plays, poetry, and other discourses that contribute to our understanding of early modern foodways in Spain, cookbooks directly link consumption of food and the consumption of the text as a commodity. Rarely read start to finish, like a conventional novel, they are nonetheless literary texts in their own right filled with authorial pride, passionate narrative voices, and acute attentiveness to the reader. Although cookbooks do not form continuous prose, most begin with a prologue and conform to some internal organization and accepted structural norms. They are generally thought of as examples of discourse colony, a type of narrative whose individual parts do not depend on one another for its meaning.[1] Cooking manuals are collections of individual units, much like books of poems or short stories, and readers most often focus on a particular section while only briefly skimming other parts of the work. Individual recipes determine crucial ingredients, but that very determination opens the dish to potentially infinite variations. They are a key site for transmitting history and memory. And when studied as a genre, cultural values emerge through the patterns of foodstuffs, cooking methods, and presentations that recur. Just as values shift within the marketplace, there is no one fixed meaning in cookbooks.

Cooking manuals from the Middle Ages and early modern period are elitist by nature but, when studied in conjunction with other discourses, reveal food habits of a wider social spectrum. This chapter looks exclusively at cooking manuals and explores notions of authorship and implied reader; the works' structures and shared culinary lexicon; strategies of imitation, from vague shared cultural tastes to cited sources; and diverse narrative voices that express pride, satisfaction, or even disappointment in describing different recipes. In addition, this chapter examines the unique and/or comparative features of each work that contribute to Spain's culinary history. To understand the culinary literature and history of Spain, one must return to these early manuscripts and books because they provide a foundation for subsequent culinary publications and, together with other discourses, offer insight into the cultural and social identity of the people of early modern Spain.

Manuscripts

Before Johannes Gutenberg (c. 1400–68) revolutionized printing with his discovery of moveable type, manuscripts of collected recipes from the Iberian Peninsula grew out of several traditions. Most notable are two manuscripts directed towards the urban aristocracy from the waning years of the Almohad dynasty (1130–1269), two works from the aristocracy of Aragon and Castile, and one woman's manual that weaves food recipes in with others dealing with home remedies, cosmetics, and general hygiene.[2] Before reviewing details of each, it should be noted that, contrary to what Martínez Montiño professes in his prologue (that all the recipes contained in his work are his and only his), no manuscripts (and subsequent published cooking manuals) are the work of any one single author. Even those that carry the name of an individual, like Ibn Razīn al-Tuğībī (1227–93), author of *Fuḍālat-al-Hiwan Fi Tayyibat al-Ta'am Wa-l-Alwan* (*Relieves de la mesa acerca de las delicias de la comida y los diferentes platos*) [The delicacies of the table and the finest of foods and dishes], are better understood as a compilation of previous works that have been amended along the way by other cooks.[3] As we will see in the works explored below, recipes overlap from one to another, sometimes word for word and at other times in a modified version that reflect changes in taste, regional shifts, or changing political and economic interests. It should also be noted that while several manuscripts may share certain common ingredients, or exhibit parallel recipes, we cannot assume that a direct influence from one to the other has necessarily taken place. There are too many unknown factors, lost manuscripts, or oral traditions that may account for overlaps in manuals. The strong possibility of an "*ur*-version," as Terence Scully reminds us in his introduction to *The Vivendier*, makes the likelihood of claiming anything more than shared cultural tastes difficult (19). Another important commonality is the actual production of the manuals, or more specifically, the errors common to scribes, copyists, and later typesetters and publishers who modified the works both intentionally and unintentionally. As Joan Santanach points out in his introduction to *Libro de Sent Soví* [Book of Sent Soví], cooking manuals, even more than literary, historical, and juridical texts, were subject to continuous modifications (*Libro* 19–20). With these commonalities and modifications in mind, we can examine the following manuscripts and begin to understand how they set the stage for early modern publications on food preparation and presentation.

Fuḍalat-al-Hiwan Fi Tayyibat al-Ta'am Wa-l-Alwan

One of the earliest manuscripts available to us today is the *Fuḍālat-al-Hiwan Fi Tayyibat al-Ta'am Wa-l-Alwan* (*Relieves de la mesa acerca de las delicias de la comida y los diferentes platos*) by Murcia-born Ibn Razīn al-Tuğībī (1227–93).[4] This work was first edited in 1960 by Fernando de la Granja Santamaría and later, in 2007, by Manuela Marín.[5] She summarizes the text's place within Arabic traditions and establishes its link with secretaries, chancellors, and other court members who aspired to define themselves by their modes of behaviour and eating habits (24–8).[6] Another manuscript, *Kitāb al-tabīj fi l-Magrib wa-l-Andalus fi 'asr al-muwahhudin li-mu'allif mayhul* (*Tratado sobre cocina en el Magrib y al-Andalus en época almohade, de autor desconocido*) [Treatise on cooking from the Magreb and Al-Andalus during Almohad period by an anonymous author], comes from the same period but is an anonymous work.[7] It was first published by Ambrosio Huici Miranda in 1961–2 as an article from a manuscript discovered by George S. Colin.[8] In 2005 Trea re-edited the work under the title *La cocina hispano-magrebí durante la época almohade. Según un manuscrito anónimo del siglo XIII traducido por Ambrosio Huici Miranda* [Hispano-Maghreb cooking during the Almohad period. From an anonymous, thirteenth-century manuscript translated by Ambrosio Huici Miranda] and included Manuela Marín's biographical introduction on Huici Miranda and his contributions to the study of Western Islamic cuisine.[9]

Although for the purposes of this study the focus of these works is their contribution to the development of Spanish cuisine, it is important to recognize that they also form part of a long-standing tradition of medieval Arab cooking manuscripts that date back to the tenth century. When Bagdad stood as one of the flourishing cultural capitals of the world, gastronomy, like poetry or music, was a sign of distinction (Huici Miranda 27). From the thirteenth century, four manuscripts are available to us today, two from the Abbasid dynasty (750–1258) in the East and the two, already cited, from the Almohad dynasty in the West. Critics agree that the manuals from Al-Andalus reflect dishes consumed by the urban elite, a group that shares class status but cuts across religious and ethnic boundaries. David Waines summarizes well when he states that "the culinary manuals implicitly represent the cooking customs of the broader-based artisan-scholar-bureaucratic segments of urban Andalusi society" (726). Furthermore, derivations of these recipes, that might include a simpler cut of meat or fewer spices, could be found at the table of the urban poor or at the country table. Likewise, a more enhanced version might be found at the tables of the more privileged.

Ibn Razīn spent his early years in his native town and continued to live there even after it converted to a *mudéjar* town.[10] But, as Christian-Muslim relations became more hostile and Muslim elite could no longer maintain their way of life in Spain, his family left Al-Andalus to move to Ceuta in North Africa (1248). In both urban centres he is part of the intellectual elite and maintains that connection throughout his adult life in Bugia, Tunis, and other Maghreb cities. In fact, throughout his life he penned various historic, literary, and poetic texts as cited both by his contemporaries and biographers (Marín, *Relieves* 21). Unfortunately the only work to have survived is his *Fuḍālat-al-Hiwan Fi Tayyibat*. It consists of an introduction and an impressive 432 recipes divided into twelve sections which the author summarizes at the end of his introduction: bread and other grain-based recipes (98), meat (90), fowl (79), Sanhagi-style recipes (3), fish and eggs (41), dairy products (13), vegetables (35), legumes (8), sweets (25), pickled and preserved food and oils (28), locust, shrimp, and snails (3), and soaps and scented powders (9).[11]

In his introduction, Ibn Razīn states in which order food should be consumed. Specifically, heavy food in need of greater digestion should be eaten first: dairy products, thick soups, harissas, pasta, fatty cuts of beef and mutton, dried beef, fish, and fried grains. Vegetables are also consumed first, not because they need the more intense digestive powers of the lower stomach but rather because they relax the digestive tract (74). Next are the other savoury items while one should finish with sweet items, fruit, and roasts. He promotes cleanliness in the kitchen, a theme repeated throughout recipe books of the early modern era. "En mi opinión, la primera exigencia del arte de cocinar es evitar para ello los lugares sucios y desagradables" [In my opinion, the first requirement of the art of cooking is to avoid dirty and disagreeable areas for cooking] (73). Citing a doctor as an authoritative source, he admonishes that red clay vessels should not be used more than once for cooking and white clay vessels, no more than five times.[12] Gold, silver, iron, and glass are the recommended materials for cooking and copper should be avoided (73).

Similar to other manuscripts in the Islamic world and in the Christian part of Spain and to later printed cookbooks of the early modern period, the *Fuḍālat-al-Hiwan Fi Tayyibat* embraces a culinary lexicon shared by cookbook writers in Europe and the Arab-speaking world (27). Ibn Razīn relies on the experience of the cook to calculate precise step-by-step instructions and cooking times (27). His recipes range from simple ones, possibly drawn from popular dishes, to very complex ones that include sophisticated procedures like deboning a hen and stuffing it without removing the skin (Marín, *Relieves* 52). Like all authors throughout these centuries, Ibn Razīn does not feel compelled to cite most sources. He proudly announces that he has created many of the recipes and that he favours Andalusian food: "me he mostrado parcial hacia la comida andalusí, proclamando que los andalusíes, en este capítulo y los relacionados con él, son gente de celo y progreso, a pesar de que hayan llegado tarde a la invención gastronómica" [I am partial to Andalusian food and proclaim, in this chapter and in other related chapters, that Andalusians are progressive people, full of zeal in spite of the fact that they were late in discovering the invention of gastronomy] (72).

Manuela Marín points out both the similarities with other Arab recipe manuscripts and the unique features of Ibn Razīn's (*Relieves* 26–7). Additionally, she identifies grains as the most important staple of the thirteenth-century urban elite diet in Muslim Spain. She also points out that of all the recipes those for grains have the most variety (*Relieves* 53). Another curiosity of Ibn Razīn's work is that he includes no less than five recipes for bread. Modern readers may think this appropriate as bread was arguably the most important food consumed in the West until relatively recently, but few, if any, medieval or early modern European cookbooks include bread recipes. The grain section is

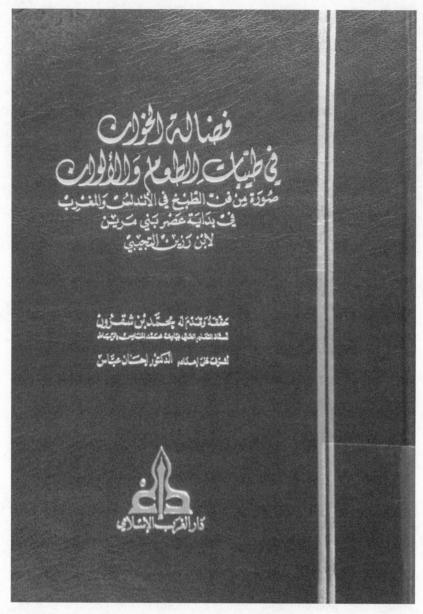

Figure 1.1. Front cover of *Faḍālat al-khiwān fī ṭayyibāt al-ṭaʿām wa-al-alwān: ṣūrah min fann al-ṭabkh fī al-Andalus wa-al-Maghrib fī bidāyat ʿaṣr Banī Marīn* by Ibn Razīn al-Tujībī (Bayrūt: Dār al-Gharb al-Islāmī, 1984).

rightly the first section of the manuscript and the most intense of all the sections because of the number of recipes, the variety of cooking methods, and the versatility of grains as corroborated by recipes made from both whole grains and flours like *panes* [breads], *sopas desmigadas* [soups and stews made with a base of breadcrumbs soaked in animal fat], *gachas* [porridge], a variety of pasta, and an endless list of grain-based pastries.[13]

Marín notes that pepper, cilantro, cinnamon, saffron, and ginger are by far the most used spices in cooking and she illustrates how expensive ingredients and elaborate modes of production distinguish elite eating habits from those of the general population (*Relieves* 30).[14] For me, this manuscript raises questions about the development of cuisine in Spain from the thirteenth century onwards. For example, the use of pasta in many forms (couscous, *fideos* [fine soup noodles], *aletrías* [angel hair noodles]) is fundamental to Hispanic-Muslim cuisine yet today few people associate pasta with this part of Spanish cultural heritage.[15] Conversely, everyone knows the connection between rice, key to Spanish culinary and economic identity today and to Muslim contributions to Spanish culinary history, but rice only appears in three recipes. Why, then, did couscous fall out of favour and rice rise in popularity?

A similar question arises when considering other individual foodstuffs. Take, for example, the eggplant, a common ingredient first to Isalmic Spain and then to the rest of the Iberian Peninsula. In *Fuḍālat-al-Hiwan* there are no fewer than twenty-two recipes dedicated to eggplant (Ibn Razīn 268–77). Later, in the early modern period it continues to be associated with Muslims. One need only look to *Don Quixote* in which Sancho confuses the narrator's name, Cide Hamete Benengeli, with the Spanish word for *eggplant* and mistakenly calls the narrator, Cide Hamete *Berenjena* (Cervantes, *El ingenioso hidalgo* 2.57), to understand that food and people are intimately connected. Yet its Islamic identity was slowly erased, its "otherness" consumed, and today eggplant is ubiquitous in Spanish cuisine. Conversely, cilantro, another food item common to Hispanic-Muslim cooking, did not find its way into Spanish culinary history; rather it was replaced by parsley.[16] Marín explains that cilantro, together with black pepper and cinnamon, were the most commonly used spices/herbs (*Relieves* 39). One wonders how rice and eggplant successfully transitioned into national food items and couscous and cilantro did not. What role might the early modern cooking manuals have played in the success of some food items and the failure of others? How might cultural and culinary values from other parts of Europe be informing the development of Spanish taste? In short, how does cultural and social capital intersect with food habits to determine national and regional cuisines? Similar questions arise with the success of almonds and the diminishment of sesame, or the similar fates of saffron and cinnamon, respectively.

Perhaps what most uniquely defines Ibn Razīn's work is his pastry section. As Marín states in her introduction, "Es en este capítulo ... donde se encuentran muchas de las recetas más típicamente andalusíes de todo el recetario" [It is in this chapter ... where many of the most typical Andalusian recipes of the whole manuscript are found] (54). In this section he introduces a wide variety of flours, fats, and sweeteners, as well as cooking methods and finishing touches. Many recipes include nuts or dried fruit and pastries are often sprinkled with sugar or drizzled with honey before consumption.

Kitāb al-tabīj

Somewhat larger and less organized than Ibn Razīn's manuscript, the contemporary *Kitāb al-tabīj fi l-Magrib wa-l-Andalus fi 'asr al-muwahhudin li-mu'allif mayhul (Tratado sobre cocina en el Magrib y al-Andalus en época almohade, de autor desconocido)* [The book of cooking in Maghreb and al-Andalus in the era of Almohads, by an unknown author] resembles a random composite of over 500 recipes from different authors.[17] As Huici Miranda states in his introduction, the recipes are "bastante desordenadas en su clasificación" [very disorganized in their classification] (46). The manuscript begins with stuffed and chopped meats, roasts, and stews, and then turns to a dish prepared Jewish-style, advice on what to eat, regional customs, what utensils to use, and how to serve dishes. Huici Miranda notes a new direction in the manuscript when it turns to lamb recipes, then *almojábanas* [fried cheese pastries], and different savoury and sweet pies.[18] In this section one finds scattered throughout a recipe for eggplant, another for stuffed eggs, meat dishes, sweet dishes, dishes for the sick, and some for the changing seasons of the year. Another chapter includes recipes from specific people, another focuses on fish dishes, another returns to pies but also includes pasta, rice, harissa, and other bread dishes, some stuffed with meat. A different section focuses on vegetable stews and includes ten different sweet dishes. This pastiche of recipes makes up 488 of the 545 recipes. The final five sections are from a different, also anonymous, text and include medicinal syrups, pastes, extracts, powders, and gels.

One of the unique features of this anonymous work is the inclusion of several Jewish recipes. Two are pheasant dishes prepared Jewish style; another is a chicken recipe. The "Plato judío relleno oculto" [Jewish dish with hidden stuffing] provides a unique take on spaghetti and meatballs. The recipe is divided into several stages. First, the meat is mashed, seasoned, and cooked with onion juice, olive oil, and rose water while covered with a heavy rag. It is then mashed again, "aromatized," and shaped into tiny meatballs that are then set aside. Two different types of pasta are prepared with eggs, salt, pepper, and cinnamon; one must be a thin pasta. Once these three parts are made, in a new pot oil is heated and one of the pastas is added and covered with the meat, which, in turn, is covered by the other pasta. Once compiled, another mixture of white flour, eggs seasoned with black pepper, cinnamon, and rose water, and what remains of the meat is poured over the top. The pot is covered and placed over medium-high heat. When done, the pot is broken; the inside is removed, placed on a platter, and garnished with mint, pistachio, pine nuts, and aromatic condiments (149–50). This and other recipes contribute to our understanding of medieval Jewish eating habits, as there are no cookbooks today that focus specifically on Jewish cuisine in medieval Spain.

Other recipes in the *Kitāb al-tabīj* acknowledge regions or specific authors. At the end of "Receta de la 'almojábana'" [Recipe for fried cheese pastries], the author identifies with Al-Andalus and mentions several of the cities where *almojábanas* are prepared: "Así lo hace la gente de nuestra tierra en el Oeste de al-Andalus, como en Córdoba y Sevilla, Jerez y otras del país de Occidente [This is how people in our land in the west of Al-Andalus make it, like in Cordoba and Seville, Jerez, and others from the country in the West] (246). At times the author acknowledges the original inventor of the dish. For example, the recipe, "Torta con carne de cordero y espinacas, leche fresca y manteca fresca" [Lamb meat pie with spinach, fresh milk, and fresh animal fat], begins with a history of the dish: "La hacía en Córdoba en los días de primavera el médico Abu-l-Hasan al-Bunani" [This dish was made in springtime in Cordoba by the doctor Abu-l-Hasan al-Bunani] (227). Other fascinating aspects of this cooking manual are the apparent inconsistencies between title and recipe. "Hechura de liebre" [Making (a dish of) hare] contains no hare (210), "Hechura de esclavos" [Making (a dish for) slaves] is a minced lamb dish made with top cuts of meat, certainly not food slaves would eat (200). Another, "Torta de vinagre, que es una de las mejores" [Vinegar pie, that is one of the best], intrigues the reader as "vinegar pie" is not at first appealing but one is drawn to read through the recipe to see what makes it "the best." As it turns out, in the end it is a couscous recipe, mounded with stewed meat, turnips, eggplant, and squash, and flavoured with the perfect amount of vinegar, "hasta que se note su gusto" [until its flavour is noted] (225). Like Ibn Razīn's manual, this one also has an abundance of eggplant (some two dozen) and other vegetable recipes. Finally, found in both manuals, and different from those of the East, are abundant recipes for beef and multiple uses of eggs. Waines notes that a popular method of finishing a recipe was to cover the dish with a layer of beaten eggs and seasonings (732–3). This use of egg batter as a finisher is also found in later, Christian cooking manuals, for example, the anonymous *Sent Soví* (c. 1324) or Maestre Rupert's *Libre de coch* [Book of cookery] (1520).[19]

The flavours of Hispano-Muslim cooking traditions are found in early modern Spanish cooking and continue to be enjoyed today. Foodstuffs such as rice, couscous, eggplant, spinach, bitter oranges, sugar, cinnamon, ginger, and saffron that were introduced and/or enhanced by Arabs, Syrians, and Berbers when they came to the Iberian Peninsula prevail in both cooking manuals and literature of the early modern period. In the major recipe manuals of the sixteenth and seventeenth centuries by Nola, Granado, and Martínez Montiño, we see the use of rose water in sauces, sweets made from sugar and nuts, recipes for couscous, pasta, and egg dishes that are shared with both the *Fuḍālat-al-Hiwan Fi Tayyibat* and the *Kitāb al-tabīj*. But before jumping ahead, we must examine the culinary manuscripts of the fourteenth and fifteenth centuries, ones written in Christian Spain that provide continued insight into the food habits of the Iberian Peninsula.

Libre de Sent Soví

Libre de Sent Soví (1st half of 14th c.) is an anonymous work most undoubtedly compiled from the kitchens of multiple cooks. As is the case with the anonymous *Kitāb al-tabīj* and most other medieval cooking manuals, critics agree that the author of *Sent Soví* collected recipes from earlier sources and brought them together to form a singular text. As Joan Santanach explains in his introduction to the Spanish edition of the text, "Lejos, pues, de ser obra de un solo autor, se trata de un texto que refleja buena parte de las preferencias y de los conocimientos culinarios de toda una etapa de la historia de la gastronomía catalana"

[Far from being the work of a single author, we are dealing, then, with a text that reflects a large part of the culinary preferences and knowledge of an entire stage of the history of Catalan gastronomy] (*Libro de Sent Soví* 18).[20] Santanach reports that at one point the *Sent Soví* probably contained nearly one hundred recipes – considerably more modest than the Hispanic-Muslim treatises – but that the manuscript available today shows seventy-two recipes. However, of those seventy-two only fifty-eight are consistent with prior *Sent Soví* manuscripts (17–19).

One of the commonalities most medieval and early modern cooking manuals share is a prologue to the text. Generally, prologues explain why the text was written, for whom, and under whose authority. The *Sent Soví* is no exception. In this case, the anonymous author explains that he is writing the book so squires and others who serve nobility can prepare meals in an appropriate way. The author's brief prologue ends with confirmation that others who have experienced these recipes (squires, cooks, ministers, servants, subjects of lords) agree with their excellent quality (*The Book of Sent Soví* 40).[21]

To the untrained eye, this collection of recipes may seem haphazard but Joan Santanach argues that "en su composición hubo una intervención deliberada, quizá a veces un poco intuitiva, que favoreció la creación de núcleos de recetas afines" [in its composition, there was a deliberative, and perhaps an intuitive, arrangement that favoured the creation of groups of related recipes] (32). Santanach points out that of the fifty-eight initial recipes, some twenty deal exclusively with the preparation of all types of sauces: white, camel, lemon, half-roast, goose, game meat, any kind of meat, parsley, vinegar, fish, mushroom, garlic cheese, green sauce, cheese, eel or onion (32). Other groupings are found for preserving meat, broths, dishes appropriate for Lent, stuffings, fried pastries, and vegetable and bean dishes. Santanach also notes that the first forty recipes are eaten from a bowl with bread or a spoon and that they are grouped separately from the remaining recipes which are meat or fish dishes that are roasted, grilled, breaded, fried, poached, or boiled (34).

In comparing this Catalan manuscript to the Arabic ones written in the previous century, one finds curious and significant differences as well as similarities. The most obvious difference is the inclusion of two pork recipes and the use of lard in several others in the *Sent Soví* that reflects the accepted religious eating practices of the respective groups. What is more intriguing is that in the *Sent Soví* parsley has replaced cilantro. In fact, there are three different parsley sauce recipes that find no comparison in the earlier texts. Additionally, the herbs marjoram, sage, basil, and oregano are used throughout this cooking manual and are not significantly present in the earlier ones. However, the *Sent Soví* does continue the use of the popular spices found in the Hispanic-Muslim cooking manuals: black pepper, cinnamon, ginger, and saffron. The one spice that is noticeably absent is coriander, which, because it is the seed of the cilantro plant, coincides with the lack of cilantro. The exception to this is a singular recipe in the *Sent Soví* called "Celiandre" [Coriander]. This recipe, designed for the ill, grinds together coriander with peeled almonds, cinnamon, ginger, clove, and white sugar. Later, the spices and sugar are mixed with verjuice and sweetener – bittersweet pomegranate juice is recommended – and served with a roasted chicken or pheasant (*The Book of Sent Soví* 88).

A similar situation is found with the use of nuts. As with the spices, in the fourteenth-century manuscript we see a strong continued use of almonds and almond milk.[22] However, hazelnuts, which are not found in the earlier manuscripts, also play a significant role. For example, in "Salsa verd" [Green sauce], toasted hazelnuts are added to the parsley, cinnamon, ginger, clove, and black pepper (*The Book of Sent Soví* 82). Other ingredients – sugar, pine nuts, oranges, and lemons – appear significantly in both the Catalan and the Arabic texts while vestiges of important ingredients from the thirteenth-century manuals – spinach, eggplant, semolina, and rose water – also appear in recipes in the *Sent Soví* but to a lesser extent. All three works use eggs in a similar way, add sugar to both sweet and savoury dishes, include fried pastry and candied nut recipes, are flexible in what type of meat can be used in certain recipes, and include references to recipes for the sick and recovering while not dedicating exclusive sections to them.[23]

In addition to the use of parsley and pork, the *Sent Soví* brings to the peninsula a mushroom sauce not seen in previous cooking manuals.[24]

Si vols fer salsa a bolets perbullits e premuts e sosengats ab oli, fes aital salsa: pren ceba, juivert, vinagre, espècies, e destrempa-ho ab vinagre e un poco d'aigua. Fes peces d'ells, que els sosengues, o en dóna ab sosenga, e puis mit-los en sa salsa o els dóna cuits en brases ab sal e oli. (*The Book of Sent Soví* 76)

[If you are going to make a sauce with boiled, pressed mushrooms sautéed in oil, prepare it thus: take onion, parsley, vinegar, and spices, grind them all together and mix them with vinegar and a little water. Mince the mushrooms, sauté them or add them to the sauté, and then add them to the sauce and serve them boiled or braised with salt and oil.]

The inclusion of this recipe draws attention to a parallel with Italian cooking manuscripts in which mushroom recipes also appear. In contrast to France and England, where we see none until the fifteenth and sixteenth centuries, respectively, mushrooms find their way into Spanish and Italian cooking manuals centuries earlier. One final similarity to *Fuḍālat-al-Hiwan* and *Kitāb al-tabīj* that reference regional areas of Al-Andalus and acknowledge cooking styles of the East, the *Sent Soví*, in its mustard recipe, acknowledges a French style of preparation: "Si la'n vols fer francesa, destrempa-la ab vinagre" [If you are going to prepare it French style, mix it with vinegar] (*The Book of Sent Soví* 80). Both here and in the Hispano-Muslim manuals, authors display their sensitivity to regional and national dishes.

Recipes from *Sent Soví* appear in the Catalan cooking manuals *Llibre de totes maneres de potatges* [The book of every kind of dish] and *Llibre d'aparellar de menjar* [The book of food preparation] (*Libre de Sent Soví* 18–19). Additionally, critics have made strong connections between *Sent Soví* and the first cooking book published in Spain, *Libre de coch* (1520), by Mestre Rupert. This work, and its translation into Castilian five years later, has been recognized as the axis that brings together the earlier Catalan manuscript with the early modern cooking manuals of Spain. However, before turning to the work of Mestre Rupert, or better known in Spanish as Roberto de Nola, we must first become familiar with two other manuscripts from the late medieval period that, although they are not technically cooking manuals, contribute significantly to the understanding of Spanish culinary history and the different voices that contributed to it.

Arte cisoria

Ironically, one of the most important food manuals of fifteenth-century Spain contains no recipes nor is it concerned with preparation in the kitchen; rather it focuses on how food is served. In 1423 Enrique de Villena authored *Arte cisoria* [The art of carving] at the request of Sancho de Jarava, official carver for Juan II of Castile.[25] Contrary to many of the authors of medieval, Renaissance, and early modern cooking manuals, much is known about the life of Enrique de Villena (1384–1434). He was the son of Doña Juana, the illegitimate daughter of Enrique II, and of Don Pedro, a direct descendent of Jaime II of Aragon. He authored several other works, the most famous of which is *Los doze trabajos de Hércules* [The twelve deeds of Hercules] (1417).

Although no recipes are included in this treatise, Villena's work is important to culinary history in several ways. First, in chapter 6, *De las cosas que se acostunbran cortar segúnt las viandas de que usan comer en estas partes* [Of things typically carved according to foods usually eaten in these parts], Villena catalogues thirty different fowl; twenty-four quadrupeds; forty-seven fish and shellfish; three reptiles; twenty-two types of fruit; and thirty-one vegetables, herbs, and spices (83–4). These foodstuffs serve as connectors between time periods and regions as they link food items in earlier works with those in later works, or in some cases, provide evidence for shifts in changing tastes. He specifically mentions the regions of Aragon, Granada, and Mallorca as areas rich in francolins (pheasant family), water buffalo, and mouflons (wild sheep), respectively (83). The inclusion of Aragon and Mallorca are logical given his own origins but his insertion of Granada, and earlier of the Almoravid influence in Spain, could imply a respect for the culinary traditions from Al-Andalus that are likewise acknowledged in the works of Nola, Granado, and Martínez Montiño.

Villena exhibits his awareness of these historic shifts when he writes, "Viandas diversas usaron en España, segúnt la diversidat de las gentes que la señorearon, mudaron los usos dellas, siguiendo la costunbre de las tierras donde viñieron, así como los almorávedis, los alanos, los suevos, los alaricos, godos, estragodos, griegos, romanos e marines" [In Spain diverse foods were consumed, depending on the diverse groups that conquered her, changed how (food) was consumed by maintaining the customs of their own lands, like the Almoravids, Alans, Sueves, Alarics, Goths, Ostrogoths, Greeks, Romans, and Phoenicians] (83). This chapter also includes a curious list of foods consumed for improving health, and includes regional and class divisions (84–6).

However, the majority of his treatise is dedicated to the performance of carving and includes detailed descriptions of a carver's proper instruments and how to use them. Among the essentials are a set of five knives, three types of forks, a holder for paring fruit, and a shell shucker. Of particular interest is his explanation of forks for both carver and diner. Made from gold or silver, forks take three distinct forms, one with two prongs, one with three prongs, and one with a long handle designed for use over the fire. He suggests that the two-pronged fork

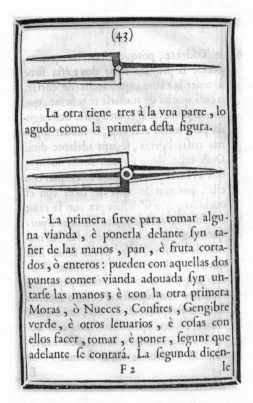

Figure 1.2. From *Arte cisoria* Madrid, 1766, 43. Photos courtesy of Dennis Sears, UIUC Rare Books Library.

sirve para tomar alguna vianda e ponerla delante syn tañer de las manos, e pan e fruta, cortados o enteros. *E pueden con aquellas dos puntas comer vianda adobada syn untarse las manos*, e con la otra punta moras o nueces, confites, gengibre verde e otros letuarios e cosas con ella fazer, tomar e poner. (71–2, emphasis added)

[is useful to pick up food and place it in front (of someone) without dirtying one's hands, the same for bread or fruit, cut up or whole. And with the two-pronged forks, *one can eat prepared food without getting one's hands greasy* and with the other prong one can do other things, pick up and put down berries or nuts, sweets, green ginger, and other electuaries.]

I draw attention to this passage because the use of the fork will later become a marker of refinement, an indicator that separates social classes by way of eating habits.

Another point of interest in Villena's treatise is his emphasis on professional training and standards.[26] In *Arte cisoria* he devotes chapters to standards on the profession, training, hiring and firing practices, distinctions within the profession, and consequences of abusing the position. The importance of sound training for those who work in the kitchen and the responsibility of those who train them appear in virtually all early modern cooking manuals. Drawing from the juridical authority of the day, Alfonso el Sabio's *Siete Partidas* [Seven partidas] (specifically, the Second Partida, title IX, law XI), Villena dedicates a chapter to training good servants: "Cómo deven ser criados moços de buen linaje acostunbrados, para tomar dellos para el ofiçio del cortar" [How boys of good lineage should be raised in order to be selected for the office of carving]. Villena asserts that both the boys' unquestionable lineage ("de fidalguez non dubdosos") and apprenticeship are key to becoming an excellent servant (121). Because of its explanation of foodstuffs and its attention to those who prepare and serve food, Villena's *Arte cisoria* is fundamental for understanding the development of food practices in Spain.

Manual de mugeres

Three aspects of the *Manual de mugeres en el qual se contienen muchas y diversas reçeutas muy buenas* [The manual for women in which is contained many very good and diverse recipes] (1475–1525) immediately engage the reader.[27] First, the appearance of *reçeutas* [recipes] in this and other titles (mentioned below) suggests how the evolution of the word passed from its medical to its culinary usage. Historically it signified a medical prescription or instructions for curing the sick and appears in this title because it contains both food recipes and health-related recipes. Later sixteenth-century manuscripts that deal with general chores carried out in the kitchen also include the word. But typically, in the cooking manuals of the day the words, *orden* [order] and *procedimiento* [procedure] were used instead of *receta*. Its first appearance to signify exclusively cooking instructions came sometime after the 1747 publication of Juan de Altamiras, *Nuevo arte de cocina* [New art of cooking].

The second fascinating point, closely related to the first, is that this manual brings together food, health, and hygiene in ways that the other recipe collections do not. Instructions for making sausage, preserving peaches, and baking chicken pie share pages with remedies for earaches and ointments for rashes as well as instructions for making shampoo and tooth powder. This unique collection of 145 recipes, of which twenty-nine are food related, focuses on the multiple kitchen tasks a woman undertakes and is better classified among an entire series of unedited manuscripts that were written specifically for woman who governed large households and estates. Other works similar to *Manual de mugeres* include *Livro de receptas de pivetes, pastilhas e vvas perfumadas y conserbas* [Book of recipes for incense, tablets, and perfumes, and preserves] (16th century) with 108 "household" recipes; *Recetas y memorias para guisados, confituras, olores, aguas, afeites, adobos de guantes, ungüentos y medicinas para muchas enfermedades* [Recipes and other memoirs for stews, preserves, fragrances, waters, cosmetics, skin softeners, ointments, and medicine for many illnesses] (16th century), with 207 recipes of which 150 pertain to food; and *Receptas experimentadas para diversas cosas* [Experimental recipes for many things] (late 16th–early 17th century).[28] This latter work is enormous and contains over 700 recipes that deal with food preparation as well as beauty, hygiene, and health.

The third point, also interconnected with the previous two, is that the target audience is unique compared to other cookbooks. Here, the manual is written for women in charge of an entire household and who are responsible for many kitchen tasks. The others are written for cooks, with the exception of *Arte cisoria*, and focus exclusively on dishes to be consumed at the table. These shifts in lexicon, content, and audience are directly tied to one another and bring a substantially different perspective to the history of Spanish culinary manuscripts and books through 1700.

Manual de mugeres as well as the other unedited manuscripts follow a long established tradition of treatises written to maintain or improve one's health that began in antiquity with Hippocrates and Galen, carried through the Middle Ages with Arabic treatises by Persian giants such as Haly Abbas and Avicenna, and continued in Latin with the *regimina sanitatis* genre in Europe.[29] The anonymous *Regimen Sanitatis Salernitanum* [Salernitan rule of health] also known as *Flor medicinae* [Flower of medicine] (12th–13th century] is an extensive poem on hygiene and health that was translated into almost every European language during the Middle Ages. In fact, translators at the Escuela de Traductores of Toledo like Gerardo Cremona and Juan Hispano were responsible for many of the *regimina sanitatis* works available to scholars both in Latin and in Castilian (Cruz Cruz, *Dietética medieval* 18–21).

One of the most important works from the "Rule of Health" genre is by the Jewish philosopher Moshé ben Maimón, better known today as, Maimonides (1135–1204). He authored *Tractatus de regimine sanitatis* (1200), which dealt directly with an illness of a sultan's son but more broadly with the promotion of good health. Later, the Catalan Arnau de Vilanova (c. 1238–1311), who was personal physician to the Aragon kings Pedro el Grande, Alfonso III, and Jaime II, wrote his version of the *Regimen Sanitatis* (1307) under the auspices of Jaime II.[30] It was later translated to Castilian in 1606 by Jerónimo de Mondragón.

In the opening table of contents of the *Manual de mugeres*, the recipes are organized into seven different categories: medical remedies (22+1), fragrances (24), facial cosmetics (31), waters and other recipes for the hands (10+1), washes and other remedies for the mouth (13), food recipes (29), and treatments for the hair (13+1) (30).[31] However, in the manuscript they do not follow said order; rather recipes from each section are scattered throughout. Of those dealing with food, twenty of the twenty-nine are grouped together at the end of the manuscript while another seven are grouped in an earlier part of the text. The overwhelming majority are sweet recipes, nineteen of twenty-nine; these include pastries, fried doughs, sweets, preserves, and one sweet soup recipe. As to be expected, the main ingredients are sugar, egg yolk, and almonds or almond milk. Flour and honey are also common and there are occasional references to pine nuts, walnuts, one reference to hazelnuts (in the turrón recipe), rose water, and orange blossom water. A representative recipe is the "Reçeuta para pasta real" [Recipe for royal paste]:

> Las almendras mondadas cortarlas heis en quartos como piñones. Y luego tomaréis açúcar molido; y para dos escudillas de açúcar tomá una de agua rosada. Y junto todo, pondréislo a cozer; y como sea cozido, es hecha la pasta real. (85)

> [Chop peeled almond into quarters, the size of pine nuts. And then add ground sugar and for every two cups of sugar add one of rose water. Once mixed, cook together and once cooked you will have royal paste.]

Of the eight savoury recipes, the two pork dishes and three dishes with clear ties to Muslim cooking are representative of the ways in which Spain's two religious traditions come together in its culinary heritage. "Reçeuta para hazer un obispo de puerco" [Recipe for seasoning bishop blood sausage] is flavoured with clove, cinnamon, and black pepper (81). Although the flavouring draws from established Muslim traditions, the main ingredient, pork, as well as the use of the word *bishop* in the title signal a culinary assimilation of incorporating "Muslim" spices into "Christian" meat dishes. The "Olla morisca" [Moorish stew] (58–9) and the "Caçuela de arroz" [Rice casserole] show their ties to Hispanic Muslims in the titles. The latter dish includes instructions for the rice to be cooked in "caldo de carne gruessa" [stock from fatty meat] and to later add "la carne que quisiéredes" [meat of your choosing] (84). This flexibility in choice of meat is common to recipes found in both the *Fuḍālat* and *Kitāb al-tabīj*. A third recipe, "Reçeuta de un manjar dicho viafora" [Recipe for a dish called *viafora*] consists of a strained stock prepared from fatty pieces of mutton or chicken and shredded, toasted almonds. Shredded lamb is added and the dish is seasoned with sugar, cinnamon, and a little ginger. Martínez Crespo notes that although the meaning of *viafora* is unknown, it could be related to the many *tafaya* dishes that appear in Hispanic-Muslim treatises (84n276).[32]

Manual de mugeres contains one recipe for a beverage, the spiced wine hippocras, and one barley-chicken broth recipe for the sick. The only fruit dishes are for quince and peaches; there are no fish dishes, and, with the exception of recipes that call for the meat of choice, no beef references. As in the *Sent Soví*, there is no mention of the popular cilantro and coriander of the Hispanic-Muslim works although cinnamon, ginger, and black pepper are still common spices. *Manual de mugeres*, together with the other two Christian cooking manuals of the late medieval period, are relatively modest in size, less than a quarter of the recipes compared to the Hispano-Muslim works. All three show similarities with the more extensive cooking manuscripts of thirteenth-century Muslim Spain and, like their predecessors, value therapeutic aromas, cleanliness, and the connections made between health and eating habits.

The recipes in all the manuscripts, whether written for diners at court, or for those living in a large estate, whether written for men or women, or for healthy or the convalescent, do not focus on specific quantities of ingredients. Generally, meat dishes from large mammals are prepared according to the type of meat but not its quantity, although at times a recipe may include the cut of meat, for example, "a leg of lamb." For fowl, fish, and smaller mammals, recipes often begin with preparing one animal, for example, "take one hen," but may also begin with instructions for using whatever amount desired or an unspecified quantity of the animal. This lack of specificity is also found in recipes for vegetables, grains, and other dishes, for example, "take as many eggs as you want ..." Other directions for quantities are equally vague. In the *Sent Soví*, for example, instructions for one of the many sauces reads, "amesura-ho de cascú" [put in just the right amount of each ingredient] (*The Book of Sent Soví* 82). In the *Manual de mugeres*, this practice continues: "Queso fresco massado con harina, y claras de huevos y açucar" [knead fresh cheese with flour, egg whites, and sugar] (85). But there are exceptions to this general line of reasoning in all of the manuscripts and occasionally a recipe will specify the weight or the exact number of ingredients for making a dish. This approach to remaining flexible towards the number of diners, for whom the cook is preparing a meal, continues through the seventeenth century. Even in Domingo Henández de Maceras's university cookbook (1607), which is specifically written to attend to students who live in the Oviedo Residence Hall at the University of Salamanca, the author tends to explain the dishes without insisting on specific quantities for the different ingredients. Assumptions are made that readers of the cooking manuals will have a sufficient level of cooking experience to know how to balance quantities in the different recipes. The exception to this rule is found in the health and hygiene recipes in the *Manual de mugeres*. Instead of following the same informality, very detailed weights and measures are provided for each ingredient. A recipe for an ointment for abscesses begins: "Media onça de pepitas de menbrillos puestas en remojo en quarto onças de agua de açahar, media día" [Soak half an ounce of quince seeds in four ounces of orange blossom water at midday] (41).[33]

These characteristics will continue to develop in future cookbooks. By incorporating new foodstuffs (such as pork and parsley) and by referencing international cooking styles, they provide evidence for a new turn in the manuals that will continue in the court cookbooks of the early modern period.

Printed Sources

Two moments significantly mark the history of early modern cooking manuals in Spain: the publication of Mestre Ruperto's *Libre de coch* (1520) and that of Francisco Martínez Montiño's *Arte de cocina, pastelería, vizcochería y conservería* [The art of cooking, pie making, pastry making, and preserving] (1611). These two cookbooks are central to understanding the history of Spanish gastronomy as the former is the first published in Spain (first in Catalan, then in Castilian) and the latter is the most famous and dominated cookbook publications for over a century and a half. Curiously, between these two pieces that define early modern Spanish court cooking, another cookbook appears, Diego Granado's *Libro del arte de cozina* [Book on the art of cooking] (1599). His work is monumental, fifteen sections that include 755 recipes. He brings to early modern Spain a more moderate use of spices, scientific cooking techniques, and significant regional and international influences. Yet, *Libro del arte de cozina* only sees two subsequent editions before completely disappearing until 1971. Why did Granado fail when Nola and, later, Martínez Montiño succeed? The answer to this question reveals the direction of Spanish cooking would take for centuries to follow.

Libre de coch

Libre de coch is the first cookbook ever published in Spain; written in Catalan probably in the mid- to late fifteenth century, the first extant edition is from 1520.[34] As the first cookbook published in Spain it claims a historic place in Spanish cookbook history. The 1525 translation into Castilian marks another significant moment because it was published eleven times in Castilian in less than fifty years.[35] Together the Castilian and Catalan editions influenced future cooks and cookbook authors throughout the sixteenth century. In the first Castilian version the publisher assigned the author the last name "de Nola" that does not appear in the original Catalan version.[36] Structurally, the recipe book contains chapters on ten different kitchen and dining room positions, on cutting meat and serving food, on medical advice, and 243 recipes for soups, stews, baked, boiled, and simmered dishes, and sauces. In addition Nola includes a section on Lent and on food for the convalescent.

Although not much is known about Ruperto de Nola's life, most agree that he was either Catalan or born of Catalan parents relocated to Naples. Nola served under Don Ferrante, illegitimate son of Alfonso I (previously Alfonso V of Aragon), who ruled Naples from 1458 to his death in 1494. The book was written, as the author clearly states in the opening words, to teach young men how to be virtuous and learn how to serve:

> Como sea cosa muy necesaria a los mozos de tierna edad aprender el camino de las virtudes, mayormente a los que se deleitan en querer servir a los señores y personas de estado y caballeros y otros de menor estado y condición para tomar crianza y aprender otras cosas de gentileza, que conviene que sepan los hijosdalgos para ser más valerosos y saber cómo han de tratar a cualquier estado y condición de gentes, y se muestren a sufrir trabajos. (233)[37]

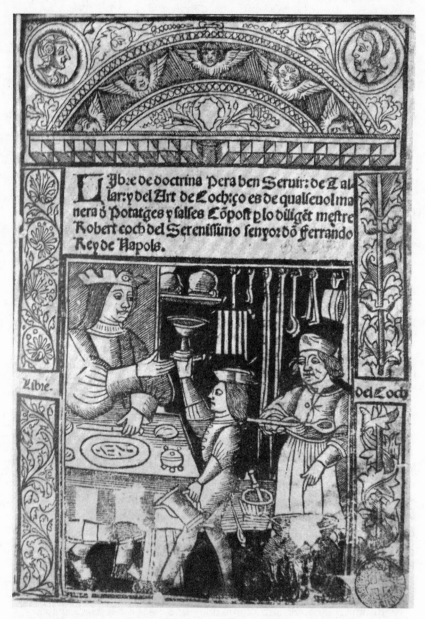

Figure 1.3. Cover of *Libre de Coch*. Reproduced in *Libro de guisados*, ed. Dionisio Pérez (Madrid: Pedro Sáinz y Rodríguez, 1929), xvi.

[As it is imperative for youths of a certain age to learn the path of virtue, in particular for those who take pleasure in wanting to serve lords, men of rank, gentlemen, and others of lesser rank and station, and be raised and learn other points of good manners, it is advisable that the sons of nobles learn how to be more effective and treat each rank and status of persons, and demonstrate how to execute their position.]

In this way, learning about a position in the kitchen and dining hall would lead to a life well lived.

The language of Nola's cookbook reveals a consciousness of the cook's social standing and in his portrayal of those who prepare food Nola shows his "modern" sensitivity to his art form. He clearly articulates that he is writing the cookbook at the king's request and for future cooks to better serve his majesty. His language suggests both a certain pride and humility regarding his station:

Puesto que haya otros mayores oficiales en mi oficio que yo, y de más habilidad, ninguno, por experiencia y uso y crianza, sabrá los apetitos y viandas y guisados que son más agradables al gusto de vuestra voluntad como yo. (231)

[There might be other (court) officials with higher ranking than my own and perhaps even those with more skill, but none by way of experience, practice, or manners knows the appetite, food, and dishes that prove most favourable to your liking as I do.]

There is no doubt that this cookbook is first and foremost a cookbook in the modern sense; the bulk of the text is recipes. But it is also a manifesto of sorts that lays forth appropriate behaviour and presentation for kitchen staff and other household positions: "contiene alguna manera de doctrina acerca del servicio y de los servidores y oficiales de las casas de los reyes y grandes señores y caballeros y otras personas de menos estados" [(the cookbook) contains a sort of doctrine on serving, for servers and officials of the residence of the king, grandees, gentlemen, and men of lower rank] (232). Many times Nola repeats this combination of humility and pride as he refers to his "humble" status while as the same time he describes cooking as a respected art form.

Within the pages of his cookbook, one finds echoes of previous works. For example, the humorous title, "Leche mal cocida" [Badly boiled milk] (298) first appears in the anonymous *Sent Soví* (*The Book of Sent*

Soví 158) although the two recipes have not much more in common than the title. In the *Sent Soví*, eggs and some bread are added to milk that is being heated. When it comes to a boil, it is removed from the heat and served. But in Nola's recipe, there is no milk. Rather, ground almonds and breadcrumbs are quickly sautéed together with beaten eggs to give a visual result of something that resembles curdled milk but that tastes delicious. We see Nola's personal touch when he finishes the recipe by stating, "y si pusieres el migalón de pan en remojo en agua rosada no puede ser sino mejor; aunque basta lo otro: la agua rosada siempre es buena en muchos manjares" [and if you soak the breadcrumbs in rose water, it could not be better, even though without it, the recipe is acceptable. Rose water is always good in many dishes] (298). Nola also measures time through prayer as is done in many of the earlier manuscripts. He references two when he describes the finishing time of a beef or fish empanada: "Tornarla al horno por espacio de un *Pater Noster* y un *Ave María*" [Put it back in the oven for as long as it takes to say an *Our Father* and a *Hail Mary*] (322, emphasis mine).

Nola's cookbook serves as a model for future writers as it signals the direction that cookbooks will take. *Libre de coch* sheds the exclusive late medieval character of former cooking manuscripts and reveals a Renaissance character. Like Miguel de Cervantes with his publication of *Don Quixote* over a century later, the work contains a "modern" sensibility. In his introduction Nola highlights the valued position of the cook and that cooking is a culinary art. Among his many stew recipes, we find the "Potaje *moderno*" [*Modern* stew] (299, emphasis mine) and "Otro potaje *moderno*" [Another *modern* stew] (299, emphasis mine) that reveal Nola's awareness of changes to cooking styles and ingredients.

Like the *nuova cucina* movement in parts of Italy, Nola's work emphasizes regional and international cooking and in doing so, aids in developing a distinct national style, another modern quality. The work contains regional Aragonese, Genoese, and Venetian recipes like "Toronjas de Xativa que son almojávanas" [Xativa grapefruits which are cheese fritters] (323), "Rosquillas de fruta que llaman casquetas en Valencia y en Barcelona" [Fruit rings called *casquetas* in Valencia and Barcelona] (323–4), "Torta a la genovesa" [Genoese cake] (320), or "Xinxanella a la veneciana" [Venetian jujube] (320–1). The recipe for Venetian jujubes is actually a broth with pasta. The pasta is made with cheese, fine breadcrumbs, eggs, saffron, and other herbs, pressed through a large grater that forms the dough into gnocchi-sized shapes that are then served in a broth. *Xinxanella* is a variant of *guinja*, synonym of *azufaifa* or *jujube*, the red, tear-drop shaped fruit of the jujube tree. Thus, the title of the dish, like so many others in the text, reflects its form, a visual image, rather than its content. Nola also underscores the contributions of other cultures, specifically Moorish and Jewish, in the development of Spanish gastronomy. Like *Arte cisoria*, Nola references several food items and dishes that are inspired by Arab and Jewish culinary traditions found throughout Spain and that form such an essential part of the country's heritage: *mirrauste* [roasted poultry with toasted almond sauce] (266), "Potaje dicho morteruelo" [Hot paté stew] (275), three recipes for "Potaje de culantro llamado primo" [Coriander soup called the first] (275–6),[38] "Salsa Granada" [Granada sauce] (313), "Berenjenas a la morisca" [Morisco-style eggplant] (285–6), and "Calabazas a la morisca" [Morisco-style bottle squash] (287). The "Salsa Granada" recipe is for a chicken liver purée thickened with egg yolk and flavoured with orange juice and spices. It had previously appeared in the Catalan manuscript, *Sent Soví* but in his *Libre de coch*, Nola omits all references to *tocino* of which no less than four appear in the *Sent Soví* version. Comparing the two *a la morisca* recipes, one finds that the label refers to a finishing style of adding finely grated cheese, ground spices that may include coriander, cumin, and/or caraway, and whipped egg batter. Even the "Toronjas de Xátiva" mentioned earlier show the Muslim influence in the recipe's second name, *almojávanas*, which comes from the Hispanic-Arabic *almuǧábbana*, meaning *made with cheese*, which comes from the classical Arabic, *ǧubn*, or *cheese*.

Almost 500 years later, we know the names of cooks who served kings, queens, and nobles: Sardinas, cook to don Álvaro de Luna; Jotxim, cook to Ferdinand the Catholic; Lopera, cook to Doña Juana; Bañuelo, cook to Charles I (later Charles V of the Holy Roman Empire); Luis el Negro, cook to Gonzalo of Cordoba; and Suárez, cook to Felipe II (Bennassar 142). But none of them left behind a written legacy; we know nothing of how they prepared their dishes, named them, or described them for others. Nola's work is unique in this respect; through the written word, his legacy endures. *El libre de coch* was the definitive cookbook throughout the sixteenth century, an era in which Spain began to define its national and regional gastronomies. It was also a time when those aspiring to improve their social standing could more easily access recipes written and published for nobility and kings. By reading and recreating dishes, they sought to validate their position in society and improve the fare at their table. For these reasons Ruperto de Nola's *El libre de coch* plays a key role in moving from medieval into early modern Spanish cooking.

Libro del arte de cozina

Generations later, one of Nola's admirers draws from Nola's masterpiece in the creation of his own cookbook. In 1599 Diego Granado published his enormous work *Libro del arte de cozina* in which parts of Nola's work appeared under Granado's name – the opening chapters on how servants should present themselves, how to cut different quadrupeds and fowl, and forty-nine recipes. Granado's work is monumental, 763 recipes divided into fifteen sections:

Especias (30)
De diversas suertes de pasteles y tortas (118)
De diversas maneras de tortas, o tortadas, que llaman en Italia
    "costratas," y en Nápoles "copos" (141)
Las maneras de hacer diversos tortillones hojaldreados y por hojal-
    drear, rellenos y vacíos (156)
De diversas viandas y guisados de pescado, platos y potajes cuares-
    males (163)
Escudillas de pescado, y otras viandas para días de Cuaresma (255)
Para hacer pasteles de varios tipos de pescados y otras materias
    para días de ayuno (280)
Tortas o tortadas y tortillones de pescados y otras cosas para Cu-
    aresma (300)
De diversas maneras de tortas y costradas de frutas y legumbres
    para días de Cuaresma y cosas de leche a la usanza de Italia (307)
De cómo se han de hacer yelos (geles, gelos, gelatinas) y salsas de
    diversas maneras para días de carne y de Cuaresma (327)
Tablero de cocina para convalecientes y enfermos (342)
Diversas maneras de asados de aves (358)
Para hacer diversos caldillos o broetes (363)
Para hacer diversas escudillas de hierbas (372)
Para hazer diversas maneras de conservas (380)[39]

[Spices (30)
On diverse types of (savoury) cakes and pies (118)
On diverse ways of (making) pies and medium pies that are called
    "costratas" in Italy and "copos" in Naples (141)
Ways of making diverse, big, flaky pies and for making flaky shells
    for filling or leaving empty (156)
On diverse food and fish stews, Lenten dishes, and soups (163)

Fish soups and other food for Lenten days (255)
To make various types of fish cakes and other things for fasting
    days (280)
Small, medium, and large fish pies and other things for Lent (300)
On different types of fruit and legume pies and turnovers for
    Lenten days and dairy products as used in Italy (307)
On how gels, jellies, and gelatins and different types of sauces are
    made for meat days and Lenten days (327)
Kitchen station for the sick and the convalescent (342)
Diverse ways of roasting fowl (358)
For making diverse broths and clear soups (363)
For making diverse vegetable dishes (372)
For making diverse types of preserves (380)]

We know virtually nothing of Granado beyond his name and the cookbook he left behind.[40] From his work it seems that he may have spent time in Italy and may have travelled through Germany or other parts of northern Europe. Multiple recipe titles would seem to substantiate this claim or at least point to the availability of northern European recipe books for this elusive author: "Para ahogar el lomillo de vaca a la tudesca" [German-style tenderloin] (65), "Para hacer platos de leche vulgarmente llamados hungarescos" [Cream soups that are ordinarily called Hungarian] (90), "Para guisar truchas a la tudesca, a la alemana" [German-style trout] (209), "Para hacer huevas de sollo al horno, que se pueden comer luego o/y guardarlas para otros días" [Caviar in the oven that can be eaten at once or saved for another day] (175). In 1598 Granado was at court in Madrid where he requested permission to print the book but Val believes he is not a native of Madrid as his name does not appear in the usual catalogues of writers and other definitive sources (xviii).

One of the frequent comments of scholars regarding Granado addresses his plagiarism of previous cookbooks. For example, Joaquín del Val, who has done the most extensive research on Granado to date, notes his blatant plagiarism: "Sin ningún escrúpulo Granado plagió una gran parte del contenido del *Libro de guisados*, sin nombrar jamás a Roberto o Ruperto de Nola ... Granado copió casi integramente la primera parte" [Without any scruples whatsoever, Granado plagiarized a big part of the content of the *Book of Cookery* without ever citing Robert or Rupert de Nola ... Granado copied almost word for word the first part] (xxiii).[41] There is no doubt that Granado stole from Nola, yet Val overstates the case. Granado's work is three times the size of Nola's, 755 recipes compared to Nola's 243, and of those, Granado selected and revised forty-nine recipes for his own work. To be sure, Nola was influential for Granado but Granado certainly drew from several and varied sources, the most significant being the Italian Bartolomeo Scappi.[42] Here, in Granado's manipulation of Scappi's opus, one can find an abundance of plagiarized work or "borrowed" material. I do not mean to understate Granado's plagiarism. Today, taking just one recipe without citing the source is a violation of copyright and grounds for a lawsuit. But this sensibility does not transfer to earlier eras. I will return to this important point momentarily but first, let us examine how Granado treats his most primary source.

Bartolomeo Scappi's *Dell' arte del cucinare* [On the art of cooking] (1570) is nothing short of a masterpiece of the early modern kitchen. It is a six-volume work that contains over 1000 recipes and twenty-eight illustrations divided into sections on meat, fowl, fish, pasta, diets for the infirm and convalescent, and recipes for Lent. Scappi cooked for five different popes and was the private cook of Pope Pius V. For over two months in late 1549–early 1550 he prepared meals for the conclave that chose Pope Julius III as successor to Paul III (Dal Col and Gutiérrez Granda 13–14). He was also responsible for the coronation feast of Charles V as Holy Roman Emperor in Bologna for which 780 dishes were prepared.

Scappi's love of his art form is apparent right from the opening pages when he describes the qualities of a good cook:

Bisogna adunque, che un prudente, et sufficiente m. Cuoco… volendo havere buon principio, meglior mezzo, et ottimo fine, et sempre honore della sua opera, faccia come un giuditioso Architetto, il quale dopo il suo giusto disegno, stabilisce un forte fondamento, et sopra quello dona al mondo utili, et maravigliosi edifitii. (1v)

[It is necessary, therefore … that a skilled and competent Master Cook, wishing to have a good beginning, a better middle and a best ending, and always to derive honour from his work, should be as a wise Architect, who, following his careful design, lays out a firm foundation and on it presents to the world useful and marvelous buildings.] (98–9)[43]

Dal Col and Gutiérrez Granda argue that Scappi's most important innovation and contribution to modern cooking was his awareness of controlling temperature: cooking off the flame, low flame, when flame should be both above and below, when pots should be covered, when dishes should be wrapped in paper to avoid excessive heat, when pots should sit in the embers, when to use a *bain marie* (35). But most, if not all, of these cooking techniques were already included in the Hispano-Muslim cooking manuals. What I find so alluring about his work is the passionate way he describes food and his commitment to the smallest details. Before entering into a formal discussion of making a dish, Scappi discusses seasonal ingredients and how to recognize good quality. He incorporates vivid descriptions of cooking techniques and is very particular about how to present the food. His tone is consistently positive. Finally, as a closing for many recipes, he offers variations to accommodate changing seasons and different tastes.

To examine how Granada uses Scappi's material, we must first look at the quantitative evidence. Of the 755 recipes that make up Granado's *Libro del arte de cozina* 556 are from Scappi (almost 75 per cent).[44] That said, Granado does not simply "cut and paste." He has revised, sometimes substantially, oftentimes in more subtle ways, the vast majority of Scappi's recipes. These revisions can be categorized into five groups:

1 delete explanation of Spanish lexicon/add explanation of Italian lexicon;
2 eliminate seasonal references;
3 delete/add/alter ingredient;
4 eliminate alternative ingredients/approaches to recipe; and
5 change order of information.

In transferring material from a cookbook written in one language and one country to another, names of ingredients (for example, types of cheeses, and variety of vegetables) have to be adapted. In one recipe Scappi uses two different local cheeses, *Parmesan* and *Riviera* (Dal Col 540). Granado replaces them with cheese from Tronchón and a creamy cheese from Pinto (152). Also understandable to some extent is Granado's decision to delete seasonal information on food products as seasons may vary slightly from Italy to Spain. On this point, Scappi is meticulous. He details hunting seasons and growing seasons alike. In "Per soffriggere, et far diverse fricassee de lepri" [Fricassées of hares], Scappi clarifies that while rabbits and hare are available throughout the year, their season begins in May and lasts until the end of August (44v, 183). In his recipe "Per far minestra di lattuca con brodo di carne in diversi modi" [Various ways to prepare a thick soup of lettuce in a meat broth], Scappi begins, "piglisi la lattuca nella sua vera stagione, la qual' e del mese de Marzo per tutto Maggio, anchor che in Roma se ne trovi d'ogni tempo" [get lettuce in its proper season, between March and the end of May, although in Rome you can get it throughout the year] (76v–7r, 240). Granado consistently eliminates this type of detail.

More fascinating is how Granado adds, deletes, and alters specific ingredients in the recipes. In one dish Scappi uses peas, garbanzos, onions, rice, chestnuts, and kidney beans; Granado chooses to eliminate the peas and the rice (Scappi 65r–v, 216; Granado 82–3). Scappi usually closes out a recipe with alternative ingredients or ways to prepare a dish, but in Granado's effort to scale back recipes, he purges them of possible alternatives and instead opts for a briefer, singular approach to preparing the dish. These conscious decisions to alter Scappi's work are also present in the way Granado structures the text. For example, in his section on recipes for sauces for Lent, Granado transfers twenty-seven consecutive recipes from Scappi. However, in the following section on food for the sick and convalescent, Granado has thirty recipes that intersperse recipes from two sources: twelve from Scappi, two from Nola, eleven from Scappi, two from Nola, and three from Scappi. Other times, while including a series of Scappi recipes, Granado deletes a recipe or two from the series or he changes the order in which they are presented. In at least one instance he combines ideas from both Nola and Scappi to create his version. This is certainly the case for "Hordiate para dolientes (agua de cebada para enfermos)" [Barley water for the ailing (barley water for the sick)] (360) for which Granado combines ideas from Nola's "Ordiate para dolientes" [Barley water for the sick] (304) and Scappi's "Per fare orzata d'orzo mondo" [Gruel of hulled barley] (403v–4r, 560–1).

Upon careful study, it is obvious that Granado's "plagiarism" must be reevaluated. His conscious selection of recipes from previous masters and his decisions to include or exclude them point to the culturally accepted theory of imitation more than to today's understanding of plagiarism. As Granado borrows from those he admires, he follows the ideals of an eclectic imitation, one that embraces drawing from a variety of models and validates his own work by associating himself with the giants of the past. In this same way, Nola drew from Enrique de Villena's *Arte cisoria* for his sections on carving meat and cutting fruits and vegetables (Val xxiii). This type of eclectic imitation was praised by Luis Vives, Garcilaso de la Vega, and other early modern writers. The acknowledgment of sources is not yet the responsibility of the writer but rather that of the erudite reader who must know the sources well enough to understand how the writer has changed them and who must then evaluate the choices each author makes. In his selection process, Granado creates his own unique work that historicizes his contributions in a line of established cookbooks. Early modern readers would not expect to find the names of Nola or Scappi so blatantly announced in Granado's work. They understood that readers themselves bring to the table the knowledge to reveal sources within. Granado's use of Scappi and Nola as two sources for his cookbook would not detract from the original popularity of his text. To understand why Granado's work ceased to be published after the 1609 and 1614 editions, we must look at the language of another cookbook author who followed him.

There is no doubt that Granado's 1599 publication introduced to Spain the creative kitchen of Bartolomeo Scappi, including new dishes like pizza and caviar and innovative cooking methods. And for a decade his work met with relative success. But, twelve years later, the subsequent publication of Francisco Martínez Montiño's cookbook sealed Granado's fate. The two court recipe books could not live together and with the appearance of *Arte de cocina, pastelería, vizcochería y conservería,* Granado's worked disappeared.[45]

Arte de cocina, pastelería, vizcochería y conservería

As with so many cooks of the early modern period, little is known about Francisco Martínez Montiño's life. He was possibly Galician and worked his entire life in kitchens, beginning as a humble kitchen boy [*galopín*] and moving his way up to head chef for Felipe III, and Felipe IV. In the opening pages Martínez Montiño alludes to having served in the kitchens of Felipe II's sister, Doña Juana, in Portugal. María de los Ángeles Pérez Samper notes that he then moved to the royal kitchens in Madrid and began serving Felipe III in 1585. He then worked for Felipe IV until his retirement or death in 1629 when records show he was replaced by another cook (*La alimentación* 29–30). Martínez Montiño's work is recognized as the most published Spanish cookbook before the twentieth century, with over twenty-five editions.[46] It is separated into two chapters – one on cleanliness of the kitchen staff and banquets, and the other on pastries, cakes, and preserves which contains 448 recipes – and two memoirs on conserves and jellies with twenty and thirty-three recipes, respectively.

Martínez Montiño shares many recipes with Granado including regional and international dishes. Both authors include ingredients and recipes that reflect Spain's Hispanic-Muslim past.[47] Internationally, Granado brings to Spain more Italian influences and Martínez Montiño, more French and Portuguese. They also share a similar sense of herbs and seasoning, a consciousness of varying cooking temperatures, a wide range of cooking verbs, a lack of seasonal references, and a more somber tone than is found in either Scappi's or Nola's cookbook.

Martínez Montiño, like Scappi, includes personal commentary as part of the recipe but his voice is sterner. For example, in his recipe on how to dress turnips, he begins by stating: "Los navos no es muy buena potagería: yo trato de ellos de mala gana, porque soy muy enemigo de ellos, porque en qualquier platillo donde cayere algun caldo de navos se hecha à perder" [Turnips do not make good soups. I reluctantly included them because I am their enemy as any dish that has turnip broth is surely a waste] (259). Conversely, he was a squash enthusiast and included at least eight separate squash dishes (252–9). But even here, there is none of the lightheartedness of Nola's cookbook or intense enthusiasm that defines Scappi's work and at times trickles into Granado's. So why, then, does this vast difference exist between the fame of Martínez Montiño and that of Granado?

The biggest single factor that may have contributed to Granado's failure comes from Martínez Montiño's own work. In the very prologue he attacks Granado's cookbook:

El intento que he tenido en escribir este Librito ha sido no haber libros por donde se puedan guiar los que sirven el Oficio de la Cocina, y que todo se encarga à la memoria: solo uno he visto, y tan errado que basta para echar à perder à quien usáre de él, y compuesto por un Oficial, que casi no es conocido en esta Corte: y así las cosas del Libro no están puestas de manera que ningun Aprendiz se pueda aprovechar, à lo menos los Españoles, antes si se siguieren por él, lo erráran, y echarán à perder la hacienda. (prologue)

[My intention in writing this little book has been that no books can be found that guide those who serve in the Office of the Kitchen and that everything must be memorized. I have seen only one and it is so flawed that whoever uses it will be ruined. It is composed by an official that hardly anyone at this court knows. Things in the book are not organized in a way that any apprentice could use to his advantage, at least Spaniards, who if they follow it, would err and ruin their fortune.]

He then mounts his own case by pointing out the originality of his recipes and that he has tested each one. Finally, he returns to attack specific recipes found in Granado:

en el capítulo de las Tortas, que está escrito en el otro Libro, hay muchas suertes de tortas, que no solo no son buenas, ni se deben hacer, mas antes es impertinencia escribirlas como son las de castañas, y otras de higos, y de turmas de tierra, y de navos, y de zanahorias, y de patatas, ni de cerezas. (prologue)[48]

[in the chapter on pies that is written in the other book, there are many types of pies that not only are no good nor should they be made, but moreover it was impertinent to write them at all like those with chestnuts, and others with figs, truffles, turnips, carrots, sweet potatoes, or cherries.]

Like Cervantes who in his prologue to *Don Quixote* 2, attacks Avellaneda for his blatant and pitiful plagiarism without ever mentioning his name, so too does Martínez Montiño write scornfully of another cookbook author whose name he cannot lower himself to mention. Granado is simply not worthy of forming part of Martínez Montiño's own opus. This diatribe against his predecessor is certainly not the sole explanation for the success of this 1611 cookbook or the failure of Granado's 1599 text, but it does distance the two works, and at the same time reveals a self-consciousness of both the role of the author-cook and the advances an individual can make within the culinary arts.

The first modern advancement for which Martínez Montiño claims responsibility is the attention to cleanliness and organization within the kitchen. While writers of culinary manuscripts and books consistently comment on the importance of cleanliness, Martínez Montiño differs in his almost obsessive attitude. The first chapter opens with a declaration on the importance of sanitation:

Pienso tratar en este capítulo de la limpieza que es la más necesaria, e importante, para que cualquier cocinero dé gusto en su oficio. Y para esto es necesario guardar tres o quatro cosas. La primera es, limpieza; y la segunda, gusto; y la tercera presteza, que teniendo estas cosas, aunque no sea muy grande Oficial, gobernandose bien, dará gusto a su señor, y estará acreditado. (1–2)

[I plan to discuss cleanliness in this chapter as it is most necessary and important for any cook to be able to please in his profession. And for this, it is necessary to observe three or four things. The first is cleanliness; the second, taste; and the third, celerity. If you observe these three things and work hard, even if you are not a high-ranking official, you will please your lord and gain a favourable reputation.]

He gives details on the importance of light in the kitchen, sparkle on all surfaces and equipment, daily trash removal, clean cloths and kitchen linens, separate stations for cleaning meat, and hand washing. In fact, he emphasizes personal hygiene with a separate towel reserved exclusively for drying clean hands. "Pondrás una costumbre, que todos los oficiales, y mozos que entraren por la mañana en la Cocina, lo primero que han de hacer sea … lavarse las manos, y limpiarse en una toalla, que estará colgada par esto, y trabajar con mucha limpieza" [You should insist as a general habit that the first thing that all officials and kitchen hands do as they enter each morning is … wash their hands and dry them with a towel, hung for this very purpose, and work with much cleanliness] (7–8). In his work Martínez Montiño also defines more fully kitchen spaces and utensils. For each recipe he names the specific equipment needed: for couscous, the couscous pan; for cream puffs, the cream puff pot; specific ovens for specific types of baking; and dozens of utensils each designed for a specific purpose (Restrepo Manrique).

In comparing the work of Nola, Granado, and Martínez Montiño, we begin to understand more fully how the authors met different destinies. Nola stands apart from the latter two. He has earned his position within Spanish culinary history both because his book was the first ever published in both Catalan and Castilian and because his kitchen instructions and recipes have inspired those who followed in his footsteps. In the case of *Libro del arte de cozina*, Nola's presence is uncontested as Granado virtually lifted his opening advice and specific recipes and placed them in his own work. In comparing Granado to Martínez Montiño, it is clear that while both authors share types of recipes, cooking techniques, and a sensitivity to modern cooking, Martínez Montiño's descriptions of sanitation, utensils, and kitchen layout set this author-cook apart from his colleague. In spite of his often harsh tone throughout the cookbook and assault on his predecessor (or perhaps due to it), the legacy of Martínez Montiño carried through three centuries. However, we live in a world that roots for the underdog; Diego Granado, not Martínez Montiño, has received more critical attention in the last fifty years. Granado's cookbook was republished in 1971 and 1990, both with critical introductions, while a critical edition of Martínez Montiño's cookbook has yet to see the light of day. Other scholars have weighed in on Granado's contributions to early modern cooking and, without exception, have criticized his "plagiarism." The adage "Even bad press is good press" has certainly rung true for Granado. By comparing the authors of the three early modern Spanish court cookbooks, we can begin to understand how their successes, along with their choices of language, tone, structure, and selected recipes have affected their places within Spanish culinary history.

Libro del arte de cocina

Moving away from court and toward institutions of learning and faith, an important cookbook surfaces that provides recipes used in university kitchens. Domingo Hernández de Maceras, cook in the Colegio Mayor de San Salvador de Oviedo at the University of Salamanca, compiled the work *Libro del arte de cocina* [Book on the art of cooking] in 1607. As he states in his dedication, he has worked in the kitchen since his youth and for over thirty years (177).[49]

Like the court cookbooks, Hernández de Maceras takes enormous pride in his position and in his knowledge and skill. However, his work differs from the others in its intended audience. In his note to the reader, Hernández de Maceras explains that he has collected only the most essential recipes for those who would like to prepare them: "Y así el autor ... quiso limitarle poniendo solamente los más usuales y necesarios a la [*sic*] mesas de los Príncipes y Señores, para los que quisieren usar y ejercer este arte en menos tiempo y con facilidad se puedan hacer capaces, leyendo este breve volumen" [And so the author has tried to limit (his selections) putting only the most common, essential ones for the table of princes and lords, so that for those who try to use and put into practice this art, they could do so in less time and more easily by reading this brief book] (178). As explained by the author, this book is intended for those without the same specialized knowledge as the author. Different from the court manuals, it is written for a less experienced audience and, although still intended for an elite audience, reaches out to a wider range of kitchens than those of the court.[50]

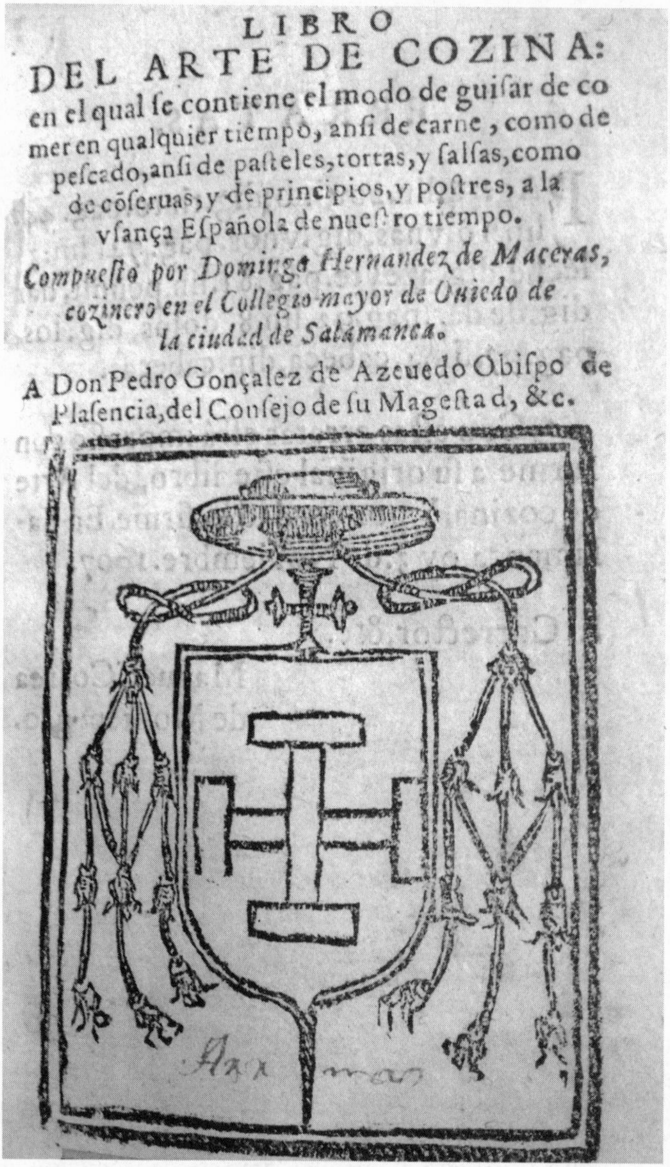

LIBRO
DEL ARTE DE COZINA:
en el qual se contiene el modo de guisar de co
mer en qualquier tiempo, ansi de carne, como de
pescado, ansi de pasteles, tortas, y salsas, como
de cóseruas, y de principios, y postres, a la
vsança Española de nuestro tiempo.

Compuesto por Domingo Hernandez de Maceras,
cozinero en el Collegio mayor de Ouiedo de
la ciudad de Salamanca.

A Don Pedro Gonçalez de Azeuedo Obispo de
Plasencia, del Consejo de su Magestad, &c.

Figure 1.4. Cover of Domingo Hernández de Maceras's *Libro del arte de cozina*.
Photo by author with permssion of the University of Chicago Special Collections Research Center.

Another difference between the court cooking manuals and this university cookbook is the decided organization of Hernández de Maceras's work. More than the works of his contemporaries, Granado and Martínez Montiño, Hernández de Maceras divides the cookbook into introductory chapters that comment generally on seasonal foods, salads, and desserts; a chapter on how to carve different meats and fowl; and three major sections on regular food days, partial abstinence days (Saturdays), and full abstinence days (Lent, Fridays, and special holidays).

The opening chapters offer many unique features not found in the court cookbooks. Chapter 1, for example, divides food seasonally and recommends that specific fresh fruit – cherries, sweet limes and oranges, sloe berries, plums, melons, figs, and grapes – and custard be eaten in summer while butter from Baeza, dried peaches, raisins, almonds, escarole, and a fairly elaborate dish of roast carrot salad be eaten in winter. His predilection for fruit and vegetables continues in the following three chapters that focus on salads and dessert. The salad of chapter 2 is comparable to today's chef's salad but without the lettuce. Here, one chops vegetables, adds capers, and tosses with oil and vinegar. It is then served on individual plates to which are added slices of fatback, tongue, trout or salmon, hard boiled egg yolks, and candied fruit as well as bitter herb, sugared pomegranate, and, as a garnish, borage blossom. The daily salad, which is almost humorous in its simplification of the former, features cooked capers with oil, vinegar, and sugar. This contrast of elaborate and simple recipes is characteristic of Hernández de Maceras's cookbook.

In book I.26, the recipe "Cómo se ha de armar un conejo" [How to assemble rabbit] includes instructions for deboning a rabbit. Later, a mixture of minced leg of lamb, fat back, spices, and verjuice or vinegar is added to the rabbit meat which is then put back on the bone, covered in a pot with marrow rounds and quartered hard boiled yolks, and set to bake at a low temperature. Contrasting this complexity is I.36 "De otro guisado de palominos" [Another young dove dish]. Here, Hernández de Maceras writes instructions for boiling young doves, seasoning with salt and pepper, and then finishing them either by sautéing or roasting. The fourth opening chapter, "De los postres" [On desserts] again brings forth both the seasonal and the regional as Hernández de Maceras describes what desserts to eat when. "En tiempo de la cuaresma se come por postres camuesas, y peros agrios y aceitunas Cordobeses, y queso, y nueces, e higos. De verano cerezas y peras y melocotones, y albérchigas, albaricoques, y cermeños" [During Lent Camueso apples, sour apples, olives from Cordoba, cheese, walnuts, and figs are eaten for dessert. In summertime, cherries, pears, peaches, apricots, and Cermeño pears] (187).[51]

Although Hernández de Maceras dedicates these opening pages to fruit and vegetable dishes, animal-based recipes dominate his work. There are 116 recipes for quadrupeds, fowl, and fish while only sixty-one on fruits and vegetables grown or collected in the wild. After his chapter on how to carve different cuts of meat and fowl, which is reminiscent of court manuals reaching back to *Arte cisoria* and almost identical to Nola's opening chapters in *Libro de guisados*, the *Libro primero* [First book] begins with a classic meatball recipe and a chopped meat and egg dish that is baked until the eggs set. What follows these two opening pieces are twelve mutton recipes, indicating the importance of this meat in the university dining hall; some ten beef, pork, and general meat recipes; almost twenty fowl recipes sprinkled with random rabbit and hare dishes, one mutton, and one pork dish; four goat recipes; he finishes with a mixture of stew, pork, fowl, and two dessert recipes. Even within the section on fowl, Hernández de Maceras maintains an organized hierarchy beginning with recipes for young doves and continuing with those for partridge, capon, turkey, young doves again, chicken, hen, pheasant, and ending with the recipe, "De todo género de aves pequeñas" [On all types of small fowl].

After this book on select meats and fowl, the next section is dedicated to foods eaten on Saturdays, indicating the partial abstinence that was observed in seventeenth-century Spain. These nineteen recipes focus on organ meat: the head, tongue, knuckles, liver, lung, kidney, and brain but also include one recipe for ventral tuna simmered in white wine. As was apparent in book I, the focus here is on sheep, but at times the author adds final instructions that include the possibility of using another type of meat as is seen in "Cómo se han de hacer manos rebozadas" [How to make deep fried knuckles] in which he explains that the sugar and cinnamon topping is also appropriate with other types of fried knuckles: "y con esta misma salsa se puede dar el cabrito rebozado, y cualquier género de rebozado, como manos de ternera, de puerco, y de cabrito, y otras cualesquiera manos" [and this same topping can be served over deep-fried goat or any type of deep frying, such as beef, pork, or kid knuckles, or any other knuckle] (224). Hernández de Maceras's organizational prowess is also apparent as he cross references recipes from the previous section. In II.6 "Cómo se han de lamprear" [How to (prepare a dish) *lamprea* style], the author writes, "En el capítulo diecisiete del libro primero, dijimos cómo se han de lamprear las lenguas, y con qué aderezo, y así me remito allí para que se vea" [In chapter sixteen of book I, we explained how to prepare tongue *lamprea* style and with what type of seasoning, and so I will refer to that to be looked at] (223).[52]

In the third book, Hernández de Maceras concentrates on fish, eggs, stews, and other abstinence dishes. Before the first recipe, he includes an introductory paragraph that explains the types of food typically consumed during Lent. He then lists twenty-three recipes for these grains, nuts, and vegetables and then turns to nine egg dishes (with one cucumber recipe slipped in between), thirty-eight fish recipes (including salt fish, frogs, barbel fish, young eel, conger eel, lamprey eel, tuna, shad, red snapper, hake, sardines, grouper, needle fish, cuttle fish, lobster), twenty-seven pies and preserves, mostly made from fruit (cherries, pears, quince, apples, peaches, grapes, and melons). He also includes a few pie recipes for borage (something similar to rhubarb), custard, farmer's cheese, pumpkin, and carrots. This section contains two unique recipes. The first is "De tortada de manjar blanco de gallina o pescado" [For a chicken or fish blancmange pie] but the instructions are for making sweet crepes with a sugar-egg filling and topped with more sugar (261–2). The section closes with "De zanahorias rellenas" [On stuffed carrots] that are boiled and filled with a mixture of ground almonds and walnuts, sugar, orange blossom water, pepper, clove, and cinnamon. The carrots are then dipped in egg wash, deep fried, and sprinkled with cinnamon sugar (266). While other cookbooks include carrot recipes, this one is unique to Hernández de Maceras.

Although Hernández de Maceras organizes his cookbook around eating habits grounded in Christian doctrine, the work also contains clear indications of Hispano-Muslim influences in its predilection for lamb, beef, and goat over pork; in its use of nuts in dessert recipes; in its use of specific ingredients like spice combinations of coriander, saffron, and black pepper, orange blossom water, and rice; and in its lexicon. For example, at the end of the recipe "Cómo se han de hacer bollos de clauonia" [How to make clavonia buns], he explains, "éstos se llaman también bollos maimones" [these are also called maimones buns] (217). The word *maimones* comes from the Arabic, *maímun* [happy]. One lamb dish called "Albujávanas" [Albujavanas], which is essentially a recipe for minced lamb patties served with an *egg-vinegar golden* sauce, takes its name from Arabic origins but includes lard in its ingredients. This addition of pork fat exemplifies how dishes adapted over time to the regional, cultural norms.

Other Works on Food and Drink

In the early modern period, manuscripts and published material on food and drink abound. Topics include drinks, especially cold drinks and wine; sweets and confections; agriculture and plants; New World products like chocolate and tobacco; and food for children including a 1629 discourse written by Juan Gutierrez de Godoy on the benefits of breastfeeding.[53] Following the thread of works written on drinks, the titles alone indicate how drinks were perceived and their positive and negative connotations. In 1490 Lluis Alcanyis writes *Regiment preservatui e curatiu de la pestilencia* [Rules on protection from and cures for the plague] in which he dedicates a section on what to drink. In the sixteenth century, there appear several works on the fashion of using snow for cold drinks. Some of the more popular drinks include horchata, barley water, and lemonade.[54] For example, in 1576 Francisco Micón publishes a 146-page work entitled, *Alivio de los sedientos, en el qual se trata de la necessidad que tenemos de bever frio y refrescado con nieve, y las condiciones que para esto son menester, y quales cuerpos lo pueden libremente soportar* [Relief for the thirsty in which is treated the need we have to drink cold and refreshing drinks with snow and the necessary conditions to do so and what kind of body can easily handle it]. That very same year, Alonso Díez Daza writes a book on drinking water called *Libro de los provechos y dannos que provienen con la sola bevida del agua. Y como se deva escoger la mejor. Y retificar la que no es tal, y de como se a de bever frio en tiempo de calor sin que haga daño* [Book on the benefits and harm that come from just drinking water and how to choose the best and purify what is not and on how to drink cold (drinks) in the heat without causing any harm]. Wine, of course, commanded much attention within the publishing world. Texts on the harm that comes from drinking wine cold (Andrés Laguna, 1555), on cultivating grapes for its production (Diego Gutiérrez de Salinas, 1598), on wine's curative powers (Jerónimo Cortés, 1614), decrees ordering tavern owners to serve good quality wine, briefs on taxing wine, royal letters on wine exemptions, poems and plays that extol wine's virtues all indicate the central role wine played in the early modern diet.

Sweets and confections appear in all cooking manuals in Spain from the *Fuḍālat-al-Hiwan* to Martínez Montiño's *Arte de cocina, pastelería, vizcochería y conservería*. Beyond these works with individual recipes or specific sections on, for example, fruit preserves, there also exist entire works dedicated to the preparation of sweets. Pérez Samper notes that these works differ from other cookbooks as they came out of the guilds and served as apprentices' textbooks as they studied for exams and memorized recipes (*La alimentación* 35). There are two significant works that date before 1700. The first is an anonymous Catalan work, *Llibre de totes maneres de confits* [Book on all types of candied fruit], from the fifteenth century.[55] The second is Castilian, written by Miguel de Baeza and published in 1592, *Los quatro libros del arte de confitería* [Four books on the art of confection].[56] In book 1, Baeza discusses sugar in all its forms, varieties, and ways of preparation, bringing in Arab and Andalusian influences and discussing where the best sugar comes from. In book 2 he treats different pastries; in book 3, sugar and honey-based preserves; and in book 4, marzipan, nougats, and similar sweet pastes. Pérez Samper lists other manuscripts that provide similar sweet recipes such as candy, jams, jellies, fruit preserves, sponge cakes, and sweet pastes (*La alimentación* 44–9).

Important works on geoponics extend back to tenth-century Spain with the *Calendario de Córdoba* [Calendar of Cordoba] (961) that explains what type of agricultural work needed to be done each month of the year. In the thirteenth century Gerardo de Cremona translated the work into Spanish at the School of Translators in Toledo. Many other agricultural treatises appeared in Al-Andalus before the early modern period.[57] Suffice it to name Ibn Wafid (1008–74) who wrote *Tratado de Agricultura* [Treatise on agriculture], the work that heavily influenced Gabriel Alonso de Herrera, author of *Agricultura General* [General agriculture] (1513). Alonso de Herrera's work was the definitive publication on agriculture throughout the early modern period and well into the twentieth century. It also contained treatises on veterinary medicine, food and health, and meteorology and earned him the epithet, the father of modern agriculture.

From the early letters of Christopher Columbus to writings of other explorers and missionaries, Europeans began to learn about plants and food items from the New World. One of the early works that comments on the reception of food from America is by the court chronicler Francisco López de Gómara, *Historia general de las Indias* [General history of the Indies] (1552). Although López de Gómara writes some fifty years after the event, he describes products that Columbus brought back to Spain and Fernando and Isabel's supposed reactions to them:

> Probaron el ají, especia de los indios, que les quemó la lengua, y las batatas, que son raíces dulces, y los gallipavos, que son mejores que pavos y gallinas. Maravilláronse que no hubiese trigo allá, sino que todos comiesen pan de aquel maíz. (50)

[They tasted chilies, a spice of the Indies, that burned their tongues, and sweet potatoes, that are a sweet root, and turkeys that are better than peacocks or hens. They were surprised that there was no wheat there and that instead they all ate bread made from that corn.]

Gonzalo Fernández de Oviedo, who penned *Sumario de la natural historia de las Indias* [Summary of the natural history of the Indies] (1526), Bernal Díaz, *Historia verdadera de la conquista de la Nueva España* [True History of the conquest of New Spain] (16th c.), and Francisco Hernández's *Quatro libros de la naturaleza y virtudes de las plantas y animales que están recibidos en el uso de medicina en la Nueva España* [Four books on the nature and virtue of plants and animals that have been received for medical purposes in New Spain] also discussed New World products.[58] Finally, Nicolás Monardes wrote a series of works from 1569–74 on the medical implications of products brought to Spain from the New World called *La historia medicinal de las cosas que traen de nuestras islas occidentales* [Medical history of things brought from our western islands].

Chocolate appears in many of the sixteenth-century works but later, in the seventeenth century, there is a surge of treatises that focus on the benefits and damages of drinking hot chocolate, for example, Juan de Barrios's *Libro en el cual se trata del chocolate, que provechos haga, y si sea bebida saludable o no...* [Book on chocolate, its benefits and whether or not it is a healthy drink...] (1609) and Bartolomé Marradón's *Diálogo del uso del tabaco, los daños que causa, etc. y del chocolate y otras bebidas* [Dialogue on the use of tobacco, the damage it causes, etc., and on chocolate and other beverages] (1618). Additionally, a heated debate on the morality of drinking chocolate and whether it breaks the fast or not was the focus of several other works. Included in these publications are ones by Antonio de León Pinelo (1636) and Manuel Caro Dávila (1699).

This chapter outlines the most significant cooking manuals leading up to and including those of the early modern period. Through the food products, preparation instructions, and personal comments of the authors, they provide evidence of what people ate and how they viewed these dishes. The chapters that follow contextualize cooking manuals with other discourses that include novels, poems, plays, dietary manuals, legal documents, and travel narratives. Together they offer fascinating images of food's role in society and the development of foodways in early modern Spain.

Chapter Two

"Una olla de algo más vaca que carnero": Privileging Meat in the Early Modern Diet

Vaca y carnero, olla de caballero

[Beef and mutton, gentleman's stew]

Popular saying

Everyone is familiar with the opening line of *Don Quixote*, "en un lugar de la Mancha, de cuyo nombre no quiero acordarme ..." [In a village of La Mancha, the name of which I rather not recall ...] (1.69).[1] But, what of the novel's second sentence in which the narrator describes the hero through the food he eats?

> Una olla de algo más vaca que carnero, salpicón las más noches, duelos y quebrantos los sábados, lantejas los viernes, algún palomino de añadidura los domingos, consumían las tres partes de su hacienda. (1.69–70)

> [A stew made of more beef than mutton, cold salad on most nights, abstinence eggs on Saturdays, lentils on Fridays, and an additional squab on Sundays consumed three quarters of his income.]

With the opening of this phrase, "una olla de algo más vaca que carnero," the narrator states that Alonso Quijano regularly ate one-pot meals made of more beef than mutton. The first questions that come to mind are, what does it mean that Alonso Quijano regularly ate meat? How does meat figure into the diet of Spaniards of different regions and socioeconomic classes during the early modern period? Why does Cervantes serve up these two meats, prioritizing the one over the other? What message did this send his contemporary readers? The second issue revolves around the *olla*, or one-pot stew. Again, by defining the hidalgo in these terms, what can we learn about his social and economic circumstances? This chapter explores the meaning of this simple phrase by examining multiple discourses that together give a general understanding of meat's privileged position over vegetables and specifically of society's preference for mutton over beef. Through cookbooks, novels, plays, travellers' logs, and legal accounts we can understand how meat was regulated and consumed at different economic and regional levels of society and how it became a type of cultural capital which defined social status and played out even in the lives of fictional characters like Alonso Quijano. Meat is, without a doubt, a cultural marker of social status but upon careful study of who ate what meat and how often we find that meat preferences also present what Stephen Mennell terms "diminishing contrasts" between social classes. The chapter also addresses the other mainstay of any Spanish table, bread, and again, through a variety of discourses explains its place in the diet and social life of Spaniards living in the sixteenth and seventeenth centuries.

Meat before Vegetables

With respect to consuming meat on a regular basis, the predilection for animal products over vegetables is found in cooking manuals, literature, medical and dietary treatises, and even lawsuits. For instance, in *Libro del arte de cocina* [Book on the art of cooking], Domingo Hernández de Maceras writes nearly double the number of recipes (116) on raised and hunted animals and fish than on gathered and cultivated vegetable products (61). In literature and medical treatises writers continually praise meat and admonish the harmful effects of fruits and vegetables. The medical doctors Bernardo de Gordonio, Alonso Chirino, and Francisco López de Villalobos, respectively extol the uses of beef broth for an upset stomach, beef juice for an earache, and dung and beef lard for making a plaster for swollen or otherwise painful joints.[2] Likewise, in dietary manuals meat plays a much bigger role in maintaining health and curing the sick than do fruits and vegetables. For example, the Renaissance gastronome, Bartolomeo Sacchi, better known as Platina, states that "meats ... nourish better and more healthfully than any other food" (229).

In the judicial system, the sheer number of lawsuits against cattle ranchers, sheep herders, and others who traversed across Spain with

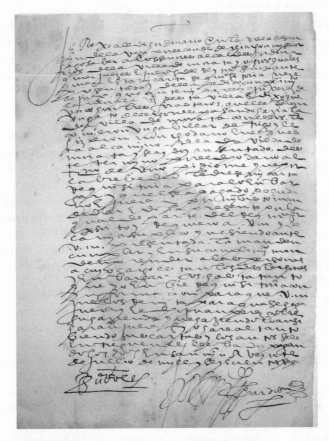

Figure 2.1. Fragment of file 913669/3286 "Una petición de un vecino para daños causados en su tripo por un hato de lechones" [A citizen's petition for damages incurred on his land by a herd of young pigs] (1606). Photo by author, courtesy of ARCM.

their herds and were protected by royal decree in spite of repeated offences in designated agricultural areas also demonstrates support for the meat industry over farmers. In the Archivo Regional de la Comunidad de Madrid [Regional Archives of the Community of Madrid] (ARCM) between 1500 and 1700 there are hundreds of orders, *autos* [judicial decrees], and requisitions like the 1606 "A petición de un vecino para daños causados en su tripo por un hato de lechones" [A citizen's petition for damages incurred on his land by a herd of young pigs], or one from the mid-seventeenth century in which a citizen presses charges against the man who allowed cattle into his vineyard.[3] These documents highlight the continued conflict between farmers and herders and the advantages the latter enjoyed. Similar lawsuits continued through the early modern period and into the nineteenth century as evidenced by an 1804 claim against cattle in a village outside the capital (ARCM, San Martín de la Vega 18390/3109 1668–1804).

Disputes of damaged lands caused by transient herds extend back as far as the Visigoth period in Spain and reached a turning point in the Middle Ages when Alfonso X created the Real Sociedad de ganaderos de la Mesta [Royal society of herders of the Mesta] and Alfonso XI began regulating it in 1347. Later the Catholic Monarchs gave this powerful guild of sheep herders absolute freedom to drive their herds through both Castile and Aragon with the idea of protecting their livelihood but also to generate needed income for the state through contracts and rights of sales. In this way both the state and the herding industry had a vested interest in all things ovine. According to Julius Klein's groundbreaking study in the early part of the twentieth century, during Isabel's reign, the Mesta was involved in over 1100 litigations (209). Later, as the Hapsburg dynasty began to fall apart, the Mesta experienced ever increasing fiscal problems with local institutions – town halls, monasteries, military orders – or private landowners. Although the institution finally collapsed in the early part of the nineteenth century, during the early modern era meat preference was directly tied to the economic gains of the state as exemplified by the Mesta's privileged position and the preference shown to pastoral land over agricultural land.[4]

A number of historians report varying information regarding meat preferences in early modern Spain that show its importance not only at court but also in cities and small villages. María del Carmen Simón Palmer observes that at court, "la carne es la base de la alimentación durante la Edad Media y continúa siéndolo en los siglos XVI y XVII. Es entonces la de carnero la más consumida, seguida de la de vaca, aves y caza" [Meat is the basis of food during the Middle Ages and continues as such in the sixteenth and seventeenth centuries. Mutton is consumed the most, followed by beef, fowl, and game] ("La cocina" 41). Ricardo Izquierdo Benito looks at regulations for meat provisions in fifteenth-century Toledo. By studying legal documents, his work shows that throughout the fifteenth century and into the early modern period meat sales were highly regulated.

En las ordenanzas de la ciudad, todo lo relacionado con el oficio de los carniceros y de los comerciantes de carne estaba minuciosamente regulado. Así, entre otras normas, se precisaba que los pesos y pesas utilizados para la venta tenían que ser de hierro y estar marcados con la señal que indicase el alcalde mayor de la justicia. Eran los siguientes: dos arreldes, arrelde, medio arrelde, tercio de arrelde, libra, media libra, tercio de libra y cuarto de libra. (cited in Izquierdo Benito 65)[5]

[In the city ordinances, everything related to the office of butchers and meat vendors was carefully regulated. So, among other norms, it was stipulated that weights and scales that were used for sales were to be made of iron and labelled with the seal that the town's court justice indicates. The following are in place: two *arreldes*, one *arrelde*, a half *arrelde*, a third of an *arrelde*, a pound, a half pound, a third of a pound and a quarter of a pound.]

Cities and villages alike took their meat seriously and through a series of ordinances tried to guarantee a stable market in which the three main staples – meat, bread, and wine – could be available on a regular basis. Izquierdo Benito shows that in fifteenth-century Toledo, meat was the most consumed product (41.1 per cent) followed by fish, wine, and other food (16.5 per cent each), and bread (9.1 per cent) (132). He also notes that the cost of an *arroba*[6] of mutton was equal to that of oil, which was also equal to a *fanega* [bushel] of rye or barley (133). These trends occurred in other Mediterranean regions as well. Massimo Montanari notes that documents in Provence, Tours, and cities in Sicily from the fourteenth to the sixteenth centuries show "notable levels of meat consumption" (74). However, studying market ordinances does not directly correlate with what was consumed at the table as people certainly acquired many foodstuffs outside the regulated markets. Purchasing meat from wholesalers or at other venues and bartering with fellow citizens and with those from outside were some of the ways people acquired food outside the state-approved markets.

Toledo, of course, is a sizeable urban centre and meat consumption there may only indicate food choices of a certain urban elite, but records from smaller villages also show significant meat consumption in early modern Spain. Similar to the city of Toledo we find that strict regulations governed meat markets in smaller communities as well. For example, in 1642, in the village of Loeches (close to Madrid) a case was brought before the court regarding billy-goat meat that was processed and sold and for which no taxes were paid. Charges were levied not only against the butcher, Alonso Delgado, but also against the shop administrator, Jusepe Milano, and the owner, Gabriel Milano.

> condeno a los dichos Jusepe Milano y Alonsso Delgado a que satisfagan a su magestad y quien huuiere de haber las sisas y impuestos lo que montare la sissa del macho de cabrío que entraran en la carnicería y más les condena a entrambos en tres mill maravedís. (ARCM Loeches 96014/26 1642)[7]

> [I condemn said Jusepe Milano and Alonso Delgado to pay His Majesty and whoever collects the charges and taxes and whatever accumulated taxes for the male kid that was processed in their butcher shop and, moreover, both are fined 3000 maravedis.]

Beyond the steep fines, the butcher was also incarcerated for not paying the appropriate taxes.

In addition to the regulation of butcher shops, laws were also in place to protect establishments, for example, *tabernas* [taverns] that could legally sell cooked meat and other prepared food from *mesones* [inns] that were only approved for lodging. Certain establishments paid for the right to sell food to travellers while others only paid for the right to prepare food that travellers brought with them. These disputes were often brought to court and settled there. For example, in 1619 Ambrosio García, village judge, heard a case that the local sheriff, Alonso García, brought before court.

> [D]enunçió a Jusepe de Morales, mesonero, vezino desta uilla, sobre raçón que estando proybido por leyes y premáticas destos reinos que no pueda tener en su mesón bodegón ni vender comida a los que allí vinieren a posar, el suso dicho en desacato de la justicia y abiendole sido mandado por ella muchas vezes que no tenga el dicho bodegón en su mesón, y siendo en perjuiçio del arrendamiento del alcabala de la taberna que está arrendada con condiçión que nengún (*sic*) mesonero pueda tener bodegón en su cassa, ni dar de comer a los güéspedes (*sic*), ni vendersela, más de solamente guisar lo que ellos truxesen ... y hallaron vna olla al fuego de carne guisada, y el dicho Jusepe de Morales estaba partiendo un pedaço de cordero para guisar. (ARCM San Martín de la Vega 913632/2551 1619)

> [(Alonso García) pressed charges against Jusepe de Morales, innkeeper and village citizen, for the reason that it is prohibited by laws and statutes of these kingdoms either to have a bar in his inn or to sell food to those who seek lodging and that the aforementioned is in defiance of the law and

having been ordered many times to not have said bar in his inn and having gone against the lease of the tax obligations of the tavern that stipulates that no innkeeper can have a bar in his establishment nor provide food to his lodgers, nor sell them any, but can only prepare what they have brought with them ... And they found a pot over the flame filled with cooked meat and said Jusepe de Morales chopping a piece of lamb to cook.]

Jusepe denied all infractions and swore that the pot was left there by other travellers. He further stated that he never prepared his food for others but only cooked what they had brought with them. When asked whether in his inn he had pots of meat, rice, and had bought fish, eggs, and other staples and if he had prepared them for others, he explained that his lodgers had given him money and had paid him for his services but continued to deny any infraction. In the end, he did jail time and was fined 1000 maravedis [mrvs], which were distributed equally between the judge, the court, and the accuser.

Jusepe's cunning character could be straight from the pages of a picaresque novel but what this case and other legal documents reveal is that meat was consumed on a regular basis in both urban centres and in small villages, even by travelling muleteers. Playwrights, novelists, and essayists all confirm that mutton and beef are meat options that many enjoyed. From villagers to gentlemen, foot soldiers to university students, actors to monks, all regularly ate meat to varying degrees. In the picaresque novel *El Guzmán de Alfarache* [Guzman de Alfarache], Mateo Alemán describes access to meat that kitchen hands had as they regularly stole from their masters:

No había mozo tan desventurado, que no ahorrase los menudillos de las gallinas o de los capones, el jamón de tocino, el contrapeso del carnero, las postas de ternera, salsas, especias, nieve, vino, azúcar, aceite, miel, velas, carbón y leña, sin perdonar las alcomenías ni otra cosa, desde lo más necesario hasta lo de menos importancia que en una casa de un señor se gasta. (189)

[No boy who worked in the kitchen was so hapless that he could not save away the hen or capon giblets, some fat back, the leftover mutton after weighing it, veal scraps, sauces, spices, packed snow, wine, sugar, oil, honey, candles, coal, and wood, nor forget about seeds or anything else from the most to the least important that was bought for a gentlemen's house.]

His description of kitchen supplies mirrors those of wealthy kitchens across the peninsula.

Regarding soldiers' fare, Alonso de Contreras describes the prices for food supplies for Spanish troops while in Mehdia, Morocco: "Y no pueden vivir sin La Mámora, porque todo cuanto hurtan lo traen a vender allí, y lo que no hurtan. Dan un carnero como un buey por cuatro reales, y una vaca por dieciséis, y una fanega de trigo por tres reales, y una gallina por medio real" [And they could not live without the Mehdia because everything they had or could steal they would bring there to sell. They paid four reals for a ram or an ox, and sixteen for a cow and three reals for a bushel of wheat, and a half real for a hen] (240). Although the market is in northern Africa, the food items noted – mutton, beef, wheat, poultry – reflect the supplies purchased for Spanish troops.

In *El viaje entretenido* [The pleasant voyage] (1604), Agustín de Rojas describes the life of travelling actors who are touring villages: "Están ocho días en un pueblo, duermen en una cama cuatro, comen olla de vaca y carnero, y algunas noches su menudo muy bien aderezado. Tienen el vino por adarmes, la carne por onzas, el pan por libras y la hambre por arrobas" [They would spend a week in a town, all cram into one poster bed, eat beef and mutton stew, and some nights those giblets were really tasty. They had wine by the sip, meat by the ounce, bread by the pound, and hunger by the ton] (154). Later, he describes a monk who gave him meat and bread in exchange for sermons: "en el monasterio de San Agustín un fraile me daba cada día un puchero de vaca y una libra de pan, porque le escribía algunos sermones" [in the Saint Augustine monastery a monk would trade me a beef stew and a pound of bread for sermons I would write] (162). Rojas presents literary food images with his usual picaresque wit but like many of his descriptions, they are grounded in the reality of actors and playwrights.

Travellers to the New World brought their preferences for beef and mutton with them. Chroniclers' logs include mutton and beef among the main staples. In 1608 Pedro de Valencia records the provisions of Zacatecas, and explains that mutton and beef, together with bread and wine and also fresh fish, corn, squash, beans, figs, and local fruit form the basis of food eaten there (Torres de Mendoza 181). It would seem, then, that meat consumption was not uncommon among most of Spain's expanding communities.[8]

Mutton and Beef

What becomes key is not whether one ate meat or not, but rather how much meat was consumed, what type of animal, and what cut of meat.

In these nuances, between prized animal and one of lesser value, between best cut of meat and worst, lie shifts in the social class structure. There is no doubt that the difference of quality and quantity in meat regularly consumed affirms a consumer's position in society. According to Pierre Bourdieu, an individual is not only distinguished by his/her aesthetic choices but by the most banal ones of eating and drinking. In any given field or social arena, people compete for resources, both material and symbolic, by using their different types of capital whether it be economic, social, or cultural. In this way, eating meat became a sort of social capital that could either reflect a deep-seated identity or indicate an attempt to change one's very identity.[9]

During the sixteenth century, Spain, like many parts of Europe, was experiencing a lot of social mobility and revolt. The elite enclosed themselves within rules and norms. They excluded and increased social discrimination between different aristocratic levels however possible, for example, by refining the table. Under Felipe III's rule, and because of the Crown's financial needs, social mobility exploded: gentlemen were granted titles, those with titles ascended to the status of grandee, and even within the grandee circle, subtle hierarchical differences were played out to distinguish one group from another. It is worth noting that while economic capital was made available to some, the cultural capital needed to achieve recognition at times was harder to obtain. "Cultural consumption [is] predisposed, consciously and deliberately or not, to fulfil a social function of legitimating social differences" (Bourdieu xxx). With the right amount of money, anyone could buy his/ her way up the proverbial aristocratic ladder but could this person acquire the recognition that comes with the newly acquired title?

One must remember that economic capital is only part of the way that a person may alter his or her social condition. Bourdieu explains that "one has to take account of all the characteristics of social condition which ... tend to shape tastes adjusted to these conditions. The true basis of the differences found in the area of consumption, and far beyond it, is the opposition between the tastes of luxury (or freedom) and the tastes of necessity" (173). This is why, for example, that when Sancho acquires his governorship, he chooses to relinquish it. His tastes of necessity, for foods which are filling by design like the *olla podrida* discussed below, so greatly outweigh the acquired tastes of luxury that come with his position.

Social ascendency was a very real issue in Hapsburg Spain. Antonio Domínguez Ortiz explains:

la categoría predominante y casi única que presidió la creación de títulos en aquel siglo, que fue la necesidad de la Corona de procurarse dinero, con lo cual, por encima de las protestas que levantara el sistema, venía a reconocerse el criterio fundamentalmente económico que, como ya queda apuntado, presidía la jerarquización del estamento nobiliario. Quien tenía dinero para comprar lugares y vasallos, llevar un tren de vida ostentoso y abonar crecidas cantidades a la Hacienda, pasaba a ser, de simple caballero, conde o marqués. (72)

[The main, and perhaps only, category that prevailed over creating titles in that century, was the Crown's need to generate revenue which, in spite of protests that doing so would bring down the system, was recognized as a fundamental economic criteria that, as already suggested, favoured the hierarchization of the nobility. Whoever had money to buy estates and vassals, maintain an ostentatious lifestyle, and credit large quantities to the Treasury went from a simple gentlemen to a count or a marquis.]

The fifty or so grandees and titled nobles during the reign of Carlos I doubled during Felipe II's rule. To those hundred, Felipe III added another twenty marquises and twenty-five counts (Domínguez Ortiz 71).

And with these dramatic increases of social ascendance came exclusionary tactics. The old aristocracy began snubbing the new by denying them entrance into certain privileged circles (Domínguez Ortiz 55), and, as Montanari points out, by supporting classist theories of nutritional privilege (82–91). According to expert opinions of the day, nobility was born with the ability to digest more easily cuts of meat that were too rich or delicate for the working class. Conversely, workers could more easily consume tougher cuts of meat than the gentry. The medical advisor to Carlos V, Luis Lobera de Ávila, explains that "las personas de negocios, grandes señores o de muy alto estado, débense evitar del mucho uso de comer vaca o buey, máxime viejo" [business men, grandees, or gentlemen of high ranking should avoid eating a lot of very old beef or ox] (74). This theory of nutritional privilege extended beyond cuts of meat to all types of foodstuffs and eating habits.

Since antiquity offering food has been a sign of hospitality and respect. In the feasting/fasting lifestyle of the Middle Ages social status and prestige were based on quantity. However, at the dawn of the modern age, the sign of prestige shifted from quantity to quality. This change evolved in part as food supplies became more regularized.

Division of labour, expansion of commerce, and competition intensified.[10] These social and economic changes clearly affected both cooking in the kitchen and eating at the table. Nobility no longer ate bigger amounts to distinguish themselves from others of a lower social class; rather, they ate better and thus, an elitist diet emerged. Montanari explains that "the consumption of certain foods (and of foods prepared in a particular way) was not simply a function of habit or choice, but rather a sign of social identity and so to be correctly observed in the interest of maintaining the proper social equilibria and hierarchies" (85). In the same way, those seeking to prove themselves could use the same theories and food practices to advance their position. As Bourdieu reminds us, "there are relationships between groups maintaining different and even antagonistic relations to culture, depending on the conditions in which they acquired their cultural capital" (4). To achieve the symbolic capital that should accompany the new social status, people could demonstrate what food products they consumed and how they consumed them. Eating, then, plays a key role in one's social identity and conversely, social identity plays a key role in what and how one eats.

The extended title of the 1529 edition to Nola's cookbook, *Libro de guisados* [Book of cooking] gives an indication of how food preparation for kings and grandees was made available to those of lesser rank in the span of a decade:

Libro de guisados, manjares y potajes intitulado libro de cozina: en el qual esta el regimiento de las casas delos reyes y grandes senores: y los officiales a las casas dellos cada uno como an de servir su officio. Y en esta segunda impression se ha anadido un regimiento delas casas delos cavalleros y gentiles hombres y religiosos de dignidades y personas de medianos estados y otros que tienen familia y criados en sus casas: y algunos manjares de dolientes y otras cosas en el anadidas: todo nuevamente revisto añadido y emendado por su mismo autor

[Book of stews, delicacies and soups entitled Book of Cooking in which are rules for the households of kings and grandees: and to the officials of each one of those houses and how to carry out their service. And in this second edition rules have been added for the households of knights and gentlemen and members of dignified religious orders and persons of middle estates and others who have family and servants in their houses: and some food for the sick and other things added: all newly revised, added, and amended by the author himself.][11]

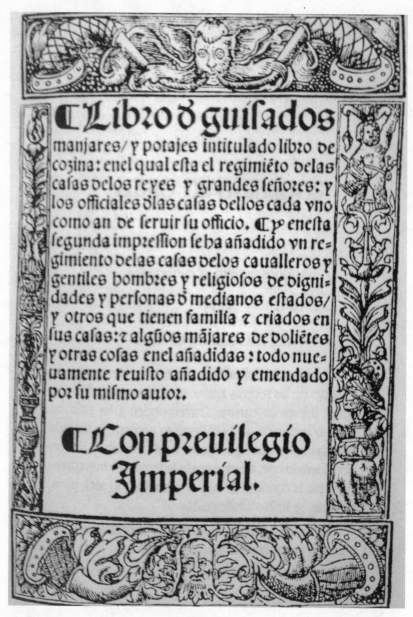

Figure 2.2. Engraving for the 1529 edition of *Libro de guisados*, ed. Dionisio Pérez (Madrid: Pedro Sáinz y Rodríguez), 2.

What was first written for court in 1520 was later made available to those of other social rankings. People of "middle estates" could then have access to prescriptive formulas for preparing and eating the same food that royalty did. In this light, cookbooks define the cultural norms for food preparation and eating and, as such, are agents of cultural capital. They also remind emerging middle classes of class privilege and that by acquiring this form of cultural capital, a person, family, or group could legitimize or ostensibly improve their social standing.

In early modern Spain, meat preferences followed a definite hierarchy with *carnero* [mutton] at the top followed by meat from *ternera* [veal], *cabrito* [kid], *puerco* [pig], *cabra* [chevon], *vaca* [cow], *oveja* [ewe], and *cabrón cojudo* [billy goat] (Valles Rojo, *Cocina* 237–8). Antonio Matilla Tascón's study on the supply of meat in Madrid during the early modern period confirms the predilection for mutton over beef. He reports that from 1481 to 1515, mutton (per *arrelde*) was consistently 30 per cent more expensive than beef and that at times it increased to 50 per cent (58). This trend certainly continued through the sixteenth and seventeenth centuries as well. Matilla Tascón also reports that in 1606 the state received almost double the tax revenues from *carnero* sales as from beef sales (67–8).[12]

What must be noted is that in early modern Spain *carnero* refers to mutton that is a year old, what today in Spain is known as *cordero pascual* [paschal lamb]. To clarify the evolution of this term, labels used today in Spain prove helpful. *Cordero lechal* [milk-fed lamb] refers to animals that are 1–1½ months old and 4–6 kilos, *cordero recental* [recental lamb], to those up to 4 months old and 13 kilos, and *cordero pascual* [paschal lamb], from 4 to12 months and no more than 8 kilos butcher weight. After 18 months of age, the slaughtered animal is considered *carnero* [mutton]. The hierarchical preference for meat from very young lambs definitively changed in the early part of the twentieth century but in the sixteenth and seventeenth centuries this was not yet the case.[13]

Early modern cookbooks have no separate word to distinguish mutton from lamb nor do the legal records of market value separate categories for *cordero* [lamb] or *lechal* [milk-fed lamb] prices. In addition, Lobera de Ávila clearly states that among all types of meat, "el carnero de un año o poco más es lo mejor" [mutton from a year old (sheep) or a little older is the best] (73). He continues by drawing support from other medical giants and further refines the best choice of meat: "Basta que la carne de carnero de un año, siendo castrado, es muy buena carne y de buena digestión" [suffice it to say that meat from a year-old sheep that has been castrated, is very good meat and easily digested] (73). When discussing in detail the different types of meats and the animals' ages, he specifies that it is healthier to eat some when they are younger but, others, like sheep, when they are older. "Estas, cuanto más son propincuas a su nascimiento, son mejores; así como ternera, cabrito, gaçapo y gamo, y al revés las flemáticas; así como cordero e lechón, etc. Cuando son más propincuas a su nascimiento son peores, e cuanto apartados mejores, como carnero, etc." [These, the closer they are to birth, the better, like veal, kid, young rabbit, and fallow deer and the opposite for the phlegmatic meat; like lamb or suckling pig. When they are closer to birth, they are worse and as they get older, they are better, like mutton, etc.] (50). For these reasons, when dealing with *carnero* in recipes I will use the term "young mutton." This phrase retains the original meaning of *carnero* while at the same time highlights the shift to a younger animal than what is defined by today's standards.

Turning to Andalucia, we see similar trends in Teresa de Castro Martínez's study on meat prices in Granada that echo those of the privileged meats at court: mutton is sold at 17 mrvs./arrelde while beef, pork, and billy goat are sold at 13 mrvs./arrelde and nanny goat and mutton from a ewe at 11 mrvs./arrelde ("Carne/3"). By comparing these prices to those of workers' wages, she concludes that as Spain moved into the early modern period, "es indudable que el consumo de carne se había homologado en todos los ámbitos, entre todas las clases sociales" [it is undeniable that meat consumption had become standardized in all circles among all social classes] ("Carne/3").

Notwithstanding, the urban elite continued to receive the best cuts of young mutton, veal, and kid. In addition, certain privileged community members were the first to choose from a selection of meats that the butcher reserved for them. In fact, in the town of Loja (between Granada and Málaga), rules were laid out in a 1491 ordinance for butchers that required them to hold aside certain cuts of meats for the most important townsmen:

quel tal obligado ... sea obligado de dar cargo cada dia al despensero del señor alcayde desta çibdad de las caderas e las carnadas e quixotes de las vacas e de la otra carne, de lo qual más quisiere;[14] e asimismo al vicario e clerigos, e alcaldes e alguasiles, e regidores e jurados e escriuanos del conçejo, e fesicos, e a sus onbres e moços dellos, so pena de vn par de gallinas. (cited in Castro Martínez, "Carne/3") [that said bound [butcher] is legally bound to release each day to the steward of this city's Lord Mayor the cow's rump, shoulder, and cheek and any other part of whatever he would want and the same for the vicar and clergy; the mayors and sheriffs; the aldermen and judges and law clerks of the town council; and magistrates and to their men or lads under penalty of a pair of hens.]

These laws inculcate the exclusionary tactics that segregated social circles. Similar ordinances led men of lesser nobility [*escuderos*] to protest as they were the object of meat discrimination and complained that the butcher's employees were not giving them meat in accordance with their social status, "no les dan segun quien ellos son" [they were not given in accordance to who they were] (cited in Castro Martínez, "Carne/3").

To understand more fully Alonso Quijano's mutton-light stew and meat consumption more generally, cookbooks contemporary to Cervantes' masterpiece also shed light on the subject. In both the court cookbook, Francisco Martínez Montiño's *Arte de Cocina, Pastelería, Vizcochería y Conservería* [The art of cooking, pie making, pastry making and preserving] (1611), and the university manual, Domingo Hernández de Maceras's *Libro del arte de cocina* (1607), young mutton and beef figure significantly but in very different ways. Using Martínez Montiño as an example, we find that he includes seventeen recipes for *carnero* dishes, the majority of them for leg of young mutton.[15] In addition, organ meat, including testicles and lung, the loin, the tail, and general *carnero* references are part of over a dozen other recipes including stuffed eggplant, couscous, and stuffed kid. Beef, on the other hand, appears in some forty recipes but only five are specific to preparing beef dishes: "Salpicón de baca" [Beef salpicon] (36), "Una empanada de pecho de vaca" [Beef brisket empanada] (187), "Un solomo de vaca relleno" [Stuffed beef tenderloin] (226–7), and two soup recipes, "Sopas a la Portuguesa" [Portuguese-style soups] (370) and "Otra sopa de vaca" [Another beef soup] (371–2). In the remaining recipes beef bone marrow figures predominately. In thirty-one of the thirty-five recipes, bone marrow is used in diverse dishes such as "Fruta rellena" [Stuffed fruit] (98–100) and "Pasteles ojaldrados" [Puff pastries] (160), and "Como se adereza la calabaza" [How to season bottle squash] (251).

Unlike *carnero*, there are two distinct words for meat from a cow based on its age: *ternera* [veal] and *carne de vaca* [beef]. In the recipe books, *ternera* is used in ways very comparable to *carnero* whereas *carne de vaca* is not. There are between ten and twenty recipes that include top cuts of veal and another dozen in which the main ingredient is offal: kidneys, liver, head, brain, knuckles, and sweetbreads. In several recipes Martínez Montiño allows for choosing either veal or young mutton for the recipe, thus aligning the way the two meats are prepared. For example in the "Fruta rellena" [stuffed fruit] recipe, Martínez Montiño provides an alternate stuffing that consists of either veal or young mutton (99). There are certain indications that point to a slight preference for young mutton over veal. In both cookbooks, young mutton comes before veal. One of Martínez Montiño's opening recipes is "Gigote de una pierna de carnero" [Leg of young mutton stew] followed by "Como se hace la Ternera" [How veal is made]. Likewise, in Domingo Hernández de Maceras's *Libro del arte de cocina*, he begins his first chapter, "De los guisados de carnero" [On young mutton dishes] with a series of *carnero* recipes before the recipes for pork, beef, veal, kid, and a variety of poultry. In his second chapter, "La comida de sábados" [Saturday food], sixteen of the nineteen partial abstinence meals are made with parts of sheep. But, generally, *carnero* [young mutton], *ternera* [veal], and also *cabrito* [kid] are often found in stew and pastry recipes with the suggestion that one meat can substitute for the other. This is not the case with beef and pork, both of which are used in very different ways.

One of the young mutton dishes that appears in the work of several authors, is *carnero verde* [green mutton stew]. In each of the three seventeenth-century cookbooks, little variations in ingredients, techniques, or explanation exist. Martínez Montiño's recipe suffices to understand how it was prepared:

Pondrás a cocer el carnero como está dicho, cortando el carnero á pedacitos, tamaños como nueces, y echalo á cocer con agua, y sal, y un pedazo de tocino gordo, y una cebolla entera: y quando el tocino y la cebolla esté cocido, sacalo al tablero, y echale cantidad de verdura, peregil, yervabuena, y cilantro verde, y picalo todo junto así caliente como está, y despues que está bien picado, y el carnero bien cocido, echa la verdura, y el tocino picado dentro de la olla ... (80)

[You can start cooking the young mutton as is stated, cutting it into small pieces, the size of walnuts, and boil it in water with salt and a piece of fat back and a whole onion. When the onion and fat back are done, take them out and put them on a cutting board and add a good amount of vegetables, parsley, mint, and cilantro, and chop it all up while still warm. After it is well chopped, and the young mutton well cooked, add the vegetables and the minced fat back to the pot ...]

Instructions follow on seasoning the dish with spices and lemon, thickening the broth with whipped egg, and serving it on a bed of sliced bread. This *carnero verde* sauce is also referenced in several other savoury dishes: "Cazuela de paxarillos" [Little bird stew] (103), "Como se adereza el sollo" [How to dress sturgeon] (272), "Otro platillo de criadillas de tierra" [Another truffle dish] (295), and "Ranas" [Frogs] (319–20).

On the stage, playwrights also reference this famous young mutton dish. Calderón uses it with erotic overtones in the opera *La púrpura de la rosa* [Purple shades of the rose] that retells Ovid's tale of Venus and Adonis. When referring to the dish Calderón plays with the connotations of *carnero-cabrón* [ram-cuckold] and *viejo verde* [dirty old man] when describing a certain type of woman:

No han de ser propias mujeres
Tanto, que con sus maridos
Desparramando placeres
A las holguras se bayan
A hablar del Carnero Verde   (240n1404–5)

[They are not so much good women/when, having husbands/ spreading pleasure/ they freely go about/ and speak of *carnero verde* (green lamb stew/dirty old cuckolds)]

The lackey in Mira de Amescua's *La mesonera del cielo y hermitaño galán* [Heaven's innkeeper and the gallant hermit] ranks *carnero verde* among other premiere foods served at the wedding banquet at the start of the play.

¿Qué has visto en ella que así,
cuando está hecha la costa,
la gente junta, amasado
el pan blanco de las tortas,
guisado el carnero verde,
sazonadas las albóndigas,
rellenos los pavos reales,
asada la tierna corza,
las perdices y conejos,

los francolines y tórtolas,
y todo tan en su punto
que a la más cartuja monja
despertara el apetito
a que sin melindre coma,
tú, necio, dejarla intentas?   (Williamsen, *La mesonera* 14–28)

[What have you seen in her that precisely/ when all is paid/ people gathered, kneaded/ the white bread for the pies/cooked up the green mutton stew/seasoned the meatballs/stuffed the peacocks/roasted the roe deer/ the partridge and the rabbit/ the francolins and turtledoves/ and everything done to such perfection/that of the most austere Carthusian nun/ her appetite would awaken/ and she would eat without holding back/ that you, fool, would try to stop it?]

The wedding food described in such detail at the opening of this play, much like the food supplies in the kitchen described in *El Guzmán de Alfarache*, is a culinary sign that creates materiality for the play and grounds the readers/spectators in the reality of the fictional moment. Knowing what *carnero verde* is and understanding what social, legal, and economic factors are behind the catalogue of privileged meat and poultry gives readers today a fuller appreciation of the food that was consumed and valued in the early modern era.

La olla

Now that we have a clearer understanding of the privileging of meat over vegetables and grains and that all meat is not created equal, we can better understand Cervantes' cultural context at the time of writing *Don Quixote* and a general perception of who ate meat and how the taste for mutton and beef fit into social eating norms. The second detail revealed in this simple phrase, "una olla más vaca que carnero" addresses Spain's gastronomic history in a different way: how meat was consumed.

It is certainly true that meat was prepared in numerous ways. Roasted, grilled, fried, braised, fricasséed, stewed, boiled, salted, and smoked are all common enough methods. Additionally, appliances and cookware such as *el horno portatil* [portable oven], *el anafe* [portable stove], *el espetón* [spit], *la parilla* [grill], *la cazuela* [casserole dish] (some with a heat source within the dish), *la olla* [pot], *tejas* [earthen tiles], even an *hoyo cavado* [hole in the ground], along with a wide range of heat sources from glowing embers to open flame and instructions on varying distances from the heat source, demonstrate the range of possibilities for meat preparation.[16] Among this diversity, one-pot meals fill the pages of the very first cooking manuals and continue into the early modern period. Generally they are oriented around one or two types of meat and vegetables. In the 1643 play *Eurídice y Orfeo* [Eurydice and Orpheus], Antonio de Solís gives a representative description of a one-pot stew:

> ¿Una olla, acaso una olla
> se ha de poner de milagro?
> ¿No ha de llevar su carnero,
> su tocino, sus garbanzos,
> su pimiento, su azafrán,
> su vaca, su punta de ajo,
> su perejil, su cebolla
> y su repollo? (191)

[A one-pot stew, do you think it/ appears miraculously?/ Shouldn't it have its mutton,/ its fat back, its garbanzos,/ its black pepper, its saffron,/ its beef, its bit of garlic,/ its parsley, its onion/ and its cabbage?]

This rhetorical question defines a classic *olla* with its meat, legumes, vegetables, and proper seasoning.

In banquets, upper classes would begin with selected roasts and one-pot meals for their first course, followed by seconds, thirds, and fruit.[17] In Martínez Montiño's court cooking manual, one-pot stews are among many first-course options that include roasts, pastries, and depending on the season, vegetables. Second courses also include roasts (both quadrupeds and poultry), in addition to stuffed meats, empanadas, and pies; and third courses are comprised of fish and eggs in addition to other roasts and savoury pies. His Christmas banquet suggestion, "Ollas podridas" [Hodgepodge stew], May menu, "Olla de carnero, y aves, y jamones de tocino" [Stew of young mutton, poultry, and fat back hams], and September menu, "Ollas podridas en pastelones de masa negra" [Hodgepodge stew in a dark-crust pie] all illustrate this practice and also exemplify the importance of one-pot stews throughout the seasons (14–19). Daily food habits and, as illustrated here, celebratory feasts were ways in which individuals could legitimize social standing or imitate the practices of those of higher social standing. Certainly the spoof of a governor's meal in *Don Quixote*, when Sancho becomes governor of Barataria and sits down to a myriad of fruit, roasted fowl, spiced dishes, and *olla podrida*, each one rapidly taken away for health reasons, also demonstrates in fiction what is seen in prescriptive texts: that the one-pot meal was enjoyed at the elite table.[18]

The classic one-pot meal in the early modern era was the *olla podrida*. Essentially, it consisted of meat, legumes, and seasonal vegetables but would also allow fowl, sausages, or anything that was available. This hardy meal varied from region to region and from table to table. Although its beginnings as a simpler stew with humbler ingredients are generally agreed upon, no one really knows its point of origin. Some postulate that it is originally Gallic or perhaps Visigoth; others theorize that the *olla podrida* comes from the Jewish *adafina* that would be prepared on Fridays to avoid cooking on the Sabbath.[19] At each table ingredients for the stew would invariably change depending on the area, season, and economic level of those cooking. But in the sixteenth century, *olla podrida* is certainly fashionable among the aristocracy, as evidenced by its inclusion in elite cooking manuals; for more than four centuries it has been served from the richest tables to the poorest. Calderón, in his *mojiganga Los guisados* [The stews], would dub the *olla*, "princesa de los guisados" [the princess of the stews] (46).[20]

Recipes would vary from one cook to the next but all agreed that the ingredients must be many and varied. Its first appearance in a cookbook, Santiago Gómez Laguna explains, is in 1570 when Bartolomeo Scappi includes the recipe "Per fare una vivanda di diverse materie detta in lingua spagnola oglia potrida" [A dish of many things as called in the Spanish language *olla podrida*] in his masterpiece *Dell'arte del cucinare* [On the art of cooking] (65–6). Gómez Laguna speculates that Scappi became aware of this stew when he provided a banquet for Carlos I in Rome in 1536 ("Aclaraciones" 10). As is explained in greater detail in chapter 1, Diego Granado, in his work *El libro del arte de la cozina* [The book on the art of cooking] (1599), translates hundreds of Scappi's recipes and holds the first written record for the *olla podrida* in Spain. He recommends the following:

> 6 libras de carnero y 6 libras de riñonada de ternera y 6 libras de vaca gorda y 2 capones y 2 gallinas y 4 pichones caseros gordos … y en otro tarro de barro o de cobre con el caldo de la sobredicha carne, cuézcanse dos cuartos de liebre trasera cortados a pedazos, tres perdices, dos faisanes, dos ánades gruesas, salvajes y frescas, veinte tordos, veinte cordonices y tres francolines. (82)

[6 pounds of young mutton, 6 pounds of veal loin, 6 pounds of beef fat, 2 capons, 2 hens, and 4 young, fat squabs ... And in another clay or copper pot with the broth of the aforementioned meat, boil two hindquarters of hare cut into pieces, three partridges, two pheasants, two ducks, fat, fresh, and wild, twenty starlings, twenty quail, and three francolins.]

The recipe contains other instructions for pork, vegetables, legumes, seasoning, and presentation but this citation begins to describe what would later become one of Spain's rich gastronomic contributions to Europe. The *olla podrida* was also enjoyed outside of Spain. Besides Scappi in 1570, Gervase Markham includes an "olla podrida" recipe in his instruction manual *The English Housewife* in 1615 (77). In 1669 Samuel Pepys writes in his journal of an "olio," his term for *olla podrida*, that was prepared by a cook who had spent time in Spain: "Sheres is to treat us with a Spanish Olio by a cook of his acquaintance that is there, that was with my Lord in Spain: and without any other company, he did do it, and mighty nobly; and the Olio was indeed a noble dish, such as I never saw better, or any more of" (509).[21] Culinary giants like Carême in his work, *L'art de la cuisine française au dix-neuvième siècle* [The art of French cooking in the nineteenth century] and Escoffier in *Le Guide Culinaire* [The culinary guide], both include the *olla podrida* as a Spanish national dish, albeit more simplified versions when compared to those of the early modern period.

Today, the *olla podrida* has evolved into *cocido*. Its rich regional variances give unique qualities to what is still a meat, bean, and vegetable one-pot delight. This dish is typically eaten in three courses: meat-based broth with noodles, garbanzos, and cabbage, variety of meats (pork, beef and fowl). The *cocido madrileño, puchero andaluz, escudella catalana, cocido de Murcia, cocido montañés* and the *cocido marigato de Asturias* are some of the regional varieties that come from the early modern tradition of the *olla podrida*.[22] The other consistent food item that, like the one-pot meal, was regularly consumed across regions and social classes, was bread. Together with meat, it defines the early modern Spanish diet.

Bread

Without a doubt, bread is the single most important food found on the early modern table, an honour that has endured up to the present.[23] Like its counterpart, meat, the type of bread consumed marked clear class boundaries. "The hierarchy of breads and their qualities in reality sanctioned social distinctions. Bread represented a status symbol that defined human condition and class according to its particular color" (Camporesi 120). The best wheat bread was reserved for the upper classes – the whiter the bread, the more valued – while wheat cut with other grains or simply other grains such as millet, rye, and barley were used to make bread for the lower classes. It was also not uncommon to find legumes or nuts ground into flour and made into bread as well.[24] Felipe III's doctor wrote that the superior bread was one that was "más fácil de partir con los dientes, y partido se mostrare por dentro más blanco que rubio" [easier to chew with one's teeth, and once split open, it was more white than golden on the inside] (Sánchez Meco 131). Fortunately, for the average worker, bread was both nutritious and affordable. Throughout the early modern period, bread was kneaded and rose at home before being taken to the communal oven for baking. An anecdote used to describe the humble life of a Jesuit captures well how bread was made in the seventeenth century. "Este Hermano era panadero, que amasaba el pan en casa, y sobre la cabeza lo llevaba al horno, donde había tantas mujercillas como las suele haber, y aguardaba allí su vez" [This brother was a baker, who kneaded his bread at home, and carried it on his head to the oven where there were so many young women as there usually were, and there, he waited his turn] (González Dávila, "Pláctica 68").

In Manuel Rubio Gago's study on the different types of bread regularly eaten in León, he writes that in the early modern period individuals would bake the appropriate amount necessary for their family for a two or three week period. Given this time frame, one can understand the abundance of recipes for *migas* (a recipe for cubed breadcrumbs and pieces of diced fat back fried together), *torrijas* (milk-soaked and sugar-laden bread dessert), and other creative ways to use older bread. The ovens were generally fired on a holiday so bread making would often times coincide with a social gathering and the roasting of an animal or additional baking. Images of a kneading trough (above) and a bread oven (below) built in Zamora, Spain, in 1920 provide an image of how bread was made and baked in the early modern era (see fig. 2.3).

The pages of early modern fiction are filled with bread imagery that promotes hospitality, displays signs of wealth, establishes cultural and social norms, highlights celebrations, reflects Christian charity and sacred acts, and performs a myriad of other functions. There is no writer who does not incorporate bread imagery in one way or another into the written text. From the pages of picaresque fiction where breadcrumbs on a jacket become the signifier for a meal never consumed, to the early

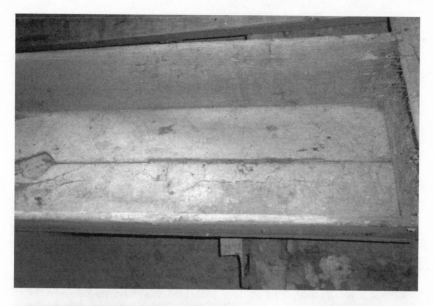

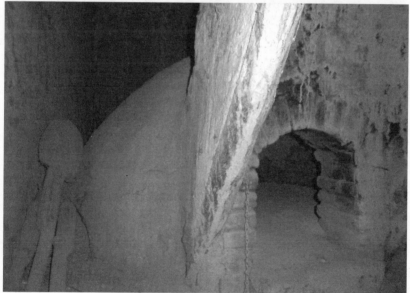

Fig 2.3 Bread oven and kneading trough in Villabrazaro, Spain. Photos courtesy of Angela and María Eugenia Madrid (Villabrazo Vivo. Web. 2 Feb. 2014).

modern plays where mountains of the whitest bread set the stage for marital celebrations, to *Don Quixote* where the knight and his humble squire take pleasure in sharing some wine, cheese and a few scraps of bread, these images exemplify the pervasiveness of bread in fiction and its multiplicity of meaning.

In Antonio de Guevara's attack on court life, *Menosprecio de corte y alabanza de aldea* [Contempt for court and praise for rural life], he provides his readers with an idyllic description of the abundance and excellent quality of bread made outside the city:

> en el aldea, a do comen el pan de trigo candeal, molido en buen molino, ahechado muy despacio, pasado por tres cedazos, cocido en horno grande, tierno del día antes, amasado con buena agua, blanco como la nieve y fofo como esponja. Los que viven en el aldea y amasan en su casa tienen abundancia de pan para su gente. (169)

> [in the village ... they eat white bread, ground at a good mill, winnowed very slowly, sifted three times over, baked in a big oven, tender from the day before, kneaded with good water, white as snow and soft as a sponge. Those who live in a village and knead in their own home have enough bread for everyone.]

Guevara's sublime description does provide us with qualities that his contemporary readers valued in bread in terms of grain selection, cooking process, colour, texture, and quantity but the harsh realities of the bread baking industry that intimately tied the village to the city are absent. Bread was regulated as much, if not more so, than meat and bakers were limited in where they could purchase their wheat and later, to whom and for how much they could sell it.

Bakers also received certain protection so that others could not undercut their business. In fact, in the Middle Ages, as bread baking became more regulated and the expectations for quality increased, women, who often ran the ovens, were replaced by men and by the second half of the fourteenth century bread baking was a respected profession (Riera Melis, "Jerarquía" 90). Following a long tradition of royal decrees that regulated bread sales, in 1571 Felipe II issued a standing prohibition for anyone kneading and selling bread or reselling grain outside of sanctioned bakers (Ávila Granados 64).[25] He also stipulated that, when necessary, the state could confiscate grain or flour from anyone and supply it to the bread makers (Ávila Granados 64).

As urban centres grew, villages had to supply bread to the cities, and in the case of Madrid, which became the capital and centre of power in 1561, the changes were enormous. Between 1561 and the end of the sixteenth century, Madrid's population rose from some 2500 houses to over 90,000 inhabitants (Castro, *El pan de Madrid* 184). The government instituted a price ceiling for grains, regulated prices, controlled grain storage and bread shipments, and imposed bread delivery obligations on local villages (Vassberg, *The Village* 33). One such example is a 1606 warning to several surrounding villages and towns advising them to make and deliver the agreed upon amount of bread to avoid heavy retribution.

Los alcaldes de la cassa y Corte de su magestad a cuyo cargo está el probeymiento de las cossas tocantes al probeymiento desta Corte, hazemos saber a bos, Benito Martínez, alguacil por nos nombrado para lo que se hará minción, que los conzejos de las villas y lugares que irán declarados an dexado de traer las cantidades de pan que yrán referidas, de lo questán obligados a traer cada semana del registro que se hizo para el probeymiento desta Corte. (ARCM San Martín de la Vega 18230 491 1606)

[The mayors of the house and court of His Majesty who are in charge of approving all things concerning the court's approval, make it known to you, Benito Martínez, whom we have named court official for what we make mention, that the councils of the villages and places henceforth named have stopped bringing the quantities of bread, henceforth cited, for which they are obligated to deliver each week according to the register recorded for the approval of this court.]

The summons continues with specific quantities for each village. For example, the village of San Martín de la Vega had defaulted on its shipment of 120 *fanegas* [bushels].

Y por la nezesidad que al presente ay de pan en esta Corte, os mandamos que luego que como este mandamiento os fuere entregado, bays (*sic*) con bara alta de justicia a las dichas villas y lugares y hareis moller con gran brebedad del trigo que hallaredes la cantidad que fuere posible, y dello y de la harina que tubieren quales quier bezinos, lo hareys masar (*sic*) y enviar en pan cozido a esta Corte a quenta de las dichas faltas, y traed presos vn alcalde y vn regidor de cada lugar por no aber cunplido con el dicho [registro?], y en ello os ocupad ocho días. (ARCM San Martín de la Vega 18230/491 1606)

[And due to the current bread needs of this court, and because you were given this responsibility, we order you to go with your staff of high court to said villages and places and make them grind as much wheat as can be found with the utmost brevity and from that and from whatever wheat the citizens may have, that they knead it and ship the baked bread to this court to go towards the aforementioned lack and that you imprison the mayor and the alderman of each place for not having fulfilled said (register?) and that they remain there for eight days.]

The warning also explains that in addition to jail time, those found negligent would have a reduced salary and a certain fine.

In spite of heavy regulation, councils across the country complained of the lack of control. The mayor of the village of Chinchón, Juan Gallo de Andrada, writes in 1606, "ay mucho excesso y deshorden en la benta del pan, bendiendolo a exçesibos presçios, y que los que lo tienen no lo quieren bender en grano, por bendello en pan coçido ... en gran daño del bien público" [There is much excess and disorder in the sale of bread, selling it at excessive prices, or those who have it refuse to sell the grain so as to sell the baked bread ... in grave detriment to the public welfare] (ARCM San Martín de la Vega 18230/496 1606), thus asserting his frustrations with the absence of fair market conditions for the sale and purchase of bread.

Additionally, the urban baking industry exploded and by the middle of the seventeenth century, Madrid was producing over 1000 *fanegas* of bread on a daily basis (Ringrose). The Catholic Monarchs and the early Hapsburg kings did not foresee the need to increase Spain's grain production, and that lack of vision coupled with the pressures from the Mesta for pasture land, loss of farmers to military demands, emigration to America, and the expulsion of the Moriscos, instigated long-term detrimental effects to agriculture and regional economies.

Although literary and legal texts attest to the primary role of bread in the early modern diet, recipes for bread making seldom appear in medieval and early modern cooking manuals, neither in Spain nor in the rest of Europe.[26] Ibn Razín is the first of the medieval manuscripts to record bread recipes in his thirteenth-century cooking manual *Fuḍālat-al-Hiwan Fi Tayyibat al-Ta'am Wa-l-Alwan* [The delicacies of the table and the finest of foods and dishes]. He opens his cooking manual with five distinct bread recipes: "Receta de pan cocido en el horno" [Recipe for bread baked in the oven], "Receta de pan cocido en el anafe" [Recipe for bread baked in a portable oven], "Receta de pan cocido en la placa o en una cazuela de hierro" [Recipe for bread baked on a sheet pan or in a cast iron pan], "Receta de pan ácimo" [Recipe for flat bread (without yeast)], and "Receta de pan de panizo" [Recipe for millet bread]. Four are made with semolina flour and one with millet. Some are baked in an oven, others on the stovetop. Different types of ovens and cooking spaces set one recipe apart from another. The first recipe is the most classic: a yeast dough that rises, is shaped, and baked in a bread oven. In the second recipe, the breads are moistened with water and stuck to the walls of the portable bread oven. The balls of dough are then covered with grape leaves soaked in water and the entire oven is sealed closed. As the breads bake, they fall to the rock-covered bottom of the oven and are then removed when done. In the third recipe, the loaves are cooked on the stovetop and flipped when needed. In the fourth recipe, the dough requires no yeast but, when rolled out, is poked with holes that are then filled with water and placed in the oven this way. The fifth recipe is made with millet and baked either in the standard oven, the portable oven, or the stovetop. At the end of this recipe Ibn Razín writes: "Esta es, de todas las clases de pan de trigo, la que más aprecian los andalusíes, y la que consumen en abundancia en la época de la cosecha del panizo" [This is, of all types of wheat bread, the one that the Andaluces like best and abundantly consume during the millet harvest season] (79). This side note, together with the five recipes, shows that while wheat was the preferred grain for baking bread, different regions and harvest seasons allowed for other grains to be ground and kneaded into bread as well.[27]

In the remaining medieval and early modern cooking manuals, bread is repeatedly mentioned in other recipes but only Martínez Montiño, in 1611, returns to include baked bread recipes in his work. In his cookbook, as in the earlier cooking manuals, bread appears numerous times toasted and sliced upon which a stew may be served or as breadcrumbs used as a thickener or filling for sausages. It is also referenced in many recipes to describe the type of yeast needed ("como para pan candeal" [as for *candeal* bread]), as a dish in and of itself, in bread recipes for *migas* [breadcrumbs] or *torrijas* [milk-soaked toasted bread] and in bread-related recipes like *bollos* [buns], *ojaldre* [phyllo], *pasteles* [pies] and *pastelones* [big pies], *empanadas* [empanadas], *rosquillas* [ring-shaped pastries], and *bizcochos* [sponge cakes]. Apart from these citations, three recipes appear for bread products: "Pan de leche" [Milk bread] (383–4), "Panecillos rellenos de conservas" [Bread rolls stuffed with preserves] (156–7), and "Panecillos de colaciones" [Bread rolls for a light meal]

(407).[28] In another recipe for blancmange Martínez Montiño makes reference to "panecillo de los de Madrid" [Madrid bread roll] when giving directions for how much salt to add (228).[29] This type of comment acknowledges that certain types of small breads were so common that all would know how much salt to add to a recipe with this simple reference.

Undoubtedly, bread and meat in the early modern Spanish diet are markers of sustenance that unite social eating habits across geographic and economic divides. Simply signalling that someone ate meat or baked bread was hardly an indication of regional identity or privileged position. As we have seen in multiple discourses, by the early modern period, some form of meat was available to all social classes and nearly everyone either prepared bread at home and baked it in a communal oven or purchased loaves from the local baker. Yet, these two food stuffs are clearly recognized objects of cultural capital. What type of meat was consumed – young mutton or beef among other choices – what part of the animal, and how often meat was eaten were all signs of privilege and position as was the colour and texture of bread. When Cervantes declares that the ingenious knight's diet consisted of "una olla de algo más vaca que carnero" he establishes Alonso Quijano's humble ranking and reveals a hierarchy of meats understood by his contemporary readers.

Chapter Three

"Salpicón las más noches": Salads, Vegetables, and New World Contributions to Spanish Fare

Comense las lechugas cozidas ... para conciliar sueño,
Y crudas ... para embotar los estimulos de Venus

[Eat boiled lettuce ... to get to sleep,
And raw ... to dull Venus's stimulation]

Sorapán de Rieros

Cervantes' description of Alonso Quijano's regular dinner, "salpicón las más noches" [salpicon most nights], reminds readers that night-time fare differed greatly from what was consumed at midday. Salpicon was something akin to a leafless salad and both then and today was prepared with either meat or seafood, marinated in vinegar, and seasoned with chopped onion. Along with the one-pot meal it is another staple of Spain's culinary heritage and vinegar, its key. When César Oudin, the first translator of the French *Don Quixote*, misidentified the dish as *salpiquet* – a warm, chopped meat dish served with a spicy black pepper or nutmeg sauce – the Spanish grammatician, Ambrosio de Salazar, in his *Espejo General de la Gramática en Diálogos* [General model of grammar through dialogue], was quick to amend his error.

> *Salpicon* dezis que es un *saupicquet*. Esso es falso ... porque *salpicon* es hecho con carne cozida y fiambre cortada menuda con cebollas y vinagre, y assi se come fria en lugar de lechugas ó otra ensalada. (cited in Morel-Fatio 159–60)

> [You say that *salpicón* is a *saupicquet*. This is false ... because *salpicón* is made with thinly sliced boiled meat and other cold meat, with onions and vinegar, and it is eaten cold in place of lettuce or another salad.]

Salazar's explanation raises important questions. What do the ingredients of a traditional salpicon and its place on the table as an alternative to a salad tell us about dinner fare in the early modern period? What are the main ingredients in a salad in the early modern period and how do they differ from our understanding of a salad today? When do key ingredients of today's salpicon and salad, namely the tomato but, to a lesser extent, the pepper and the potato, become part of the menu in Spain? And finally, how do writers across discourses describe and respond to Old World vegetables found in salpicon and salad, and New World products that are appearing in Spain for the first time? This chapter explores salpicon and salads first as night-time fare and then as examples of the diminishing contrasts between the foodstuffs consumed at socially diverse tables. It then turns to the moment of confluence where traditions of the past blend with revolutionary discoveries from the New World that not only transform what salpicon and salads mean but in the process transform food identity around the world. With the possible exception of refrigeration and industrial farming of the nineteenth century, there is no greater global food shift than that which takes place in the early modern period. As food travelled into Spain, we witness the early stages of transculturation through food that laid the groundwork for revolutionizing Spanish cuisine.

Looking carefully at Salazar's explanation of salpicon, it is clear that vinegar is what distinguishes salpicon from a simple dish of leftover meat. It not only preserves food naturally but also adds a distinctive aroma and flavour to any dish. Vinegar is one of the oldest foodstuffs produced and, along with oil and wine, it was a staple common to most village houses. Vineyards and wine and vinegar production date back to the Phoenicians, were advanced by Arabs, and played a fundamental role in both monastic and secular life in the early modern period.[1] According to David Vassberg,

> vineyards were almost ubiquitous in early modern Spain, and almost everywhere they were owned by small peasants. The reason for the widespread ownership of vines was that viticulture did not require large plots, and the work schedule of the typical Castilian peasant permitted caring for some vines, in addition to grain, which was almost everywhere the major crop. (*Land* 54)

Its importance is confirmed in registry books of villages throughout early modern Spain. For example, in 1610 the town of Fuentidueña de Tajo recorded how much wine, oil, and vinegar every household had:

En la uilla de Fuente Dueña, en primero día el mes de abril de mill y seiscientos y diez años, sus merçedes de Pedro Díaz y Juan Sánchez, alcaldes hordinarios desta villa, y Juan Pérez y Pedro Sánchez, rexidores della, justicia y comisarios del otabo y ensancha del vino, vinagre y azeyte desta villa, mandaron se notifique a Alonso Pocaranco y Gregorio Cabeza, vecinos desta villa, rexistradores y tassadores de la sisa, nombrados por el ayuntamiento desta villa, que luego vayan por todas las casas a haçer el rexistro del vino, vinagre y azeyte desta villa que ay a el presente por este año. (ARCM Fuentidueña de Tajo 13236/1048 1610–1759)

[In the village of Fuentidueña, the first day of the month of April 1610, Their Graces Pedro Díaz and Juan Sánchez, executive mayors of the village, and Juan Pérez and Pedro Sánchez, aldermen of said village, justice and superintendents of the taxes and increases of wine, vinegar, and oil of this village, ordered notification that Alonso Pocaranco and Gregorio Cabeza, citizens of this village, aldermen and tax collectors, be named by the town council to go from house to house and register the wine, vinegar, and oil of this village that is present this year.][2]

As vinegar, together with salt, sugar, and lard, was the main way to preserve food before the days of industrial canning and refrigeration, it comes as no surprise that recipes for pickling and marinating meats and vegetables are abundant in cooking manuals. For example, Martínez Montiño writes about pickling cucumbers in "Pepinos en vinagre para todo el año" [Cucumbers in vinegar for the whole year] (421), Hernández de Maceras has several recipes for pickling partridge (207), rabbit (208), eel (248), and sea bream (251). And in earlier manuals, like the anonymous *Sent Soví*, recipes appear for "Sols" [vinegar marinade].

Si vols fer sols a què et vulles, a carn o a peix, pren de la carn o del peix fruit e fets-ne trossos, e gita'ls en vinagre; e dessús gita primerament farigola.

E si vols lo sols cald, hages pebre e safrà e vinagre, e del brou de la carn o del peix, e ceba tallada; e destrempa-ho tot e gita-ho dessús. (*The Book of Sent Soví* 84)

[If you are going to make a vinegar marinade for whatever, meat or fish, take the meat or fried fish and cut it into pieces; put them in the vinegar but before doing so, sprinkle entirely with thyme.

And if you prefer a warm marinade, combine black pepper, saffron, and vinegar and some of the meat or fish broth and chopped onion and mix all together and pour on top.]

Salpicon was another of the many recipes that included vinegar as a central ingredient. In the early modern period, salpicon, like that of the one-pot meal, crossed social boundaries and was consumed by poor and wealthy alike. In the more humble kitchens, it provided a method for using up leftovers. Yet, it was also appreciated at court as recipes are found in palace cooking manuals. Martínez Montiño writes instructions for both beef and tuna. In the one for beef, he insists on adding fat back to improve the flavour:

> quiero avisar, que quando te pidieren salpicon de baca, que procures tener un poco de buen tocino de pernil, cocido, y picado, y mezclado con la baca, y luego su pimienta, sal y vinagre, y su cebolla picada, mezclada con la carne, y unas ruedas de cebolla, para adornar el plato. (36)

> [I must advise that when asked to prepare a beef salpicon, you add a small amount of good pork fat that has been cooked and diced and mixed with the beef. Later, add salt, pepper, vinegar, and minced onion to the meal and some onion wheels to garnish the dish.]

In Part 2 of *Don Quixote*, when Sancho is governor of Barataria and finally permitted to eat, he will savour salpicon as part of his dinner.

> le dieron de cenar un salpicón de vaca, con cebolla, y unas manos cocidas de ternera algo entrada en días. Entregóse en todo, con más gusto que si le hubieran dado francolines de Milán, faisanes de Roma, ternera de Sorrento, perdices de Morón, o gansos de Lavajos. (II.405)[3]

> [They served him a beef salpicon with onion and some boiled calf knuckles that were a few days old. He devoured it all with as much pleasure as if he had been served Milanese francolins, pheasant from Rome, Sorrento veal, partridges from Morón, or Lavajos geese.]

Here, salpicon advances the farce of Sancho as governor and is used as a poor man's fare to promote classist theories of nutritional privilege. Sancho surrenders his desire to govern after feasting on this cold meat dish and declaring that his stomach is not designed for rich food. In this charade of rich food-poor food, we see an elitist aversion to salpicon, particularly when it is coupled with boiled calf knuckles. Food is central to understanding the game of social ascension at play in the novel and those involved in the farce at Barataria – Sancho, the narrator, and Cervantes – all implicitly acknowledge the association between salpicon and the humble table. Returning to the opening lines of the novel, the mention of salpicon gives further weight to the humble status of Alonso Quijano in spite of the fact that it was also served at the king's table as evidenced in the pages of Martínez Montiño's cooking manual.

Salpicon, both today and in the early modern era, is considered a leafless salad. In fact, this dish is regularly mentioned with salad as typical meals served as dinner. In Baltasar del Alcázar's poem, "La cena jocosa" [The joyous supper], the poet includes both salad and salpicon as key elements of the dinner he shares with his dining partner, Inés. "La ensalada y salpicón/ hizo fin" [The salad and salpicon/finished (the meal)](vv. 41–2). And, it is clear from other sources, that in Spain, salads were eaten for dinner much more so than for lunch (L. Jacinto García, *Carlos V* 140). But can we further pinpoint what a salad is for the early modern table? In Quevedo's burlesque poem "Matraca de las flores y la hortaliza" [The clamour of fruits and vegetables], the poet suggests that watercress and cucumber are often found in salads (Quevedo, *Francisco de Quevedo* 755.41–8 and 54–60). Again in "Boda y acompañamiento del campo" [The country wedding party] Quevedo acknowledges the cucumber's love of salad: "Don Pepino, muy picado/ de amor de doña Ensalada" [Sir Cucumber, very much/ in love with Lady Salad] (Quevedo, *Francisco de Quevedo* 683.69–72), suggesting again, that cucumber is often part of a salad. Furthermore, in Vélez de Guevara's *El Diablo cojuelo* [The mischievous devil], cucumbers are used to define the diet of a stingy person: "un rico avariento ... siendo esclavo de su dinero y no comiendo más que un pastel de a cuatro, ni cenando más que una ensalada de pepinos" [a stingy rich man ... slave to his money and not eating anything more than a four-pence pie and dining on a cucumber salad] (III.63–4).

We can further approach the concept of salad in the seventeenth century by examining cooking manuals. Of the thousands of court recipes printed in Ruperto de Nola's *Libre de coch* [Book of cookery] (1520), Diego Granado's *Libro del arte de cozina* [Book on the art of cooking] (1599), and Martínez Montiño's *Arte de cocina, pastelería, vizcochería y conservería* [The art of cooking, pie making, pastry making, and preserving] (1611), only one carries the word "salad" in its title. In Martínez Montiño's "Ensalada de acenorias" [Carrot salad] he writes that dark carrots are preferable with the following specific instructions:

Lavarlas; y mondarlas de las barbillas, y cortarles el pezon, y la colilla, y meterlas en una olla, las colas por abaxo, y que estén muy apretadas; y poner la olla en el rescoldo, y echarla lumbre alrededor, y por encima, y se asarán muy bien. Luego sacarlas, y mondarles unas cascaritas que tienen muy delgadas, y sazonarlas de sal, y sirvelas con aceyte, y vinagre, y caliente; y si las quisieres echar azucar, podrás. La olla ha de estár boca abaxo. Hanse de poner estas acenorias adonde están las borrajas, y hazlas raxitas. (98)

[Wash them, scrub off the fine threads of roots, chop off the top and bottom, and place them in a pot, end down and packed together. Put the pot on the embers, fire them and the carrots will roast well. Then remove them, peel off their fine outer layer, and season with salt. Serve them warm with oil and vinegar. If you like, you can sprinkle them with sugar. The pot should be face down. Serve on a bed of borage and cut into small pieces.]

For modern readers this salad recipe would be considered more of a side dish but here it stands as the single salad recipe of all early modern court cookbooks.

In institutional cookbooks, like *Libro del arte de cocina* [Book on the art of cooking], written by Domingo Hernández de Maceras, cook in the Colegio Mayor de San Salvador de Oviedo at the University of Salamanca in 1607, we see more extensive salad recipes. Differing from the court manuals, Hernández de Maceras highlights salads in the very first chapter, "De principios de comida, y cena, de invierno, y de verano" [On beginning lunch and dinner, in winter and in summer] (181). When focusing on winter foods, he recommends endives served either raw or cooked. Like Martínez Montiño, he includes a warm carrot salad in which he describes how to prepare, roast, and serve the salad. In addition, Hernández de Maceras includes cooking time, two hours. This reference to specific cooking time is one of many indications that the author writes for cooks who might not have as much background knowledge as the professional cooks found at court. The increase in salad recipes in the university cookbook when compared to those of court cookbooks also correlates inversely with social rank. In other words, as one's social rank decreased (from king or grandee to nobleman or gentleman), one's salad consumption increased.

In the following two chapters entitled "Cap. 2. De ensaladas" [Chap. 2 On salads] and "Cap. 3. De ensalada cotidiana" [Chap 3. On everyday salads], there are additional salad recipes that do not indicate whether they are served cooked or warm. In chapter 2 "vegetables" replaces the word "carrot" suggesting a wider range of choices for the salad's main ingredient.

Tomen todas verduras bien picadas, y échenles alcaparras, y lávalas bien y échalas en un barreño, y échales aceite mucho, vinagre poco, haz de ellas tus platos, y luego ponle por encima, a cada un plato lonjas de tocino del pernil y de lenguas y truchas, o salmón, yemas de huevos y tajadas de diacitrón, maná, azúcar y granada, flor de borrajas porque parece bien. (183)

[Mince all vegetables and add capers, wash them and put them in a bowl and add a lot of oil, a little vinegar, and plate them up. To each add a slice of fat back, tongue, trout or salmon, egg yolk, slices of citron, manna, sugar, pomegranate, and borage blossoms because they look good.]

This recipe approaches the modern day *ensalada mixta* [mixed salad] with its fish and egg but instead of raw lettuce it contains sweet ingredients: citron, manna, sugar, and pomegranate.[4]

In Hernández de Maceras's third chapter, the salad recipe is simpler. "Toma alcaparras, y desálalas muy bien, y cuécelas bien cocidas, y échales aceite, y vinagre y azúcar" [Take capers and desalt them well, boil them until well cooked, and sprinkle with oil, vinegar, and sugar] (185). Given that a variety of salad recipes are present in the university kitchen, we can infer that they are also common dinner options in homes of those affluent enough to send their sons to university. However, there remains a clear distinction between what is described as salad and how lettuce is prepared and eaten.

In novels, poetry, travel journals, contemporary cooking manuals, and even works of art lettuce functions independently of salads which are more loosely understood as a mixture of vegetables that sometimes include lettuce but more often than not, do not. These salads can also include meat, poultry, or seafood and are dressed with oil and vinegar and flavoured with salt, pepper, or other seasonings. Conversely, lettuce or any of the leafy vegetables – escarole, romaine, endives, chicory, and arugula – were not limited to salads, as they are today, but rather, were cooked and served warm in soups or as wraps for stuffed food. Lettuce and other leafy greens, like those shown in figure 3.1, were generally considered beneficial to one's health although when eaten too frequently, lettuce "especially dulls the keenness of vigorous eyes" (Platina 215).

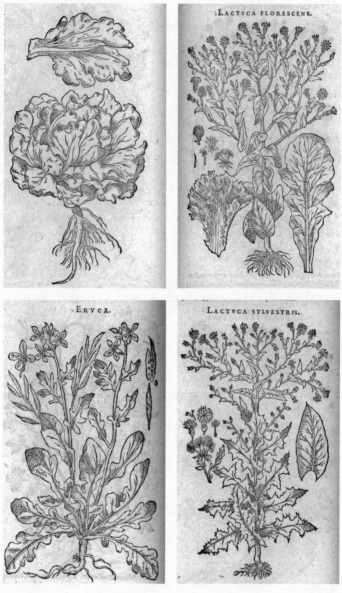

Figure 3.1. The Italian botanist Pietro Mattiolo depicts a variety of leafy greens
in his commentary on Dioscorides, *De plantis epitome utliissima* 1586: 298–306.
Photos by Dennis Sears, courtesy of the University of Illinois, Urbana-
Champaign Rare Book and Manuscript Library.

In the 1513 *Obra de agricultura* [Treatise on agriculture], which continued through the early twentieth century as a highly regarded reference
manual on the influence of food on health, Alonso de Herrera writes,

> Las lechugas se llaman assi deste nombre de leche, o porque tienen mucha
> leche, y entonces no valen ellas nada para comer, mayormente crudas,
> porque si las mugeres que crían las usan comer les hace tener abundancia
> de leche. Dan sueño: crudas, o cocidas, son buenas un poco estrujadas del
> agua para ensaladas para personas delicadas, y enfermas, y viejos, con
> aceite, y poco vinagre, y sal, o azúcar, y para templar su frialdad mezclenle
> un poco de canela molida ... las lechugas mientras más verdes son mejo-
> res, porque son más nuevas. (cited in Valles Rojo, *Cocina* 253)

> [Lettuce is called such because of its association with milk {*leche/lechuga*}
> either because it contains so much milk and is therefore not worth eating,
> especially raw, or because when nursing women eat it, they overproduce
> milk. It makes one tired, raw or cooked. For the weak, sick, or elderly, it
> is good when the water is mostly removed and served as a salad with oil
> and a little vinegar, and salt or sugar. And, to reduce its cold nature, mix
> in a little cinnamon ... The greener the lettuce, the better, as it is younger.]

Herrera suggests that its very name comes from its association with
milk and that lactating women may overproduce if they eat lettuce. The
quote contextualizes the use of lettuce for the sick and the elderly and
declares its cold nature. Since antiquity, cooked lettuce was thought to
be more nutritious than raw and also helped to distract one from sexual
contact. Bartolomeo Platina carries these ideas into his own writing
when he writes, "This food induces sleep, soothes a cough generated
by a warm humor, moves the urine, slows passion and moves the bow-
els" (215). Both Platina's reference to slowing passions and Herrera's
annotation regarding the cold nature of lettuce recall what was part of
the collective memory of seventeenth-century Spaniards, that lettuce
was an anti-aphrodisiac and aided in refraining from sexual activity.
This was certainly true in Quevedo's writing. In "Pendencia mosquito"
[Drunkard's brawl], a burlesque poem about swindlers and whores
getting drunk at a tavern, he writes:

Un cogollo de lechuga
fue el violón de este sarao:
que el que es bailarín castizo
no repara en lo templado.   (*Francisco de Quevedo* 861, 13–16)

[A lettuce heart
was the double bass of this soirée
for the one who is the real Castilian dancer
does not heed restraint.]

In this poem lettuce, which functions like the double bass does in an orchestra by controlling the music's bass line, is debunked by the dancer, or in the case of the poem, the swindler, who will not be moderate or restrain himself in any way. In a similar fashion, in *El buscón* [The swindler], Quevedo transmits this cultural norm by creating a double meaning for the verb *desmayarse*. It traditionally means "to faint," but Quevedo also creates the notion of removing oneself (*des-*) from erotic thoughts that are typically associated with May (*mayo/mayarse*) and springtime. When one of the students at the Viveros inn boasts of the relative that he and the main character's cohort have in common, he describes how the mere sight of lettuce would affect him. "[U]n agüelo tuvo v. m., tío de mi padre, que en viendo lechugas se desmayaba; ¡qué hombre era tan cabal!" [Your Grace had a grandfather, uncle to my father, who, at the sight of lettuce, would faint. What an upstanding man!] (*La vida* 25). In this way the grandfather/uncle figure faints or distances himself from erotic "May" thoughts at the very sight of lettuce.

Lettuce does not appear in salad recipes in the major cookbooks of the day, yet there are other indications that suggest lettuce was often consumed raw, without any dressing. In Albert Jouvin de Rochefort's section on Spain in *Le voyageur d'Europe* [The traveller in Europe] he records his observations on dinner in Spain, "no cenan a no ser una ensalada u otro refresco, como frutas, o algunas lechugas sin aliño" [for dinner they eat only a salad or some other refreshing thing, like fruit, or some lettuce without dressing] (cited in Díez Borque, *La vida española* 65). In Quevedo's poem "Boda y acompañamiento del campo" [The country wedding party], Quevedo suggests that lettuce is best when not dressed:

La Lechuga, que se viste
sin aseo y con fanfarria,
presumida, sin ser fea,
de frescona y de bizarra.   (*Francisco de Quevedo* 683 vv. 17–20)

[Lettuce who is dressed
without dressing but with fanfare
Thinks herself, without being ugly,
Very fresh and dashing.]

Finally, in *Dinner at Emmaus* (c. 1620, shown in figure 3.2) the Italian painter Bartolomeo Cavarozzi, who lived and worked in Spain in 1617–18, includes a head of lettuce as an emblem of charity in his interpretation of this biblical scene.[5] Here, the viewer infers that all food placed on the table is to be consumed in its current state. Lettuce, like the fruit, is eaten raw, and without dressing as both Jouvin and Quevedo suggest in their writing.

Although not as a salad ingredient, lettuce does appear in cooking manuals in many different recipes. In Diego Granado's "Para hacer platos de lechuga con caldo de carne de diversas maneras" [Several different lettuce dishes with beef broth], the author provides a typical example of how lettuce was prepared: "Con las dichas lechugas se pueden poner a cocer rellenos de hígado, papada de puerco y tajadas de pernil y pollos rellenos y pichones de media pluma (tiernos) y cuando estuviere cocido, sírvase caliente todo con su caldo" [With said lettuce, one can cook them stuffed with liver, pork jowl and ham slices, and stuffed chicken and young, tender pigeon and when they are cooked, serve them warm in their broth] (108). Martínez Montiño provides recipes for "La sopa de lechuga" [Lettuce soup], "Las lechugas rellenas" [Stuffed lettuce], and "Las lechugas rellenas en día de carne" [Stuffed lettuce for non-abstinence days] (242–4). Hernández de Maceras includes two recipes with the same title, "Cómo se ha de rellenar una lechuga" [How to stuff lettuce], but prepares them in very different ways (cited in Pérez Samper, *Alimentación* 211–12, 237). In the first recipe, shown in figure 3.3, lettuce is stuffed with ground mutton seasoned with mint, parsley, and spices. When the lettuce is cooked, it is sliced and presented in rounds and garnished with lemons or verjuice.

The second recipe is for a sweet dish. One first cooks together borage, parsley, and mint, chops them fine, and adds either oil or lard. Then, the recipe states that one should combine "piñones, pasas, y azúcar, y dos o tres huevos, y una poca de canela, y azafrán, y mételo todo en la lechuga, y átala, y ponla a cocer. Servirásla con azúcar y canela" [pine nuts, raisins, sugar, and two or three eggs, and a little cinnamon and saffron, fill lettuce with this mixture, tie it, and boil it] (237).

Based on these numerous sources, we can conclude that lettuce was appreciated for its anti-aphrodisiac quality and eaten among all social classes. It holds little connection to salads, as we know them today; indeed, what was then called salad would today be considered cold marinated vegetables or cooked vegetables served as a warm side dish. Lettuce becomes part of regular salad recipes in the eighteenth century as seen in its first appearance as a salad's main ingredient in Juan de

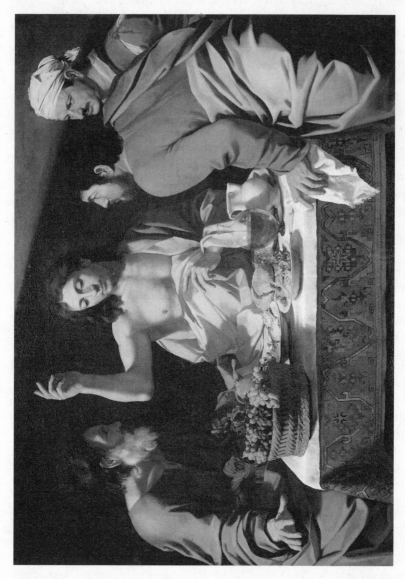

Figure 3.2. *Dinner at Emmaus* by Bartolomeo Cavarozzi, c. 1620. Courtesy of J. Paul Getty Museum, Los Angeles.

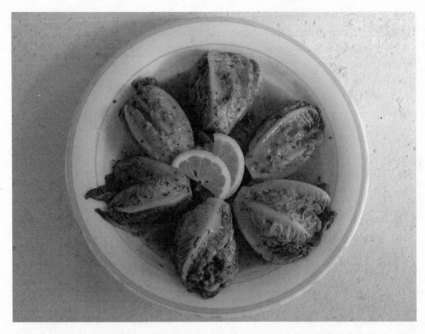

Figure 3.3. Lettuce stuffed with minced lamb, adapted from cap XL of Hernández de Maceras's *Libro del arte de cocina*. Photo by author.

la Mata's 1747 cookbook, *Arte de repostería en que se contiene todo género de hacer dulces secos, y en líquido, bizcochos, turrones, natas, bebidas heladas de todos géneros, rosolís y mistelas, con una breve instrucción para conocer las frutas y servirlas crudas* [The art of confectionary baking in which is found how to make all types of dry and liquid sweets, sponge cakes, turron, creams, all types of iced drinks, liquors and punches, and with brief instructions on recognizing and serving raw fruit] (162). However, during the early modern period, lettuce was incredibly versatile. It was used to make soup, often stuffed with a variety of meats or dried fruit and other vegetables and then cooked and served in its broth or with a flavourful sauce. It was served either raw or cooked, could stand as a main course or be combined with a meat dish, and was prepared either as a savoury dish or as a sweet one.

Today's classic Spanish salad is served cold, like Don Quixote's salpicon, but consists of lettuce, tomato, and onion, dressed with oil and vinegar and seasoned with salt. From the cooking manuals, one could surmise that the tomato had still not been incorporated into any type of salad or salpicon. But evidence found in poems, plays, and paintings indicates otherwise. To consider more fully the tomato's place in Spain's history, we must diverge from foods long established on the peninsula to those that were first introduced in the early modern era.

When Christopher Columbus made his four separate voyages in search of an alternative sea route to India, his explorations forever changed world history and instigated a gastronomic revolution. Arrival of these food products to Spain catalyzed contact between popular, indigenous communities of the New World and both popular and courtly communities of Spain and later, the rest of the world, in unique ways. Mary Louis Pratt coined the term "contact zones" to identify those "social spaces where disparate cultures meet, clash, and grapple with each other" (4).[6] Where Pratt goes on to examine European travel literature and, when possible, self representations of the conquered and their conquerors in Latin America (and Africa), in this chapter the contact zone centres on food exchanges and the force of the New World products in transforming Old World cuisine. Pratt deliberately reconfigures the "domestic subject of Euroimperialism" to include not only the Western metropolitan authoritative voice but also multiple voices from the colonial periphery. Her study on the transculturation of European constructions of subordinated others that have been shaped by those others allows us to understand New World foodstuffs entering the Old World as another transcultural contact zone.

New World food products – including potatoes, tomatoes, corn, avocado, pineapple, haricot, kidney, and butter beans, lima beans, scarlet runners, French beans, chocolate, peanuts, vanilla, red and green peppers, tapioca, turkey, tobacco, chewing gum, and quinine (Tannahill 197–276) – become agents of the periphery. They are signifiers of the subordinated other that invade and transform the Old World in much the same way as wheat, sugar, and a myriad of animal products brought from Spain transform the agricultural map of the Americas. When Columbus and later Cortés and other explorers returned to Spain with these "peripheral" products, these exotic edibles transform the "metropolitan" Western world in unprecedented ways.[7] Although all of the above-mentioned New World products were introduced into Spanish cuisine and from there into other national cuisines, tomatoes, peppers, potatoes, and chocolate are by far the four foodstuffs that impact Spanish cuisine in the most significant of ways.

In keeping with a universal reluctance to change eating patterns, Spain did not immediately incorporate New World products into its dietary habits. The earliest references appear in travel journals, and then migrate to works of fiction before finally appearing in published recipes over two hundred years after the first European encounter with the New World. References to these products in works of fiction are key to understanding their role in the transformation of Spanish cuisine because the texts shed light on how the general public understood them. For example, from the passages in literary works, we can rightly assume that consumption of these foodstuffs occurs in Spain sometime between their appearance in travel journals in the late fifteenth and early sixteenth centuries and literary texts that begin to reference them as early as the mid-sixteenth century, and certainly well before their regularized appearance in cookbooks in the mid-eighteenth century. In works of fiction, the treatment of New World foodstuffs as exotic promoted the romanticization of the cultural other, and functioned in the context of the bigger colonial and imperialist project of oppression and exploitation in the New World. But what is unique to these foodstuffs is that their exploitation informs a culinary revolution that forever changes how Spaniards and eventually the rest of the world eats. These products and their uniquely Spanish culinary treats, *gazpacho andaluz*, red *piquillo* peppers, *tortilla española*, and *chocolate con churros* would take centuries to become established within the Spanish gastronomic system but once introduced, these exotic culinary gems set off one of the biggest gastronomic transformations the country has ever experienced, second perhaps only to the industrialization of agriculture and the era of refrigeration in twentieth-century Spain.[8]

In the mid-sixteenth century, Bernardino Sahagún was among the first Europeans to describe the tomato when he recorded the many varieties found in the Mesoamerican marketplace.[9]

El que trata en tomates suele vender los que son gruesos, y también los menudillos, y todos los que son de muchos y diversos géneros, según se trata en el texto, como son los tomates amarillos, colorados y los que están bien maduros. (613)

[The one who deals in tomatoes normally sells the ones that are large and also the small ones and all of the many and diverse types that are dealt with in the text, like the yellow tomatoes and the reddish ones and the ones that are very ripe.]

In 1544 the Italian botanist Pietro Mattiolo also wrote about tomatoes and provided an accompanying image as seen in the woodcut in figure 3.4. He described tomatoes in the following way.

Portasene a i tempi nostri un'altra specie in Italia, le quale si chiamano pomi d'oro. Sono queste schiacciate come le mele rose, y fatte a spichi, di color prima verdi, y come sono mature in alcune piante rosse come sangue, y in altre di color d'oro. Si mangiano pur anch'esse nel medesimo modo. (502)

[Another species brought to our times in Italy is called golden apples. They can be milled like pink apples or segmented into wedges of spring-green colour, and when mature, some plants are red like blood, while others are golden. They are then also eaten in the same way.]

In Italian, the phrase *pomi d'oro* evolved into *pomodoro*, the word still used today for *tomato*. At the end of his description, "in the same way" refers to his earlier explanation of how eggplant is eaten: "Mangiansi volgarmente fritte nell'olio, con sale, e pepe, come i funghi. Questo tutto disse Hermolao [They are commonly eaten fried in oil, with salt and pepper, like mushrooms. All this Hermolaus said].[10] In these few lines, Mattiolo captures the essence of the tomato: a fruit that is eaten like a vegetable.

Antonio Garrido Aranda notes Prieto Garramiola's research on the registry of the House of Aguilar in Montilla, 1659.[11] Garramiola discovered lunch menus that included "pollos con tomates" [chicken with tomatoes] and "cazuela de tomates con huevos duros" [stewed tomatoes with hard boiled eggs]. He also noted how often tomatoes appeared on their shopping list (Garrido Aranda 207). As early as 1608 the Hospital de la Sangre in Seville bought large quantities of tomatoes (Garrido Aranda 209).

Tomato references are found on the stage, for example, in Tirso de Molina's *El amor médico* [Love the doctor] (1618–20), and it is here where we begin to see the treatment of these products as something more than just food. The comic figure and servant Tello says, "Oh, ensalada de tomates/qué coloradas mejillas/dulces y a un tiempo picantes" [Oh, tomato salad / how rosy your cheeks/at times sweet, at times hot]. Here and in other Tirso plays, the tomato is a referent for the erotic. This comes as little surprise as the tomato's bright red colour and sweet and spicy flavour quickly evoke in the reader's mind (and for the audience

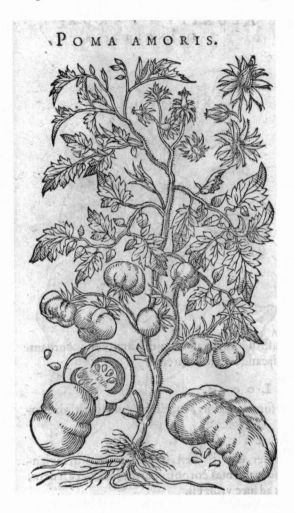

Figure 3.4. One of the first images of the tomato or, as some called it, the "poma amoris" [apple of love] from Mattiolo's *De plantis epitome utliissima* (Frankfurt am Main: [J. Feyerabend], 1586), 821. Photo by Dennis Sears, courtesy of the University of Illinois, Urbana-Champaign Rare Book and Manuscript Library.

viewing the performance) passion and love. And later, in the middle of the seventeenth century, Lope de Vega's daughter, Sor Marcela de San Félix (1605–87), uses the image of the tomato as she brings Appetite to life in the spiritual verses "Muerte del Apetito" [Appetite's Death]. In this play, Sor Marcela presents an allegory of the Soul who ultimately defeats Appetite after being tempted by his catalogue of mouth-watering dishes that includes roasted hen, olives from Cordoba, blood sausage, and a refreshing tomato-cucumber salad: "cosa fiambre/quisiera, y una ensalada/ de tomates y pepinos" [Some cold cuts/ I would most enjoy, and a salad/ of tomato and cucumber] (1369–71).[12] This passage is particularly striking as it references a tomato-cucumber salad as both an object of gluttony and as a dish as familiar and sought-after as olives, poultry, and sausage. As we see from the tomato's appearance on the stage, as early as 1620 writers created images of the tomato as part of a salad that whetted the viewers' appetite.

Finally, Bartolomé Murillo incorporates tomatoes into his genre painting *La cocina de los ángeles* [The angels' kitchen] (1646). As seen in the highlighted area of figure 3.5, Murillo includes a still life of squash and tomatoes in front of seated cherubs. They are assisting the Franciscan cook, who is currently experiencing a mystical moment, with his preparation. Their placement next to different squashes recalls the later eighteenth-century recipe "Calabaza de otro modo" [Squash another way] that bakes slices of squash with chopped tomatoes covered in breadcrumbs (Altamiras 110). From these and other references, we clearly see that tomatoes were eaten in salads, both cold and warm, throughout the seventeenth century.

Although it is clear that tomatoes were one of the most consumed New World products in Spain during the early modern period, no recipes for tomatoes appear in the early seventeenth-century cooking manuals. Because no new cookbooks are published between 1611 and 1740, it is difficult to assess when and to what extent the tomato was integrated into the diet of different classes and regions. However, in 1740 María Rosa Calvillo de Teruel pens *Libro de apuntaciones de guisos y dulces* [Book of notations on stews and sweets]. In this work of 100 recipes for soups, sauces, cold cuts and organ meats; meat, poultry and fish dishes; vegetables, pies, preserves, and many desserts written for a middle-class Andalusian audience the author includes over a dozen recipes with tomatoes. These recipes include tomato sauce, dishes with zucchini, wild mushrooms, potatoes, eggplant, and several poultry and meat dishes. It is clear that by the mid-eighteenth century, the tomato is fully established into Spanish cuisine.

Again in 1745 the Franciscan Juan Altamiras pens *Nuevo arte de cocina* [The new art of cooking], a cookbook written specifically to feed the poor. He too includes more than a dozen recipes for stews, organ meats, poultry, fish, eggs, rice, and vegetables that include tomatoes among their ingredients. In his recipe "Abadejo con tomate" [Haddock with tomatoes] he highlights the importance of the tomato:

> freirás cebolla, y tomates con abundancia; compondrás las raciones en una vasija ancha, cubre la primera superficie de ella con las raciones, sobre que echarás la cebolla, y tomate, perejil, y pimienta, ajos machacados ... este no necesita de otra especie, por cuanto, suple el tomate; es así muy gustoso y cómo conservarás los tomates todo el año, verás más adelante. (87)

> [Fry onions and a lot of tomatoes; place the portions in a wide pot and cover the bottom with the portions. Place on top the onion, tomato, parsley, pepper, and mashed garlic ... This dish needs no other spice in so far as the tomato provides it all. It is very tasty and later on you will see how to preserve tomato throughout the year.]

Two years later, Juan de la Mata, in his book *Arte de repostería* [The art of confectionary baking], publishes recipes for tomato sauce. The first recipe, "Salsa de tomates a la española" [Spanish-style tomato sauce] indicates that the Spanish style differs from another style, most likely one from the Americas that combined tomatoes and chilies as Bernardino Sahagún described in his writings. In Mata's recipe the tomatoes are first roasted, their skin removed, finely chopped and then parsley, onion, garlic, salt, pepper, oil, and vinegar are mixed together and added to make the sauce. In the second recipe, "Otra manera" [Another way], the tomatoes are seasoned with oregano and cumin (165). It is also worth noting that gazpacho recipes do not yet contain tomatoes but rather focus on garlic, bread, and typical salad ingredients such as lettuce, escarole, onion, or celery.[13]

Like the tomato, another food product from the New World that transformed cuisine around the globe was the fruit of capsicum plants. In his diaries, Columbus confuses green and red peppers with the *piper nigrum* [black pepper] native to India. During his first expedition, he writes in his 15 January entry, "También hay mucho ají, que es su pimienta, della que vale más que pimienta y toda la gente no come sin ella, que la halla muy sana" [There is also a lot of *ají*, which is their black pepper, and which is more valuable than black pepper, and no one eats without it as they find it very healthy] (Cristóbal Colón 191). Critics

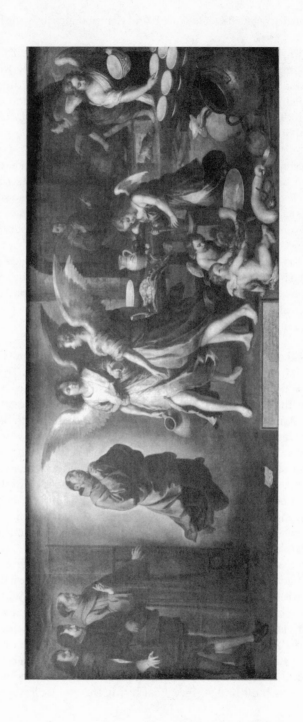

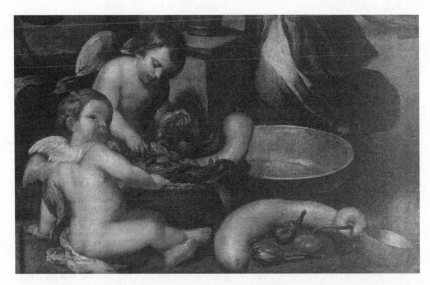

Figure 3.5. Squash and tomatoes in *La cocina de los ángeles* [The angels' kitchen] by Bartolomeo Murillo (1646). Courtesy of ©RMN-Grand Palais, Musée du Louvre, Gérard Blot.

speculate that Columbus brought seeds from the new world to the monastery of Guadalupe and from there, they rapidly travelled to Yuste, other monasteries throughout Spain and Portugal, and from Portugal on to India and the rest of the world (Abad Alegría 21–2). Cultivated and eaten raw, fried, roasted, stewed, sauced, stuffed, and even jellied, peppers were also dried and pulverized and used as a spice in the early part of the seventeenth century.[14]

The poet Gabriel Lobo Lasso de la Vega, who served both Felipe II and Felipe III, included peppers in two of his ballads published in *Manojuelo de romances nuevos y otras obras* [Little bundle of new ballads and other works] (1601). In one of the burlesque poems, peppers are included in a catalogue of a king's provisions: "Docientos de berenjenas,/ tres hanegas de garbanzos,/ doce sartas de pimientos,/ y dos costales de nabos,/ de pepinos tres arrobas,/ y berzas para su año" [two hundred (baskets) of eggplant,/ three bushels of garbanzos,/ twelve strings of peppers/ two sacks of turnips,/ cucumbers, some three dozen kilos,/ and cabbage for the whole year] (179). Here, readers can infer that these peppers were strung up to dry so that they could later be chopped or ground and used as a seasoning in the way that black pepper was consumed. In a historic ballad on El Cid, Lobo Lasso de la Vega includes a Moor pepper vender as one of the characters: "un triste morillo/ que vino a vender pimientos" [a sad, little Moor/ who came to sell peppers] (182). While included to add humour to the poems, Lobo Lasso de la Vega's incorporation of peppers into his verses reveals that peppers were fully established on the Iberian Peninsula at the start of the seventeenth century. They also appear in Cervantes' 1613 short novel *Rinconete y Cortadillo*, when Monipodio and his gang enjoy a basket of stolen food that includes "alcaparrones ahogados en pimientos" [marinated giant capers and peppers] together with cheese from Flanders, bread from Gandul, and other local delights. Finally, several authors, including Quevedo and Moreto, name characters Pimiento to highlight sarcasm or comic relief in their texts.[15]

The *Diccionario de autoridades* [Dictionary of authorities] references the 1680 Pragmática de tassas [tax ordinance] that explicitly states how much ground (red) pepper costs. It also defines how pepper tastes and is commonly used: "Tiene el sabor mui acre y picante, y tostado en el horno y hecho polvos, se usa de él para sazonar las viandas, como de la pimienta fina, y se llama pimiento molido" [It has a spicy, acrid taste and when it is toasted in the oven and ground, it is used to season food, like finely ground black pepper, and it is called ground pepper] (273). This notation makes clear that ground capsicum pepper was also definitely established on the peninsula by the late seventeenth century; its process evolved over the next century into paprika, a spice familiar to many regional cuisines across the country that has become the fifth largest producer of peppers in the world today (Abad Alegría 91).

Like the tomato, it is not until well into the eighteenth century that peppers surface in cooking manuals. In Calvillo de Teruel's *Libro de apuntaciones de guisos y dulces*, almost 25 per cent of the recipes include pepper. The author often distinguishes between green and red peppers and also between whole peppers and ground pepper that are used as a spice. One recipe, "Estofado con salsa negra" [Stew with black sauce] clarifies that *pimiento colorado* dulce [*sweet* red pepper) be used (32, my emphasis). A common technique found in many of the dishes is to grind together roasted peppers and garlic, this mixture, called *majado* [mash], is then added to the dish along with other seasonings. Calvillo de Teruel is the first to document the use of pepper in any Spanish cookbook.

In *Arte de repostería* Mata includes two recipes for candied and pickled peppers. "Los pimientos no se diferencian de las Frutas precedentes en el modo de confitarlos; solo se deberá observar se han de escoger los que no estuvieran inclinados al color encarnado, que sean pequeños, verdes, y de hermosa vista" [Peppers are no different from previous fruit in the way they are candied; but one should pay attention to select those that are not already turning red, that are small, green, and are a beautiful sight] (49). Later he explains how to pickle them. "Los pepinos, y pimientos se han de elegir los que no estén de todo punto maduros, y comienzan a fin de agosto, o a principio de septiembre: échanse en una vasija para conservarlos con vinagre, sazonados de sal, y pimienta molida, y algunos clavos es especia, cubriéndola muy bien" [One should select cucumbers and peppers that are not completely ripe, and that start at the end of August or beginning of September: place them in a pot to preserve them by completely covering them with vinegar, seasoned with salt and ground pepper and some cloves] (162). This idea of pickled peppers aligns with the cooking practices of the salpicon that Alonso Quijano regularly consumed; vinegar once again plays a key role in the way that both peppers and tomatoes are prepared.

The potato, or *solanum tuberosum*, is more difficult to track in the early modern period as there exists a linguistic confusion with the sweet potato, *ipomoea batatas*.[16] In the sixteenth and seventeenth centuries, historians and poets alike refer to the *batata* [sweet potato] as *patata* [potato] but also, although less frequently, write about the potato as *patata*. The sweet potato was native to the Caribbean and Mexico when Spaniards arrived and was one of the items that Columbus brought back to Spain after his first voyage. The potato, on the other hand, was not one of the foodstuffs among the late fifteenth-century New World explorations. In fact, it was not until Gonzalo Jiménez de Quesada travelled the Colombian altiplano in 1537 that Spaniards came across "una especie de trufas" [a type of truffle] when they entered homes of those who had fled the Bogotá region (Terrón 99). The following year Cieza de León would write his *Crónica de Perú* [Chronicle of Peru], published some fifteen years later in Seville, and describe in detail typical provisions of Indians that included potatoes (cited in Terrón 90). Garcilaso de la Vega, El Inca, pens the third key document related to the *solanum tuberosum*. In his *Comentarios reales de los incas* [Royal commentaries of the Incas] (1608) he describes how potatoes were frozen, their water removed and then preserved (cited in Terrón 101). In his exhaustive study on the potato, Eloy Terrón provides examples of the linguistic confusion in the early modern period between the potato and the sweet potato. He draws from the works of Quevedo, the anonymous author of *Esteban González*, and Moreto to exemplify how frequently authors confused the *patata* with the *batata*. More recently, in a study on the *batata de Málaga*, another term for the sweet potato, María Isabel Amado Doblas traces how the word *patata* was confused with the sweet potato until the nineteenth century. She examines the work of many major authors, including Santa Teresa de Jesús, Luis de Góngora, Mateo Alemán, Lope de Vega, and others and concludes that all, with the exception of Góngora, use the term *patata* to describe the sweet potato (944).[17]

Foreigners who travelled through Spain also noted the presence of the potato. In fact, according to James Howell in a letter he wrote to Lady Cottington in 1630, potatoes were standard fair in the *olla podrida*. "The *Olla podrida* hath intellectuals and senses; Mutton, Beef, and Bacon, are to her as the Will, Understanding, and Memory, are to the Soul; Cabbage, Turnips, Artichoaks, Potatoes and Dates, are her five Senses, and Pepper the Common-sense" (229). His description continues with details of marrow and fowl but what calls one's attention, apart from his curious metaphor for stew as a living being, is that the potato figures in the dish with other long-standing vegetables such as cabbage and turnips, as if it had always been essential to this one-pot meal.

In the sixteenth and seventeenth centuries, there is a singular reference to the potato in all the early modern cooking manuals and it is unclear whether the author is referring to the potato or to the sweet potato. In his prologue, Martínez Montiño attacks an earlier published work, possibly by Diego Granado, and contends that certain recipes should never have been written. Among them, he cites a potato pie:

en el capítulo de las Tortas, que está escrito en el otro Libro, hay muchas suertes de tortas, que no solo no son buenas, ni se deben hacer, mas antes es impertinencia escribirlas como son las de castañas, y otras de higos, y de turmas de tierra, y de navos, y de zanahorias, y de patatas, ni de cerezas. (prologue).[18]

[in the chapter on pies that is written in the other book, there are many types of pies that are not only no good, nor should even be made, but furthermore it is insolent to write them at all like those with chestnuts, and others with figs, truffles, turnips, carrots, potatoes, or cherries.]

There is no recipe for potato pie in Granado's work, although Martínez Montiño may have had available to him another version of the work or he may have been critiquing a different work entirely. And while Martínez Montiño does not include other references to the potato in his cookbook, its appearance in his prologue among other common fruits and vegetables suggests that it had incorporated itself into the Spanish diet.

In the eighteenth-century, we begin to see more clearly evidence of both the sweet potato and the potato in Spanish cookbooks. In *Libro de apuntaciones de guisos y dulces*, Calvillo de Teruel has one recipe, "Cómo se guisan las papas" [How to cook potatoes], in which chopped potatoes are cooked with onion and tomato sautéed in butter together with appropriate seasonings of clove, black pepper, saffron, and cinnamon (37). The other recipe, "Pudin de patatas" [Sweet potato soufflé], is made with sweet potatoes, sugar, egg yolks, and lemon juice. Eggs whites are later folded in and it is all placed in a pie pan and baked with low heat.

In *Arte de repostería*, a book dedicated to sweets and desserts, Juan de la Mata rightly includes two recipes for *batata de Málaga* [Malaga sweet potato] and none for the potato. And in *Nuevo arte de cocina* [The new art of cooking], one has insight into the personality and humor of Juan Altamiras in his recipe for truffles when he quips:

Las patatas se componen del mismo modo; y si comes muchas te advierto, estarás de tan buen aire, y tan favorable, que con el aire que soples puedes componer embarcación para ir al Papa, si no es que sea tan fuerte, que por romper las velas sea necesario su reparo, que no se hace a costa de patacas. (115)

[Potatoes are made the same way; and if you eat a lot, I must warn you that you will have such good and favourable air, that with the wind you blow, you can set sail to see the pope unless it's so strong that you rip your sails and have to mend them, in which case I hope you don't use potatoes.]

In this final note to the recipe, the author plays with other words for the potato – *papa*, a homonym for the pope, and *pataca*, the Portuguese and Galician word for potato – to describe its *windy* effects.

Chocolate differs considerably from tomatoes, peppers, and potatoes in its popularity, production, and consumption. On his last voyage to the New World, Christopher Columbus came across cocoa beans without knowing what they were when his men intercepted a Mayan shipment on route from the Yucatán to Guanaja. Among the inventory noted, cocoa beans are called almonds.

y muchas almendras que usan por moneda en la nueva España, las que pareció que estimaban mucho, porque cuando fueron puestas en la nave las cosas que traían, noté que, cayéndose algunas de estas almendras, procuraban todos cogerlas como si se les hubiera caído un ojo. (Hernando Colón 294)

[and many of those almonds that the people of New Spain use as money, the ones that they seemingly hold in high esteem because when we were loading them on our ship with their things, I noticed that when one of those almonds fell, everyone would immediately bend down to pick it up as if their eye had fallen out.]

Almost a hundred years later, Juan de Acosta, in *Historia natural y moral de las Indias* [Natural and moral history of the Indies], also emphasizes the monetary value of the cocoa bean in Mexico. "Sirve también de moneda, porque con cinco cacaos se compra una cosa, y con treinta otra, y con ciento otra, sin que haya contradicción; y usan dar de limosna estos cacaos, a pobres que piden" [It is also used as a coin, because with five cocoa beans you buy one thing and with thirty another, and with a hundred another, without there being any contradiction; and these beans are given to the poor who beg for them] (266).

Cocoa beans' arrival to Spain is often credited to Hernán Cortés when he presented Mexican treasure to Carlos V in 1528. However, in their study on the history of chocolate, Sophie and Michael Coe explain that cocoa beans and chocolate were not among the gifts, which included humans, animals, weapons, and accessories but no plants or seeds (130). Rather, Coe and Coe write that the first recorded appearance of chocolate in Spain is in 1544 when Dominican friars arrived with Mayan nobility who presented gifts to the young Prince Felipe that included whipped chocolate (133). Thus, while tomatoes and potatoes became part of Spanish cuisine from the bottom up, chocolate took a different route. It moved from the elite, religious circles of the Aztec empire to the monasteries and court of Hapsburg Spain. Throughout the sixteenth century it maintained its elite status; only the seasonings changed from the hot chili pepper and ear flower of Mexico to cinnamon, anise, or black pepper, the more familiar flavours of the Spanish palate, that were added with sugar to sweeten the drink.[19]

It was not until the close of the sixteenth century that records from merchant vessels begin to reveal shipments of cacao with any regularity. In her study of chocolate (and tobacco) in the Americas, Marcy Norton writes that in 1591 Pedro de Mendoza, one of the wealthiest merchants in Seville, shipped from Guatemala one hundred pounds of cacao and four years later ordered that another shipment be made that included both cacao and *xícaras* [lacquered gourds] that were used as chocolate drinking vessels (144). Other merchants who shipped chocolate from the Americas included Rodrigo de Vadillo and Antonio de

Armijo (Norton 145–6). Together with other merchants, this wealthy elite controlled the merchant guild and maintained a monopoly on the commercial imports of cacao but imports were dauntingly small in comparison with other goods they controlled (Norton 148). Then, in the early part of the seventeenth century a change occurred as "members of the merchant oligarchy shifted to actively enter the market as traders as well as consumers" (Norton 148). And it is at this time that chocolate begins to appear in plays, poems, and beyond.

Chocolate not only begins to appear in works of fiction, but doctors and monks also fiercely debate chocolate's merits soon after its arrival to Spain. For example, in 1591 Juan de Cárdenas in his work *Problemas y secretos maravillosos de las Indias* [Problems and marvellous secrets of the Indies] dedicates three entire chapters to the medical benefits and detriments of consuming chocolate and argues that drinking hot chocolate does not break the fast. Later, in the seventeenth century, more authors contribute to these discussions. Juan de Barrios's *Libro en el cual se trata del chocolate, que provechos haga, y si sea bebida saludable o no...* [Book on chocolate, its benefits and whether or not it is a healthy drink ...] (1609) and Bartolomé Marradón's *Diálogo del uso del tabaco, los daños que causa, etc. y del chocolate y otras bebidas* [Dialogue on the use of tobacco, the damage it causes, etc., and on chocolate and other beverages] (1618) are just two of the works that contain medicinal aspects of this New World product. Additionally, the heated debate on the morality of drinking chocolate and whether it breaks the fast or not was the focus of several other works including publications by Antonio de León Pinelo (1636) and Manuel Caro Dávila (1699).[20]

Chocolate's connection to breakfast is one of the most fascinating aspects of its introduction to Europe. Prior to chocolate, breakfast was not a communal event as lunch and dinner were, but rather defined more singularly as a function of peasants' work (the intake of energy to work throughout the morning) or religious mores (as an end to the previous evening's fast). In fact, in the highly successful work *La antipatía de franceses y españoles* [The antipathy between the French and the Spanish] (1617), Carlos García explains that Spaniards most commonly ate two meals: lunch and dinner (240). In early modern novels and plays, *desayunar* [to have breakfast] is most often used to describe breaking the fast rather than naming a specific early morning meal. Characters commonly mention bread or cake soaked in wine, eaten with preserves, sweets, cream, fresh cheese, lard, and oranges. Sometimes, as we find in picaresque novels, breakfast might be a few leaves of cabbage, some garlic, or whatever characters could get their hands on. It was also common to drink breakfast in the form of spirits or wine or even chocolate and as chocolate became increasingly popular, so too did breakfast.[21] In Moreto's *La fuerza del natural* [The force of nature], Aurora suggests chocolate as a breakfast item at court that will reinvigorate one of the main characters, Carlos. However, breakfast is absent from cooking manuals through the nineteenth century. Health and dietary treatises discuss how much to eat at lunch and dinner, what types of foods should be eaten before others, how much time to allow between the two meals and between eating and sleeping but none specify rules on food for the morning.

In terms of breaking the fast, many doctors – from Galen to those of early modern Spain – prescribed a series of healthy activities before eating. Carlos I's medical advisor, Luis Lobera de Ávila, explains that his health treatise, which primarily concerns the health effects of foods consumed, encompasses "el modo y manera que se ha de tener desde que la persona se levanta, hasta que se acuesta" [the ways and means a person should have from the moment one arises until one goes to bed] (38). His first chapter, "En el cual se contiene la orden que un hombre ha de tener después de despertarse en la cama, hasta la hora de comer [In which is found the order in which a man should proceed after he wakes up in bed until mealtime] (39) provides specifics for the morning routine: "Cuando el hombre se quisiere levantar por la mañana de dormir, ha de extender las manos y los pies y los otros miembros, porque los espíritus vitales se atraigan a los miembros exteriores y se asutilen los espíritus de celebro" [When a man wants to awaken in the morning after having slept, he should stretch his hands and feet and other appendages so that the vital spirits will flow to the appendages and awaken the brain's spirit] (39). His advice includes dressing; washing hands, face, and eyes with cold water; and combing one's hair. A man should also brush his teeth "porque de no hacerlo se seguiría hedor en el aliento y corrupción en los humores y pertubación en el celebro" [because if he does not he would continue to have bad breath, decaying humours, and an unclear head] (40). These practices of eliminating "bad humour" buildup and stagnant spirits occur before ingesting any food, and thus imply that attention to health extends beyond what is consumed. Lobera de Ávila then closes his chapter by reminding those who are privileged to attend to his words that these actions are "limpieza de nobles hombres y los hace diferir de otros de no tanta suerte" [cleanliness of noblemen and it distinguishes them from others not as fortunate] (40).

Beyond chocolate's connection to breakfast, it was also fashionable as a mid-afternoon or late night snack. Mariana de Caravajal, in her collection of eight short novels, *Navidades de Madrid y noches entretenidas* [Christmas in Madrid and entertaining nights] (1663), finishes her work with hot chocolate and platters of sweets at the end of the week-long dinner party. The host Don Antonio insists that his guests not depart without having consumed hot chocolate to protect themselves against the cold winter air. "No será razón que salga ninguno de lo abrigado de salas tan apacibles, sin que primero tome defensas para el sereno, que las noches desta Pasqua han sido rigurosas, y assí suplico a Vuesas Mercedes me den permiso para que se les sirva chocolate" [It would not be right for anyone to leave the warmth of these peaceful rooms without first defending oneself against the night air, as this Christmas has been particularly harsh, so I ask that my honourable guests allow me to serve you hot chocolate] (249). The hot chocolate and the platters of sweets served with it are clear markers of Don Antonio's status as noted in his guests' response: "Aplaudieron todos su buen gusto, renovando en la opinión de todos lo merecedor que era del renombre de cortesano" [Everyone applauded his good taste, confirming their opinion of how deserving his fame as courtier was] (249).

Madame d'Aulnoy also writes about chocolate in her *Memoires de la cour d'Espagne, Relation du voyage d'Espagne* [Memories of the court of Spain, account of the voyage to Spain]. She includes the presentation of a variety of chocolate drinks during an afternoon snack:

> Presentaron después el chocolate, cada taza de porcelana sobre un platito de ágata, guarnecido de oro, con azúcar en una caja de lo mismo. Había allí chocolate helado, otro caliente y otro con leche y huevos. Lo toman con bizcochos o panecillo tan secos como si estuviesen fritos y que los hacen expresamente. (cited in Díez Borque *La sociedad española* 100)

> [They then served hot chocolate. Each porcelain cup on a marble saucer trimmed in gold, with sugar in a matching box. There was frozen chocolate, hot chocolate, and another with milk and eggs. They drink it with cakes or rolls so dry they seem fried, which are made specifically for the occasion.]

Madame d'Aulnoy's description of this event brings to mind the modern day chocolate and churros. It also highlights the importance of how food and beverages were served. Throughout Europe, domestic goods that enriched interior spaces, specifically serving dishes and tableware, were clear markers of refined consumption, a desire for luxury, and a certain social rank.[22] Sometime in the seventeenth century, the Marquis of Alella commissioned Lorenzo Passoles to create an enormous tile piece entitled *La chocolatada* [The chocolate party]. In a large semicircle piece, a detail of which is shown in figure 3.6, the artisan depicts an afternoon gathering in a stately garden. Across the tilework, Passoles portrays guests arriving, couples conversing, servants making and serving chocolate, and a group of nobles seated around a table enjoying hot chocolate and sweets. This visual depiction echoes what Mariana de Caravajal and Madame d'Aulnoy both describe in their writing.

Recipes for making chocolate appear in seventeenth-century treatises. For example, in 1631, Antonio Colmenero de Ledesma includes several ways to prepare this novel beverage in his *Curioso tratado de la naturaleza y calidad del chocolate, dividido en quatro puntos* [Curious treatise on the nature and quality of chocolate, divided into four points]. He suggests substituting New World spices when they are not available (or perhaps not desirable), using milk instead of water, or adding eggs or bread and having it for breakfast. But, like those for virtually every other New World product, chocolate recipes are absent from cooking manuals until the eighteenth century and then they appear in full force. Juan de la Mata includes dozens in his *Arte de repostería*. Recipes for chocolate drops (70, 122–3), cakes (86–7), marzipan (105), hot chocolate (144), and a whipped cold chocolate drink (158) fill the pages and exemplify how important chocolate has become at all levels of society.

From kitchens of kings to monastic refectories to Alonso Quijano's humble table, salpicon, salads, and pickled foods were served to one and all. Different social classes ate similar salads, vegetables, and pickled fare and as such they signify a diminishing contrast between social classes, much like we saw with meat consumption in chapter 2. Another diminishing contrast is reflected by the structure of meals. At all levels of society people ate collectively lighter in the evening than at midday and rarely considered breakfast as a social, organized meal but rather a reflection of religious practices or as a form of energy to start the day. Cooking manuals, literary texts, medical and historic documents, and town hall registries reveal that all levels of society followed similar food practices. That said, distinctions of quality certainly continued to exercise a dominant social force, particularly through the receptacles in which the food was served, and also regarding who served the food and where it was consumed.

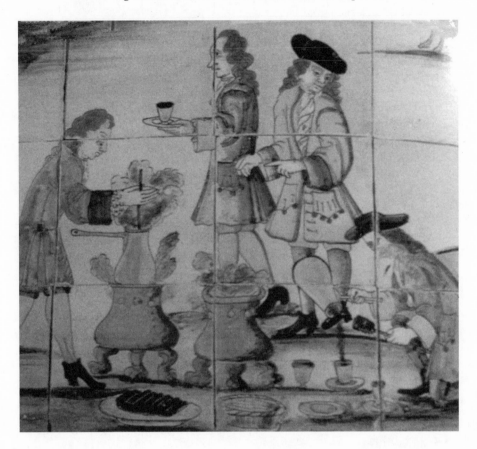

Figure 3.6. *La chocolatada* [The chocolate party] 1710. Tilework. Museu del Disseny, Barcelona. *Museo de cerámica, Palacio de Pedralbes, Barcelona* By Trinidad Sánchez-Pacheco, M. Antonia Casanovas and Maria Dolors Giral. (Zaragoza: Ibercaja, 1993): 40.

Beyond the social implications of eating habits, salpicon, salads, and pickled foods bring to light the history of particular foodstuffs, both those that are new to the Iberian Peninsula and those that have been part of the eating habits through multiple generations. For example, from the early seventeenth-century texts we learn that salads often refer to warm, roasted vegetables and that lettuce was eaten without any dressing or was used as a wrap for chopped meat or other vegetables. In the eighteenth century we see that lettuce becomes a dominant salad ingredient and that the incorporation of new world products begins to substantially mark Spanish cuisine. In spite of the imperialist project of imposing Spain's grandeur on "inferior" cultures, the state could not control the impact of New World foodstuffs and the transformation of Spanish identity they provoked. Transferring food across culture takes time and this is certainly the case with products brought from the New World at the end of the fifteenth and start of the sixteenth centuries. Though not always entirely accurate, the various discourses of food found in novels, poems, cookbooks, travellers' journals, and legal documents throughout the early modern period exhibit an increasing interest in New World vegetables and seeds. These revolutionary food items contribute significantly to the evolution of salpicon, salad, and other dishes common to Alonso Quijano and other early modern eaters. In contrast to this fickle relationship with the arrival of New World food, the following chapter examines in detail how the acceptance of specific foodstuffs and foodways shifted from the Middle Ages to the early modern period as some Jewish and Muslim food practices became absorbed into mainstream culture while others disappeared from Spain's culinary map.

Chapter Four

"Duelos y quebrantos los sábados": Jewish and Muslim Influences on Early Modern Eating Habits

Los jamones y las lenguas de cerdo tienen fama en este país

[This country is known for its ham and pork tongue]

Madame d'Aulnoy

With the description of what Alonso Quijano eats each Saturday, "duelos y quebrantos" [pain and suffering], Cervantes accords us the most discussed culinary reference of the entire early modern era. Curiously it does not appear in any early modern recipe book yet authors like Lope and Calderón write about it as a very popular dish. In the *mojiganga, El pésame de la viuda* [Sympathy for the widow], Calderón describes the ingredients of this dish when he writes:[1]

Para una cuitada,
Triste, mísera viuda,
Huevos y torreznos bastan
Que son duelos y quebrantos.   (69–72)

[For a grief-stricken,
Sad, miserable widow,
Eggs and fried pork fat are enough
Which are pain and suffering.]

Torreznos, or pieces of fried pork fat akin to today's bacon only fattier, mixed with scrambled eggs, has been one of the dominant interpretations of this dish throughout the centuries. This chapter explores the various interpretations of the phrase, examines the significance of pork for Spain, and reveals the Jewish, Muslim, and Christian practices that contributed to Spain's evolving gastronomy in the early modern period.

"Duelos y quebrantos"

Since 1614, when César Oudin translated "duelos y quebrantos" as "deuils et brisures" and explained that in Castilian the phrase refers to "des oeufs au lard" [eggs with bacon] (1556n1), critics have been debating the significance of "duelos y quebrantos" and even today, continue to weigh in on the discussion (Francisco Rodríguez Marín, Agustín de la Granja, Antonio Gázquez Ortiz, and Jesús Moreno Gómez). Of particular importance is a 1907 article by Clemente Cortejón, "Duelos y quebrantos (I, Cap. 1) Comentario a una nota de la primera edición crítica del 'Don Quijote'" [Duelos y quebrantos (I, Chap 1) Commentary on a note in the first critical edition of *Don Quixote*], in which he sides with Oudin and argues in favour of eggs with fried pork fat. Rodríguez Marín studied critics' references from 1614 through the middle of the twentieth century and again supports the theory that the dish refers to scrambled eggs with fried pork fat (434).

However, other critics propose that this is not the case. Scholars who disagree with Cortejón and Rodríguez Marín on the interpretation of scrambled eggs with diced pork fat put forth that the dish is made of scrambled eggs and organ meat, typically goat brain. This position is supported by the *Diccionario de autoridades* [Dictionary of authorities] where "duelos y quebrantos" is defined as a dish made of "tortilla de huevos y sesos" [tortilla of eggs and brain] (2.346). Partial abstinence laws that were in effect in Spain further bolster the theory. On Saturdays, animal extremities, such as head, tongue, or knuckles were permitted as were all organ meats: liver, lung, kidney, intestines, and brain. In fact, in the *Diccionario de autoridades* the expression "carne de sábado" [Saturday meat] refers to "extremos, despojos y grosura de los animales comestibles, por ser lo que se permite en esse día" [extremities, guts, and organs of edible animals because that is what is permitted (to be eaten) on this day] (3.S1). But on visiting Valladolid, the Portuguese professor Thomé Pinheiro da Veiga notes that Saturday meat also includes *tocino* [lard] from which *torreznos* are made (cited in Díez Borque, *La vida española* 105). Thus, either theory for "duelos y quebrantos" is supported by Spain's singular case of consuming offal, intestines, and extremities on Saturdays. One seventeenth-century French traveller notes, "Encuentro bastante singular el que coman ese día [sábado] las patas, la cabeza, los riñones, y que no se atrevan a comer otra cosa del mismo animal" [I find it rather peculiar that on Saturdays they will eat the feet, the head, and the kidneys but not any other part of the same animal] (cited in Díez Borque, *La sociedad española* 99). While fasting and abstinence go back as far as the creation of the church, the idea of limiting meat intake to animal innards on Saturdays was introduced into Spain in 1212, when Christian forces won a defining battle in the fight for dominance over Muslims in the Iberian Peninsula (Moreno Gómez 285). This custom continued well into the eighteenth century at which time Pope Benedict XIV and then Pius VI lifted Saturday abstinence laws in different parts of Spain (Moreno Gómez 285).

In Domingo Hernández de Maceras's university cookbook, *Libro del arte de cocina* [Book on the art of cooking], he dedicates almost two dozen recipes to Saturday meals, sheep being the animal of choice. To give but one example, in "cómo se han de hacer manos rebozadas" [how to make deep-fried knuckles] he explains that a sugar and cinnamon topping can be served over deep-fried goat or any type of knuckle, such as beef, pork, or kid] (224). And most readers will remember the sheep head that Lazarillo's second master, the stingy clergy, would devour on Saturdays: "Los sábados cómense en esta tierra cabezas de carnero, y enviábame por una que costaba tres maravedís. Aquélla le cocía y comía los ojos y la lengua y el cogote y sesos y la carne que en las quijadas tenía, y dábame todos los huesos roídos" [Around here they eat sheep head on Saturdays and he would send me to buy one that cost three maravedis. He would cook it up and eat the eyes, and tongue and neck and brains and whatever meat he could find in the jowls, and he would give me all the gnawed bones] (*La vida de Lazarillo* 115). With ample evidence for both positions, the question of the real meaning of "duelos y quebrantos" went unresolved; in fact, more hypotheses surfaced.

A third position, first advanced by Juan Pellicer in 1798 in his edition to the novel, offers a pragmatic explanation for the phrase:

> Era costumbre en algunos lugares de la Mancha traer los pastores a casa de sus amos las reses que entre semana se morían, o que de cualquier otro modo se desgraciaban, de cuyos huesos quebrantados y de los extremos de las mismas reses se componía la olla en tiempo en que no se permita en los reinos de Castilla comer los sábados de las demás partes de ellas ... esta comida se llamaba *duelos y quebrantos* con alusión al sentimiento y duelo

que causaba a los dueños el menoscabo de su ganado y el quebrantamien-
to de los huesos. (cited in Rodríguez Marín 431–2)

[In some areas of La Mancha it was customary for shepherds to bring to
their masters' house the remains of animals that had died during the week
or had suffered a fatal injury, and whose broken bones and carcass extremities would go into the one-pot stew in times when it was not allowed
in the kingdoms of Castile to eat other animal parts on Saturdays … this
meal was called *duelos y quebrantos* in reference to the sorrow and pain that
the loss of their herd and broken bones caused the proprietors.]

This position aligns somewhat with the first two, but goes beyond the
specifics of fried pork fat or goat brain to allow for a wider definition of
the dish by incorporating any organ, entrails, or extremity of the animal.

The last major tenant of the "duelos y quebrantos" debate allows for
an even more liberal interpretation of the phrase. Still other critics claim
that the reference included among the dishes that Alonso Quijano ate
on a weekly basis did not, in fact, refer to a specific dish at all but rather
to leftovers that a beggar may receive at the doors of a convent (Granja
223).[2]

Although we may never come to know the original meaning of this
dish, I find most compelling the position supported by Oudin and
Rodríguez Marín. First, Oudin in 1614 (and later Lorenzo Franciosini,
the first translator of the novel into Italian in 1622), have time on their
side. The later theories do not appear until more than a century after
the publication of *Don Quixote*. Second, the term "duelos y quebrantos" existed before its culinary application and with a moral meaning
as "duelos y quebrantos" literally translates as "pain and suffering."
Sebastián de Covarrubias, author of the leading dictionary of the day,
writes that this same dish, which he also interprets as eggs with fried
pork fat was also called *la merced de Dios* [mercy of God] among "old
Christians."

> güevos y torreznos, merced de Dios … si viene a deshora el güésped y no
> ay qué comer, el señor de casa dize a su muger: ¿Qué daremos a cenar a
> nuestro huésped, que no tenemos qué? Y aflígese mucho. La muger le re-
> sponde: Callad, marido, que no faltará la merced de Dios; y va al gallinero
> y trae sus güevos y corta una lonja de tozino, y fríelo con los güevos, y dale
> a cenar una buena tortilla, con que se satisfaze. Y de allí quedó llamar a los
> güevos y torreznos la merced de Dios. (668)

[eggs and fried pork fat, mercy of God ... if a guest shows up unexpectedly and there is nothing to eat, the man of the house will say to his wife: "What shall we give to our guest for dinner? There is nothing here." And he will be very distressed. The wife will answer: "Hush up, husband, there is no lack of God's mercy"; and she will go out to the hen house and bring in eggs and slice some fat back, and fry it with eggs, and give him a good tortilla and he will enjoy it. And that is where calling eggs with fried pork fat, "mercy of God," comes from.]

Américo Castro suggests that its newer name reflected eating habits of "new Christians" who showed the authenticity of their conversion through their food practices and that the expression could have reflected the physical and moral pain caused by eating pork, one of the food items prohibited both by Jewish and Muslim law (26).

Muslim and Jewish Influences

Certainly converts could prove the authenticity of their conversion through the food they ate as revealed in the poem the *converso* Antón de Montoro wrote in the fifteenth century:

Hice el credo y adorar
Ollas de tocino grueso,
Torreznos a medio asar
Oír misas y rezar
Santiguar y persignar,
Y nunca pude matar
Este rastro de confeso.   (De Marcella and Rodríguez Puértolas 75)

[I recited the creed and worshipped/ I made pots filled with fat back/ Half roasted pork fat/ I went to mass and prayed/ And crossed myself and crossed myself/ But never could I erase/ This trace of a *converso*.]

It was also clear from sixteenth-century laws laid down after Granada was taken by Christian forces that animals must be slaughtered in a Christian fashion: "matando las carnes según y por la orden que las matan los cristianos e no en otra manera" [slaughtering animals according to and in the order that Christians slaughter and not in any other manner] (cited in Valles Rojo, *Cocina* 338). Even earlier, laws had been established prohibiting Christians from buying meat from Jewish or

Muslim butchers. The fines were high for both buyer and seller: 300 maravedis for a first offence and up to 1200 maravedis and fifty public lashings for repeated offenders.[3] So, given these cultural and legal circumstances, "duelos y quebrantos," would have emphasized newly acquired eating practices of the recently converted. Some critics go so far as to speculate that perhaps Don Quixote himself was a recent convert (Eisenberg). In the novel Don Quixote is identified as being a "Christian," in contrast to Sancho who is several times referred to as a "cristiano viejo" [old Christian]. Calling the dish *duelos y quebrantos* instead of *merced de Dios*, and eating it on the Sabbath may not necessarily implicate Alonso Quijano as a *converso* but, at a minimum, it establishes the impact of Jewish and Muslim practices on the eating habits of early modern Spain.

There is no doubt that Muslims and Jews living on the Iberian Peninsula shared culinary tastes with their Christian neighbours as evidenced both in Inquisitional records, in particular for Jewish eating habits, and in the comparative study of Muslim and Christian cooking manuals in chapter 1.[4] The major differences pertained to ritualistic prayer before food preparation and consumption, food items in celebrations, and perhaps most obviously, in the dietary restrictions and distinctions of what was not consumed.[5] In the Inquisitional trials of Ciudad Real, the testimonies of witnesses regularly included food preparation as evidence of the Jewishness of the accused. In the 1483–4 trial of María Díaz, several witnesses, including Juan de Merlo, gave testimony regarding her observation of the Sabbath and kashrut practices.

> Dixo que puede aver poco mas de un año que estando en casa de Maria Diaz, la çerera, con Juan de Torres, su hermano, <vido> como la dicha çerera e Costança Dias su hija ... guisaba<n> de comer del viernes para el sabado. E que sabe que guardavan el sabado ellas y vestian camisas e ropas linpias e comian el guisado del viernes. E que sabe que escondidamente deste testigo guardaron una Pascua de judios por invierno. E que sabe que non comian carne de la carneçeria salvo si fuese degollada con çerimonia judayca. (Beinart 55)

> [He said that it was a little over a year ago that while in the home of María Díaz, the wax dealer, with his brother, Juan de Torres, he saw how said wax dealer and her daughter, Constanza Diaz, cooked food for Saturday on Friday. And that he knows that they observed Saturdays and dressed

in clean undergarments and clothes and ate food prepared on Friday. And that he knows that they secretly observed a Jewish Passover in winter. And that he knows that they did not eat meat from the butchers unless the throat was slit with a Jewish ceremony.]

Other testimonies included eating unleavened bread, lettuce, celery, thistle, and vinegar as evidence of her non-Christian practices (Beinart 58). In the end, María was condemned as a rebel and sentenced to be burned in effigy the following month.

It is common knowledge that Muslim and Jewish laws forbid the consumption of pork products. The fact that Jews were exiled in 1492 and Muslims in 1609 as the Crown sought to unify a nation under one religion, directly connects the country's religious and cultural identity with its culinary heritage of pork. Pork's position in the early modern period is a clear example of how food preferences carry hegemonic identity. And even after Spain's imperial presence faded, ham continues to inform Spain's cultural identity. From the finest restaurants to the humblest abode, from neighbourhood butchers to big box supermarkets, two varieties of ham dominate the country: Iberian and Serrano. In all regions and all social classes, Spaniards eat ham for breakfast, lunch, dinner, and snacks throughout the day. Their love of pork is not limited to the porcine hind leg; rather they consume every part imaginable.

Returning to the early modern period, ham was so valued that writers praised specific towns for their reputed pork products. In Quevedo's burlesque poem "Los sopones de Salamanca" [The beggar students of Salamanca], he describes a barmaid by her enticing thighs, comparing her "hams" to those of two Spanish towns, Rute and the then called, Algarrovillas.

Catalina de Pelares,
una gallega maldita
más apreciada de perniles
que Rute y Algarrobillas.
(Quevedo, Francisco de Quevedo 868, vv. 29–32)

[Catalina de Pelares
naughty Galician gal
(with hams) more valued
than (those from) Rute and Algarrovillas.]

Martínez Montiño cites the latter town as he begins his recipe for mutton or ham pie: "Tomarás unos torreznos de buen tocino de Garrobillas" [Take some good pieces of fried pork fat from Algarrovillas] (376). Quevedo once again repeats the allusion to Algarrovillas in his "Poema heroico de las necedades y locuras de Orlando el furioso" [Heroic poem of the stupidity and craziness of Orlando the Furious], when he describes guests by the food stereotypically associated with them: Italians and macaroni, Manchegans and breadcrumbs, Andalusians and sweet potatoes, and Extremadurans and their sausage-inspired cheer "Algarrovillas" (*Francisco de Quevedo* 875, vv. 153–80). While both towns produced excellent cured ham, as evidenced in the writings of Quevedo, Cervantes, Tirso, and others, Rute's ham fame is directly tied to its convert population in the sixteenth and seventeenth centuries.[6] At that time, it was a farming community known as much for its firewater (*aguardiente*) as for its cured ham. The Holy Office of the Inquisition condemned forty Rute citizens to 200 lashings as part of a disciplinary action tied to a "limpieza de sangre" [blood cleansing] designed to route out false converts. Whether the hams were cured to such perfection because of the new Christian status of its citizens or in response to the punishment, either way, the best hams available at the Hapsburg court were cured in Rute ("Historia").

Muslim and, to a lesser extent, Jewish contributions to Spain's culinary heritage are more significant for their concrete contributions than for noted absences or dietary restrictions that may have guided Christian eating habits towards the very foods that were prohibited. Rice, saffron, eggplant, spinach, almonds, sugar, cinnamon, oranges, and lemons are some of the most important ingredients commonly found in Spanish cuisine today that Arabs either brought to the Iberian Peninsula or extensively developed when there. Additionally, in the early modern period we also see the continued use of cilantro, black pepper, couscous, rose water, and other flavours that are less prevalent today but were significant in the early stages of Spanish cuisine. In chapter 1, comparisons between the two extant Hispano-Muslim cooking manuals, *Kitāb al-tabīj fi l-Magrib wa-l-Andalus fi 'asr al-muwahhudin li-mu'allif mayhul* [The book of cooking in Maghreb and Andalus in the era of Almohads, by an unknown author] (1228–43), *Fuḍālat-al-Hiwān Fi Tayyibat al-Ta'am Wa-l-Alwan* [The delicacies of the table and the finest of foods and dishes] (1243–1328), along with several Christian cookbooks, including the *Sent Soví* (first half of 14th century) and the works of Nola (1520), Granado (1599), Hernández Maceras (1607), and Martínez

Montiño (1611) are discussed in detail and outline both food products and cooking methods shared among the three religious groups.

Jewish influences in Spanish gastronomy are hard to document as there are no extant early modern Jewish cooking manuals available to us today. But, recipes labelled "Jewish" are found in the medieval manuals, *Fuḍālat-al-Hiwān* and *Kitāb al-tabīj*. In fact, in the former, the editor Manuela Marín notes that the only source cited in Ibn Razīn's cooking manuscript is by the Jewish doctor, Yonah Ibn Ganah (11th c.) (*Relieves* 27). He wrote *Tratado sobre la explicación de los medicamentos* [Treatise on the explication of medicine] from which Ibn Razīn borrowed a recipe on cured meat.

> El autor llama *al-namkasūd*, que es una receta de carne salada con sal machacada. La diferencia entre esta receta y la cecina es que el *namkasūd* se hace de un carnero entero o partido en dos mitades; la carne queda blanda y grasa, cuando la aprietas te untas la mano y el cuchillo la corta como si fuera carne fresca, no como se corta la cecina. Quien lo desee, puede hacerlo, y que lo experimente. (306)

> [The author calls it *al-namkasūd*, which is a meat recipe salted with ground salt. The difference between this recipe and beef jerky is that *namkasūd* is made from a whole sheep or one cut in two; the meat is soft and greasy, and when you squeeze it, your hand turns greasy and the knife cuts through it like fresh meat, not how one cuts beef jerky. Whoever wants to can do it and may experiment with it.]

Although there are no extant Jewish recipe manuals, the anonymous *Kitāb al-tabīj* offers several recipes with "Jewish" as part of the title: "Perdiz judía" [Jewish partridge] (102), "Plato de perdiz judía" [Jewish partridge dish] (104–5), "Plato de pollo judío" [Jewish chicken dish] (103, 106–7), "Plato judío relleno oculto" [Jewish dish with hidden stuffing] (109–10), and "Plato judío de berenjenas rellenas con carne" [Eggplant stuffed with beef, Jewish style] (266–7). By comparing, for example, the Jewish partridge recipes to others in which the main ingredient is also partridge, we can begin to see the overlaps in Muslim and Jewish cooking and also begin to understand some of the nuanced differences between the two food preparation styles.

In total, the *Kitāb al-tabīj* contains eleven partridge dishes; two of those eleven carry the name "Jewish" in the title.[7] Comparing the nine partridge recipes that do not directly reference Jewish tradition, we can see that, following Muslim dietary laws, instructions for slaughtering an animal are often included. Some partridge recipes begin by stating that the bird is slaughtered and hung with feathers intact the night before. The breast is almost always used for making meatballs, which are later added to the recipes. In addition to oil, vinegar, salt, and pepper, seasoning often includes cinnamon, saffron, *almorí* (barley-based flavour enhancer), and cilantro or coriander. Single entries appear for cumin, rosewater, citron shoots, fennel stalks, lavender, cloves, ginger, pine nuts, honey, peeled almonds, and caraway. The partridge recipes, with the exception of the roast partridge, are all finished with a crust of whipped egg and a combination of flour and/or breadcrumbs. The variations for partridge recipes include one with peas and garlic ("Otro plato igual") [Another like dish] (85), one with vinegar and cilantro juice ("Plato alabado en primavera para los que tienen tensión y los de sangre ardiente") [A dish praised in springtime for those with fulness and those with burning blood (131)], another with apples, fennel, onion, and rosewater ("Receta del plato de pollo o perdiz con membrillo o manzana") [Recipe for a dish of chicken or partridge with quince or apple] (85), and another with Swiss chard, olives, and cheese ("Receta del plato de aceitunas" [Recipe for a dish of olives] (90–1).

Another rule governing both Muslim and Jewish food practices is the complete removal of blood prior to preparing the meat. This can be done in a few different ways. Muslims sometimes use vinegar to draw out any remaining surface blood. In the Jewish tradition, final blood is removed either by soaking in water for thirty minutes and then salting the animal for an hour or by broiling. In an Inquisitional trial against Diego Díaz Nieto in Mexico, 1601, evidence brought against Blanca Lorenzo was based on how she prepared poultry. "[G]uardaba la ley de Moysén por tener a los judíos en su casa y por haberle visto degollar las aves y desebar la carne y echarla en agua para que se desangrase aunque no se declaró con éste ni éste con ella, no oyó decir que lo fuese" [She practised the laws according to Moses by allowing Jews in her house and by having seen her slit the throat of poultry, porge the meat, and soak it in water so that all the blood was removed even though she never declared her Judaism to him or he to her, nor had he ever heard her claim that she was (Jewish)] (Uchamany 275). This type of preparation also surfaces in Jewish recipes in the *Kitāb al-tabīj*. For example, in "Plato de pollo judío," instructions for salting the chicken before cooking it, "se sala el pollo y déjalo" [salt the chicken and let it rest] (103), remind readers of this tradition. We also see these practices in Christian cookbooks of the early modern period. In the recipe for broth for a sick person, "Una escudilla de caldo" [A bowl of broth], Martínez Montiño explains that after killing the hen, one must soak the bird in water to remove all the blood: "y echala en un poco de agua, por un quarto de hora, para que se desangre" [and then put it in a little water for fifteen minutes so that the blood can drain] (393). Likewise, in the Muslim tradition, it is common to find recipes that begin with instructions similar to the one for "Receta de su asado" [Recipe for roasting (aquatic fowl)]: "Después de degollarlo, se cuelga una noche de la pata y a la mañana siguiente se lava y se deja aparte" [After slitting its throat, hang by its foot overnight and the next morning, wash it and set it aside] (Kitāb al-tabīj 70).

In both Jewish recipes, organ meat is central to the recipes. In "Perdiz judía" [Jewish partridge], instructions include pounding partridge entrails together with almonds and pine-nuts and adding crushed almorí, oil, a little cilantro juice, black pepper, cinnamon, Chinese cinnamon, lavender, five eggs, and any additional meat that may be necessary (102). This stuffing is spread between the flesh and the skin of the bird. Anything remaining is inserted into the cavity along with two boiled eggs. The stuffed bird is then placed in a pot with oil, almorí, and salt, covered with dough, and constantly shaken while over the flame until the sauce has reduced. More vinegar is added together with citron and mint shoots and, similar to the many Muslim recipes, finished with beaten eggs and baked with coals surrounding the dish. The partridge is served on a platter garnished with hard-boiled yolks and sprinkled with black pepper, cinnamon, and sugar (102).

In the second recipe, "Plato de perdiz judía" [Jewish partridge dish], organ meat is again essential to the dish. The bird is quartered and stewed with the usual spices, cilantro juice, onion juice, almorí, vinegar, oil, and water. Similar to the other Jewish recipe, citron and mint shoots and pine nuts are also added. When the sauce has cooked down, the organ meat is removed, mashed and combined with egg batter, then added back into the pot until it has set. The dish is turned out onto a platter and covered with the egg yolks and mint shoots. It is finished with chopped pine nuts and almonds and a little rosewater (104–5).

The Jewish recipes are very similar to the Muslim ones in preparation, seasoning, the use of egg batter for a crust, and the use of egg yolks and roasted nuts as garnish. The biggest variances are the central role of the organ meat, the addition of citron and mint shoots, and the surprising lack of meatballs in the Jewish recipes. Meatballs were commonly associated with Jewish fare. In fact, David Gitlitz and Linda

Davidson point out that, "[t]ogether with the Sabbath stew, *adafina*, meatballs were – at least in old-Christian eyes – one of the defining characteristics of Ibero-Jewish cooking" (174). Recipes for meatballs fill the pages of the Muslim recipe collections, thus showing another example of the overlaps in Jewish and Muslim food choices. Although sometimes served on their own, meatballs are most often made from the meat of the animal being prepared and used as stuffing, an additional stew ingredient, or as a garnish.

Returning to the distinctive aspects of the Jewish recipes, the chicken dish also highlights the use of organ meat and uses cilantro juice, pine nuts, citron, and here, fennel shoots instead of mint (103). Again in the meat dish, "Plato judío relleno oculto," [Jewish dish with hidden stuffing] and the eggplant dish, "Plato judío de berenjenas rellenas con carne" [Eggplant stuffed with beef, Jewish style], cilantro juice, onion juice, and citron shoots appear in the recipe with mint shoots, rosewater, and pistachio and pine nuts as garnishes (109–10, 264).

When examining even more closely the Muslim dishes, mint, which appears in some three dozen recipes, is much more commonly used for its juice or as a garnish, with the exception of an eggplant recipe that also includes chopped mint. Another variant is the use of rosewater in savoury dishes. Rosewater is very popular in the Muslim tradition particularly for sweets and fowl. Regarding its use in beef dishes, no Muslim recipes include rosewater while the Jewish one does. In addition, in the entire work only two lamb recipes use rosewater, and one of them is the "Plato judío de berenjenas rellenas con carne." These minor differences, while certainly noteworthy, do not take away from the commonalities the two ethnic kitchens shared. Scholars have studied many of the dishes consumed by exiled Jews that emigrated to parts of Italy, Turkey (Cooper 122–4, 132), and the New World (Uchamany) and affirmed the similarities with those eaten in medieval Spain: meat soups, beef dishes, lentils, noodles, phyllo pastry, rice, olives and olive oil, and a wide variety of sweet pastries.

In Aldonza's Kitchen

Moving into the early modern period, Francisco Delicado's picaresque novel *La lozana andaluza* [Portrait of the lusty Andalusian woman] (1528) provides us with images of the *converso* kitchen. Generally, the work describes the underside of Rome in the early sixteenth century and the lifestyle of marginalized characters such as prostitutes, thieves, and conmen. The main character, Aldonza, who has emigrated from Andalusia to Italy, spends her time in "Pozo blanco," the Jewish ghetto of Rome.[8] At the outset of her tale, in Mamotreto II, she reminisces about her culinary upbringing, the role of her grandmother, and her personal talents in the kitchen.[9] Her food memories, combined with erotic connotations of her language, are instruments of self-fashioning and form the basis of her *converso* identity.

ella me mostró guisar, que en su poder deprendí hacer fideos, empanadillas, alcuzcuzu con garbanzos, arroz entero, seco, graso, albondiguillas redondas y apretadas con culantro verde,[10] que se conocían las que yo hacía entre ciento. Mirá, señora tía, que su padre de mi padre decía: "¡Éstas son de mano de mi hija Aldonza!" Pues, ¿adobado no hacía? Sobre que cuantos traperos había en la cal de la Heria querían proballo, y máxime cuando era un buen pecho de carnero. Y ¡qué miel! Pensá, señora, que la teníamos de Adamuz, y zafrán de Peñafiel, y lo mejor del Andalucía venía en casa d'esta mi agüela. Sabía hacer hojuelas, prestiños, rosquillas de alfajor, textones de cañamones y de ajonjolí,[11] nuégados, sopaipas, hojaldres, hormigos torcidos con aceite, talvinas, zahinas y nabos sin tocino y con comino; col murciana con alcaravea, y holla reposada no la comía tal ninguna barba.[12] Pues boronía ¿no sabía hacer? ¡por maravilla![13] Y cazuela de berengenas mojíes en perfición; cazuela con su ajico y cominico, y saborcico de vinagre, ésta hacía yo sin que me la vezasen. Rellenos, cuajarejos de cabritos,[14] pepitorias y cabrito apedreado con limón ceutí. Y cazuelas de pescado cecial con oruga,[15] y cazuelas moriscas por maravilla, y de otros pescados que sería luengo de contar. Letuarios de arrope para en casa, y con miel para presentar, como eran de membrillos, de cantueso, de uvas, de berengenas, de nuezes y de la flor del nogal, para tiempo de peste; de oregano y hierbabuena, para quien pierde el apetito. (177–9)

[She showed me how to cook; under her guidance I learned how to make noodles, mini empanadas, couscous with garbanzos, rice – whole grain, dry, fatty – little, round meatballs packed with cilantro. The ones I made, anyone knew, were one in a hundred. Look, my dear aunt, this is what my father's father, who is your father, used to say, "These are from the hand of my daughter Aldonza!" And you think she didn't make marinade? You know how many rag-and-bone men in the Jewish quarter of Heria wanted to try it? All of them, when it was a good breast of mutton. And, what honey! Just imagine, ma'am, that we had it from Adamuz, and saffron from Peñafiel, and the best of Andalusia came through my grandmother's house. She knew how to make puff pastries, honey-sprinkled fried dough, almond cookies, sesame meringues, nut- and honey-filled pastries, fried dough, phyllo treats, nut butter pastries with oil, almond-milk and simple porridges, and cumin turnips without lard; Murcia-style cabbage with caraway, and no one who ate her simmering stew could stop. And, stewed eggplant, you think she couldn't make it? Hers was marvellous! And her twice-baked eggplant casserole, to perfection; a casserole with a little garlic, a pinch of cumin, and a hint of vinegar, I could make this without anyone having to show me. Stuffings, goat tripe, fricassées, and Ceuta-style roasted kid with lemon. And dried fish with arugula sauce and incredible Morisco-style casseroles and so many other fish dishes that it would take too long to recount. Syrup-based electuaries for home and honey-based for giving [to others], like those from quince, Spanish lavender, grapes, eggplant, walnuts, and walnut flower for the plague; oregano and spearmint for when someone loses their appetite.]

Critics have primarily approached this passage in terms of the erotic and the connections between sexuality and Aldonza's *converso* status but my focus shifts to how her food memories help us understand Spain's culinary identity.

Stoler and Strassler examine food memories within the field of colonial studies to understand better constructions of the past. One of the most engaging aspects about their project is how they raise awareness of the very processes that construct those pasts. "Our work rests on a relatively simple but disconcerting observation: namely that 'the colonial' is invoked with such certitude of its effects by those studying it, and 'colonial memory' with such assuredness of its ever-presence, that both are treated as known and knowable quantities, rather than as problematic sites of query in themselves" (4). Delicado's passage that describes Aldonza's kitchen indeed problematizes how we conceive of the past. These memories of a fictional, *converso*, female character that are created by a male author, also most likely *converso*, provide the reader with a nostalgic look into the *converso* kitchen. The images recalled prompt an empathetic response to a *converso* lifestyle, specifically to the rich flavours of their cuisine. This nostalgia for cultural *converso* heritage, specifically through rich imagery of the kitchen, stands in direct contrast to and even undermines the political position of Spain's cultural heritage. These memories present a detailed and idealized image of the lifestyle of the marginalized in early modern Spain that stands in stark contrast to the position of the state. In this way we can see how

Delicado chooses to interpret and redesign, as Stoler and Strassler argue, "the conditions of possibility that account for his past, present and future" (9).

Intimate memories, such as those associated with food preparation and its consumption, reveal power relations between the colonizing and the colonized, or in early modern Spain, between majority and minority ethnicities. Stoler and Strassler show that employers and servants remember tastes, smells, textures, and sounds in completely different ways. Food memories that include specific details of how ingredients come together certainly attest to the symbolic power of food, the specialized knowledge of food preparation, and the intense daily labour involved in its production (34–5). People remember detailed menus of food eaten decades earlier and subjects are able to summon up recipes with energy and care. In the case of Aldonza, she too exhibits compelling recall capabilities as she lists the catalogue of dishes learned in her grandmother's kitchen with pride and excitement. At least five times she refers to how others acknowledged the excellence of her and her grandmother's cooking ("the ones I made anyone knew," "from the hand of Aldonza," "no one who ate her simmering stew could stop," "hers was marvellous," and "I could make this without anyone having to show me"). She proudly mentions specific herbs and spices that gave dishes their defining touches (meatballs with cilantro, turnips with cumin, cabbage with caraway, kid with lemon), and highlights her soliloquy with geographical superlatives that reinforced the quality of ingredients (honey from Adamuz, saffron from Peñafiel, the best of Andalusia). What Stoler and Strassler rightly note about the power of food memories equally applies to Aldonza's passage. "This clustering of memories around practices of cooking and eating was obviously linked to food's symbolic power and daily importance" (34). Memory, like food itself, is intimately tied to issues of identity but must also be understood in terms of its political weight. In *La lozana andaluza*, Aldonza's food memories are couched in erotic language. Readers can easily dismiss the historic food value and focus on the way a *converso* prostitute sexualizes food. In this light, these images would serve as a link between *converso* eating habits and immoral activities thus politicizing her memories and further discriminating against non-Christians and, by extension, their contributions to Spain's cultural and social identity.

However, what Aldonza chooses to remember, or rather, how Delicado constructs Aldonza's memory for his readership, tells us two important things about Spain's culinary history that, when analysed in conjunction with other discourses, primarily elite cooking manuals, offers a more complete understanding of this aspect of early modern culture. First, the memories that Aldonza privileges challenge Delicado's readers to acknowledge culinary contributions of Muslims and Jews that span back to their medieval roots. By comparing the personal, albeit fictional, memories of a Jewish *converso* to dishes found in Hispano-Muslim cooking manuals, we can begin to understand how the two ethnic kitchens overlapped. The previous examples of meatballs used in both Jewish and Muslim cooking is one clear example of this intersection. Her catalogue can loosely be divided into grain-based recipes, sweets, vegetables, spices and casseroles, and finally, medicinal pastes. Today, we can analyse these parts, compare them to extant medieval cooking manuals, and get a sense of the similarities and differences in Muslim and Jewish influences in Spanish cuisine.

Other critics have explored the connections between the protagonist and the author; Delicado, like Aldonza, fled Spain and lived in Rome during the early part of the sixteenth century.[16] As such, these culinary references are most likely grounded in the personal experiences of the author and lead to the second historical point. By comparing Delicado's picaresque novel to the medieval Hispano-Muslim cooking manuals and then looking at the early modern Christian food manuals, traces of the former become clear in the development of Spanish cooking.[17] In this way, Delicado's treatment of Aldonza's food memories is pivotal in connecting food across centuries and multiple ethnic groups. It serves as a "contact zone" within fields of cross-cultural experiences and is a material base for marking routes that both producers and consumers travel (Döring, Heide, and Muehleisen). As we shall see in *La lozana andaluza* when comparing it with culinary manuals, these texts create a map that allows us to understand the route cooks and their consumers took that influenced the evolving Spanish foodways of the Middle Ages through the early modern period.

Aldonza reminisces over the lessons learned from her grandmother and begins her catalogue with grain-based dishes – noodles, small empanadas, couscous, and rice. In this very first phrase, she acknowledges the lesser known, but primary, contributions of Muslims and Jews to Spanish fare. In the *Kitāb al-tabīj*, the author includes several noodle recipes. These are gathered together with recipes for savoury pies, couscous, rice, harissa (a dish of cheese and pulled meat, kneaded into dough), and other related recipes (223–40). The following reveals the variety of noodles common in the thirteenth century.

Receta de fideos. Esto se hace de masa y tiene tres clases: la alargada a modo de trigo, la redondeada a modo de grano de cilantro, que se llama en Bugía y su región *ḥamīṣ*, y la que se hace delgada con la delgadez del *kagīd* [hoja de papel] y es una comida de mujeres; la cuecen con calabaza, aromas y grasa; es una de los *qaṭāif*. La manera de cocer los fideos es como la de los macarrones. (Huici Miranda 228–9)

[Noodle recipe. This is made from dough in three different ways: long like wheat, round like a coriander seed, which in Bugia and the surrounding region is called *ḥamīṣ*, and the thin type which has the thinness of *kagīd* (a sheet of paper). It (the latter) is food for women, cooked with bottle squash, aromatics, and fat; it is one of the *qaṭāif* (shredded phyllo doughs). The way to cook noodles is similar to cooking macaroni.][18]

Long before Marco Polo's expeditions to Asia, many types of pasta were consumed on the Iberian Peninsula. Most noodle dishes were eaten in a broth, and, when possible, with meat. This tradition continues today and is most explicitly seen in the traditional soup served on Christmas day in Cataluña, *sopa de galets,* a clear soup with meat-filled pasta shells.

In the recipe "Hechura de la cocción de los macarrones" [The way to cook macaroni] the author cooks the broth down leaving a rich pasta dish that can be used as easily for rice or noodles as it can be for macaroni.

Se toma carne de las colas, de las piernas, del pecho, de la cintura y lo que haya de ellas que sea graso, se corta y se pone en la olla con sal, cebolla, pimienta, cilantro seco y aceite; se pone a un fuego moderado y se cuece hasta estar en sazón; luego se saca y se clarifica la salsa, se vuelve a la olla y se le añade mantequilla, grasa tierna y aceite dulce; cuando ha hervido, se ponen fideos finos en cantidad suficiente, se hierve y se agita suavemente y cuando se seca el agua y está a punto, se aparta del fuego y se deja un poco; se vierte en la fuente y se iguala hasta que se disuelva la grasa; luego se toma, si la quieres, cocida como está o frita y se alínea en la fuente, se maja algo de ello en los fideos y se espolvorea con canela y jengibre y se presenta; con esta receta se hacen el arroz y los fideos. (Huici Miranda 229)

[Take meat from the tail, legs, breast, belly, and anything that is fatty, chop it up, and place it in a pot with salt, onion, pepper, coriander, and oil, on medium heat and cook until done. Remove it and clarify the broth; then add butter, a high-quality fat, and sweet oil. When that comes to a boil, add just the right amount of fine noodles, boil, and gently stir until the water is gone and it is perfect. Remove from the flame and let it rest a little. Turn it onto a platter, let it settle and the fat dissolve. Enjoy it as is or fried and arranged on the platter. Mash some of the meat into the noodles and sprinkle with cinnamon and ginger and serve it. This recipe can also be used for rice or noodles.]

In *Libro de guisados* [Book of cookery] Ruperto de Nola acknowledges the same flexibility in trading grains in his recipe "Potaje de fideos" [Noodle stew]. He also allows almond milk to substitute for goat or sheep milk, a possible acknowledgement of the Jewish dietary laws forbidding the simultaneous consumption of meat and milk.

> y cuando comenzare de hervir el caldo, echar en la olla los fideos con un pedazo de azúcar; y desque sean más de medio cocidos echar en la olla, con el caldo de las gallinas o de carnero, leche de cabras o de ovejas, o en lugar de ello, leche de almendras, que ésta nunca puede faltar, y cuezga bien todo junto y desque sean cocidos los fideos apartar la olla del fuego y dejarla reposar un poco….mas como tengo dicho en el capítulo del arroz muchos hay que con potajes de esta calidad que se guisan con caldo de carne dicen que no se debe echar azúcar ni leche, mas esto está en el apetito de cada uno; y en la verdad, con fideos o con arroz guisado con caldo de carne, mejor es echar sobre las escudillas queso rallado que sea muy bueno. (289–90)

> [and when the stock begins to boil, add the noodles to the pot with a lump of sugar, and when it is more than half cooked, add to the hen or mutton stock, goat or sheep milk, or in its place, almond milk that is always tasty. Boil everything together and when the noodles are cooked, take the pot off the flame and let it rest a little ... as I have stated in the chapter on rice; there are many who say that stews of this quality that are prepared with meat stock should not have sugar or milk added to them, yet this is up to each person's taste and truth be told, noodles or rice prepared with beef stock are better when served in a dish with grated cheese on top; it is very good.]

Nola's insistence on not including milk again recalls Jewish food practices and the importance of acknowledging the diner's appetite. Yet, he closes the recipe with his own "Christian" preference for grated cheese instead of cinnamon and sugar, and in this way, the Jewish separation of dairy and meat products from the same animal in a specific dish

disappears from the recipes. It is impossible to know if Nola consciously included and dismissed this specific Jewish food aversion. What is
apparent, however, is that the relationship between Christian and
Jewish food practices are complicated and cannot be easily separated
even decades after Jews are exiled from Castile and Aragon. The taste
for noodles cooked in meat broth with sugar and cinnamon, that Nola
deems inferior to a noodle stew finished with grated cheese, continues
through the eighteenth century as illustrated by Juan de Altamiras's
recipe, "Fideos gruesos" [Thick noodles]. In this recipe he makes pasta
with breadcrumbs, cheese, cinnamon, sugar, eggs, and beef broth and
presses the dough through a slotted spoon into the boiling meat broth.
Later, it is served on a plate with cinnamon and sugar sprinkled on top
(73). These noodle dishes that first appear in mid-thirteenth-century
Hispano-Muslim manuals weave their way through the culinary and
literary texts of the Middle Ages and the early modern period.

Even more prevalent in Spain's culinary history are empanadas,
which fill the recipe books from the thirteenth-century Hispano-Muslim
tradition to early modern court cooking of the sixteenth and seventeenth centuries.[19] Although similar to other pie varieties – *pasteles,
pastelones, tortas, tortadas* – empanadas are generally understood as free-
standing stuffed bread. The dough itself varies. Some empanadas are
made with yeast, others are not; some use oil, others butter; some are
baked, others fried; some resemble the enclosed empanadas we know
today, others are open-faced. In the Hispano-Muslim manuscripts, fill-
ings range from poultry to fish to nothing at all. Others mix meat with
different vegetables such as eggplant, turnips, peas, or greens. There are
empanadas made of lamb, eel, or garbanzos. In one recipe, seasonings
of black pepper, cilantro, and mashed onion are sautéed in oil and water, breadcrumbs added, and all is poured onto a platter, formed into the
shape of an empanada, and served with oil or fat poured over the top
(*Kitāb al-tabīj* 192). Several other recipes are for sweet empanadas. One
resembles a Napoleon with alternating layers of thin dough and sweet
cream. These layers are then covered with a thicker crust, soaked in a
condensed milk mixture and later sprinkled with cinnamon and sugar
(*Kitāb al-tabīj* 144).

These recipes, sweet and savoury alike, are also found in the cookbooks of Nola, Martínez Montiño, and others. Martínez Montiño has
some two dozen empanada recipes. Like the earlier recipes, his dough
varies. At times he kneads flour with water, eggs, salt, and fat; other
variations include a thin batter made from rice flour, sugar, egg yolk,

and a dash of wine. In one innovative recipe, Martínez Montiño creates an empanada-encrusted roasted fowl. In "Empanadas en asador" [Rotisserie empanadas], he roasts poultry on a spit and coats the fowl with the batter as it turns. As each layer bakes, he adds more until the meat is fully covered. The dish is finished with a lard glaze and powdered sugar (40–1). Martínez Montiño also includes wild game filling for other stuffed foods, something not included in previous cooking manuals. Empanadas, like noodles and pasta in general, fully survived and continued to evolve as defining elements of Spain's gastronomy. *Canelons a la catalana* [Catalan cannelloni], *empanada gallega* [Gallegan empanada], and *fideuá* [Valencian noodle paella] are all examples of how medieval tastes have evolved and endured today.

However, the semolina-based couscous, which Berbers brought with them to the Iberian Peninsula in the eighth century and was still enjoyed at the Hapsburg court through the seventeenth century, did not fare as well. Critics, like Inés Eléxpuru, have explained that couscous fell out of favour because of its close ties with Islam. "El cuscús es el plato más prestigioso e internacional de cuantos se preparaban en aquella época, aunque paradójicamente ha desaparecido por completo de los fogones españoles debido a la persecución que sufrió durante la inquisición, como signo delator de la presencia morisca entre la población" [Couscous is the most prestigious and international dish of all that were prepared at that time even though paradoxically it has completely disappeared from the Spanish stove given the persecution Moriscos endured during the Inquisition as it was incriminating proof of Moriscos among the population] (85). But in studying the range of foods associated with Muslims or also with Jews, it is clear that many foods crossed over to Christian cuisine without any problem. If we limit ourselves just to grains, we see that rice and noodles, fully associated with Arabic influences in Spanish cooking, successfully transitioned beyond the early modern era while couscous did not.

Cooking, no less than other facets of life, reflects how Spain attempted to come to terms with its Muslim past. One sees a definite hybridity of Christian-Muslim-Jewish cooking practices in the kitchen as food items with clear Muslim ties are assimilated into the national court and institutional kitchens.[20] Eggplant and rice both exemplify this trend. Yet, other cooking practices and foodstuffs, of which couscous is the primary example, are displaced. By examining the complex preparation of this dish, we begin to understand that its absence in Spain's gastronomy may have less to do with an increasing culinary maurophobia, than with the advanced culinary skills necessary to prepare it.

In *Fuḍālat al-Hiwān*, Ibn Razīn includes five different couscous recipes. He explains in detail how this Maghreb contribution to the Almohad dynasty in Spain is made.[21] First, the grain itself is prepared and stored for later use (130). Then, in a pot seasoned with oil, salt, pepper, coriander, and chopped onion, one adds veal and its bones and covers everything with water. The author explains that seasonal vegetables are also added and suggests cabbage, turnips, carrots, lettuce, fennel, fresh fava beans, bottle squashes, and/or eggplant. Throughout the recipe the author emphasizes the tactile nature of the dish. In the initial preparation of the semolina he explains, "Se rocía con agua en la que se ha disuelto un poco de sal y se remueve con las puntas de los dedos para que la absorba. Luego se frota entre las palmas de las manos con cuidado para que tome la forma de cabezas de hormiga" [You sprinkle with water that has some salt added to it and stir it with your fingertips so that the water gets absorbed. Then you carefully rub (it) between your palms so that it forms the size of an ant head] (130). Later, at the stage when the grains are being steamed, the importance of the contact between the hands and the grains is key. "Cuando está hecho, se pone en la artesa y se frota con las manos con grasa de buena calidad" [When it is done, place in the kneading trough and rub with a good quality fat between your hands] (131). In the Middle Ages, variations on the basic couscous recipe included rubbing the couscous with ground walnut, adding heavier portions of vinegar and saffron, substituting finely grated breadcrumbs for the couscous, combining couscous with mashed fava beans, or stuffing a lamb with a couscous filling and baking it (*Fuḍālat-al-Hiwān* 130–3).

The recipe does not appear again until 1611 when Martínez Montiño, in his cookbook *Arte de cocina, pastelería, vizcochería y conservería* [The art of cooking, pie making, pastry making, and preserving], includes two couscous recipes. The first details how to make couscous from scratch, an art form that only survives today in parts of the Maghreb. The second gives a typical recipe of meat and vegetables served on a bed of couscous. Like his Hispano-Muslim predecessors, Martínez Montiño also stresses the importance of preparing couscous by rubbing carefully with one's hands the mixture of semolina (*harina floreada*) and durum wheat (*cemite*): "irás trayendo la mano estendida por encima la harina, y siempre à una mano; luego bolverás à echar mas agua con el hisopillo, y andar con la mano estendida sobre la harina; y de quando en quando meterás la mano, y revolverás la harina lo de arriba abaxo; y de esta manera irás haciendo, hasta que la harina ande haciendose muchos granillos, y que no tenga polvo" [you will pull your extended hand over the flour, always with one hand. Then you will sprinkle more water with a sprinkler and continue moving your extended hand over the flour. Every once in a while you must dip your hand into the flour and move it around top to bottom and in this way you will continue preparing it until all the flour forms little beads and no flour remains] (360–1). He also notes the specific pot necessary for preparing the dish and, anticipating that his readers may not be familiar with it, he describes it in detail: "luego echalo en su alcuzcucero, que es una pieza de barro, ò de cobre con muchos agujerillos en el suelo un poco angosto, y romo de abaxo, y ancho, y abierto de arriba" [then place it in the couscous pan, which is made of clay or copper and has a flat, narrow bottom with many small holes and is wide and open on the top] (361–2).

Several factors indicate that Martínez Montiño took great care in preparing this recipe and that he shows no disrespect for its Muslim origins. First, these two recipes are among the most extensive and detailed of the entire collection. He distinguishes the type of grains needed to make couscous, how the water should be sprinkled over the flour, and the care involved in touching the mixture. In addition, his instructions reflect an emotional attachment to the dish not characteristic of his writing. For example, for boiling the liquid, he writes, "pon la olla sobre la lumbre que cueza amorosamente" [place the pot over the flame and let it lovingly (gently) boil] (362).

While these first three food items Aldonza mentions are based on wheat, the most valued grain both for Romans and Muslims, rice, described in three different ways – arroz entero [whole grain rice], seco [all broth or water is absorbed], and grasso [cooked with animal fat] – also informs her selective memory. Around the world today there are more than 2000 varieties of rice and within Europe, Valencia is its biggest cultivator. This comes as no surprise as Muslims brought rice to Europe, via Spain and, as Ibn Razīn proudly announces in his rice purée recipe, "Este puré no es común, excepto en mi ciudad Murcia, o Valencia, Dios la devuelva [al Islam], que se caracterizan por el cultivo y abundancia del arroz, a diferencia del resto de las regiones de al-Ándalus" [This purée is uncommon, except in my city of Murcia or Valencia; may God give her (the city) back to us, which are known for the cultivation and abundance of rice, differing from the rest of the Al-Andalus regions] (103). Historians speculate that rice actually first arrived in the peninsula with the Visigoths but that in the eighth century the Arabs introduced it in large-scale production (García Sánchez, "Los cultivos de al-Andalus" 187–8). Its first literary appearance occurs in the thirteenth-century translation of *Calila y Dimna* as food prepared for hungry travellers. "Et la noche que veno a albergar con Helbed, guisóle un manjar de arroz, ca los reyes de India suelen comer mucho arroz" [And the night he came to stay with Helbed, she cooked him a rice dish since the kings of India are known for eating a lot of rice] (289).

In the Hispano-Muslim cooking manuals, a variety of rice appears, both sweet and savoury. Aldonza's passing rice reference brings to light the popularity of this grain and the multiple ways it is prepared. The three forms mentioned are not necessarily mutually exclusive. In both the anonymous Hispano-Muslim recipe manual and the Christian cookbook *Libre de coch* we find recipes made from whole grain rice, cooked just until the liquid is absorbed, and that include animal fat, like the *Kitāb al-tabīj* recipe "Hechura anarcisada de pinillo" [Narcissus dish with ground pine] (204), and Nola's "Arroz en cazuela al horno" [Baked rice casserole] (289).[22] In both, rice, cuts of marbled meat, saffron, and other seasonings are cooked and finished off with a layer of whipped eggs that form a top crust on the dish. Today, this recipe is still popular in parts of Spain, for example, "Arròs amb costra d'Elx" [Egg crusted rice, Elche style].[23] Other *arroz seco* dishes familiar to today's diner include the famous Valencian paella; *arroz negro*, a rice prepared with squid ink; and a myriad of rice dishes prepared with seafood, meat, or vegetables.

In Martínez Montiño's collection, he includes several rice dishes, many of which resemble medieval recipes in terms of sweet or savoury, *seco* or *grasso*, cooked stove-top or baked in the oven. In addition he includes a recipe for "Buñuelos de arroz" [Rice fritters]. They are made in the usual fritter method but he announces at the close of the recipe, "Son mejores de lo que parecen" [They are better than they look]. He also warns of the appropriate use of flour for dredging the rice balls when he finishes the recipe with the following alert: "La harina ponsela de una vez, y antes pequen de mucha harina, que de poca" [put the flour on all at once and better to sin by using too much flour than not enough] (234).

Among all of these authors, certain care is taken to signal the different types of liquids used for cooking rice. Water and meat stock are common enough, but across the centuries, milk was the preferred liquid and undoubtedly improved the quality of the dish. In the Hispano-Muslim recipes, sheep milk is preferred and later, in the Christian cookbooks, goat milk. Interestingly, Nola clearly indicates that when using meat stock, the addition of milk is superfluous. "Mas nota una cosa, como dije en el capítulo de la sémola: que en ningún potaje de éstos, como son arroz, sémola, faro y fideos, cuando se cuece con caldo de carne no hay necesidad de poner ninguna condición de leche" [Moreover, take note, as I explained in the chapter on semolina: in none of these stews, whether it be rice, semolina, faro, or noodles, is the addition of any type of milk necessary when using meat stock] (288). One wonders if this is merely a culinary preference or if Nola, who clearly expresses sensitivity towards Jewish and Muslim culinary contributions throughout his cookbook, is embedding in his recipes the Jewish law of not mixing animal flesh with its milk.

Beyond these grain dishes and the already mentioned meatballs, Aldonza gets excited about regional foodstuffs, for example, honey from Adamuz or saffron from Peñafiel,[24] and prides herself on the myriad of sweets and desserts that came from her grandmother's kitchen. She savours the *hojuelas* [puff pastries], *prestiños* [honey-sprinkled fried dough], *rosquillas de alfajor* [almond cookies], *textones* [sesame meringues], *nuégados* [nut and honey-filled pastries], *sopaipas* [fried dough], *hojaldres* [phyllo treats], *hormigos torcidos con aceite* [nut butter pastries with oil], *talvinas* [almond-milk porridge], and *zahina* [simple porridge] and bears witness to the popularity of the recipes found in the elite cooking manuals (178).[25] In fact, Fernando de la Granja Santamaría states that all the recipes from *La lozana andaluza* are in the *Fuḍālat al-Hiwān* (15), a cooking manual that has more recipes dedicated to sweets that any other food item, apart from meat. Arguably, what most uniquely defines Ibn Razīn's *Fuḍālat-al-Hiwān* is the pastry section. As Marín states in her introduction, "Es en este capítulo ... donde se encuentran muchas de las recetas más típicamente andalusíes de todo el recetario" [It is in this chapter ... where many of the most typical Andalusian recipes of the whole manuscript are found] (54). In this section he uses a wide variety of flours, fats, and sweeteners, cooking methods, and finishing touches. Many include nuts or dried fruit and are often sprinkled with sugar or drizzled with honey before consumption.

Aldonza's catalogue of cookies, pastries, and other sweet treats exemplifies desserts prepared both with honey and with sugar. A major Muslim contribution to Spanish fare, sugar was primarily available to the wealthy up to and throughout the early modern period. It first appears in Spain in the tenth-century document *Calendario de Córdoba* and was grown in the eastern part of Spain but, as Eléxpuru reminds us, it was not processed into powder until the thirteenth century when several treatises comment on it (96).[26] Found in Hispanic-Muslim treatises, in Catalan and later Castilian court cookbooks, in convents and universities, sugar enhanced both savoury and sweet dishes. Across ethnicities, languages, and institutions, all cooking manuals commonly included sugar as a garnish sprinkled atop a meat or poultry dish. Martínez Llopís, in his work *La dulcería española* explains that as early as the tenth century, Arabs specified a wide variety of different sugars ("sukkar"):

El azúcar áspero, sin refinar, que recibía el nombre de "kakkar surj", que cuando era cocido por segunda vez y quedaba limpio, se llamaba "sulaymani", y cuando se cocía por tercera vez pasaba a llamarse "fanid". El "khayendi" fue antecesor del azúcar cande y el "taberzad" fue el precursor del azúcar cristalizado. Las concreciones azucaradas que se producen de modo espontáneo en la caña índica, recibían el nombre de "tabashir." (21)

[Rough, or unrefined, sugar received the name "kakkar surj," and when it was cooked a second time and came out clearer, it was called "sulaymani," and when it was cooked a third time, it was then called "fanid." "Khayendi" was the predecessor to rock candy and "taberzad" was the precursor to crystalized sugar. The sugar concretions that seep out naturally from the Indian cane took the name "tabashir."]

In the *Kitāb al-tabīj* sugar appears no less that 171 times, even more than honey (135 times). Often, sugar alone is sprinkled on top of a dish but there are also recipes that call for sprinkling sugar with a mix of cinnamon and/or black pepper, as is the case with the stewed mutton dish "El plato 'Gasānī'" [The Gasani dish] (262) or the chicken soup dish "Sopa de jabīs con dos gallinas" [Mixed up soup with two hens] (109). For savoury dishes sugar is most commonly used for poultry and mutton. Additionally, it appears in porridges, creamy rice dishes, sweet breads, and pastries. The recipe "Dulce de azúcar" [Sugar sweetness] is a good example of how sugar was used as a primary ingredient.

Se toma una libra de azúcar molido y de harina candeal majada hasta que se haga como la harina de sémola, un tercio de libra; se le añade huevos y se bate con ello; entonces se pone la sartén a un fuego ligero con una libra de aceite dulce y cuando éste hierve, se vierten en él estas migas y el azúcar batido con huevos; se remueve al fuego ligero hasta que se ligue y se enfríe; se espolvorea con azúcar, espliego y canela. (274)

[Combine one pound of ground sugar with one third of a pound of white flour that has been pounded until it looks like semolina. Add eggs and beat everything together. Then heat sweet oil in a frying pan on low heat and when it is boiling, drop the breadcrumb batter into the oil and shake over low flame until it comes together and cools. Sprinkle with sugar, spikenard, and cinnamon.]

Sugar's role in later Spanish cookbooks is also significant. For example in the *Sent Soví*, sugar appears in a third of the recipes and in Nola's *Libre de coch/Libro de guisados*, it has an even more substantial presence.[27] In fact, in the mid-fourteenth century, another manuscript appeared, *Llibre de totes maneres de confits* [Book on all types of candied fruit], in which sugar prominently appears. Recipes for marzipan and fruits and nuts candied with sugar fill approximately half of the thirty-three-recipe work.[28] Additionally, in the university cookbook, *Libro del arte de cocina*, Pérez Samper also notes that either sugar or honey appear in over half of the 180 recipes (*La alimentación* 78). What Aldonza cites in *La lozana andaluza* and what early modern cookbooks demonstrate is that sugar is a primary ingredient in many sweet dishes. In "Resoles" [Fritters] from the *Sent Soví* (*The Book of Sent Soví* 128), sugar is generously sprinkled over the fritters. For "Empanadas de azúcar fino" [Confectionary sugar empanadas] Nola combines ground almonds and sugar with rosewater and ginger before frying them in sweet oil and sprinkling them with honey (322). Likewise, sugar is a secondary ingredient or a finisher in many savoury dishes, especially poultry but also in dishes with grains, vegetables, quadrupeds, and even fish. Countless recipes from the thirteenth-century Hispano-Muslim texts up through to the Christian cookbooks of the early modern period include sprinkling cinnamon and sugar as a finisher for both sweet and savoury dishes. In Lope de Vega's *Los locos de Valencia*, the lover Floriano, uses the following metaphor to complain of his unrequited love: "Pido azúcar y canela/Y daisme paja y cebada" [I asked (her) for cinnamon and sugar/ and she gave me barley and straw] (I.7), thus showing how this combination of sweetener and spice infiltrated cultural spaces beyond the kitchen.

At the close of her culinary catalogue, Aldonza remembers the variety of electuaries her grandmother created. Electuaries are pharmaceuticals, recorded as far back as Galen, that combined bitter-tasting healing herbs with a sweetener. They can take a solid, paste, or liquid form and are made primarily with fruits, vegetables, nuts, and herbs. The Arabs introduced to Europe both sugar as a central ingredient and new techniques for making electuaries (Plouvier as well as Jazi and Asli). At the start of the twelfth century, regulations were well established that forbade anyone except medical experts to sell them: "nadie venderá jarabes o electuarios, ni preparará medicamentos, si no es un médico experto, ni tales remedios se comprarán a drogueros o boticarios, que lo que quieren es coger dinero sin saber nada, y así, echan a perder las recetas y matan a los enfermos" [No one shall sell syrups or electuaries or prepare medicine without being a medical expert nor shall such remedies be sold by druggists or pharmacists if they just want to make money and have no knowledge and thus ruin the recipe and kill the sick] (Levi-Provençal and García Gómez 145).

Aldonza's grandmother prepared the ones for home use with syrup and the ones for others with honey. It is unclear whether there was sugar available to produce the syrups for the electuaries or whether these came from other sweeteners. Either way, her passage clearly acknowledges that what is meant for home differs from what is presented to the greater population. Both are made with bases of quince, Spanish lavender, grape, eggplant, walnuts, walnut flower, oregano, and mint.

In the *Kitāb al-tabīj*, the author dedicates a chapter to "Las pastas" [Pastes] and includes eleven different recipes for a sweet paste made from nuts, dried fruit, or essence of flowers boiled with honey. The recipe, "Pasta de nuez verde" [Green walnut paste] serves as an example.

Se toma una libra de nuez verde y se agujerea mucho con un pincho de hierro, luego se macera en agua tres días; se saca del agua y se toma para cada libre tres de miel limpia de su espuma, después de cocerse un poco las nueces; se sacan del agua y se vuelven a la miel y se cuecen hasta que tomen forma de pasta; se aromatiza con canela, clavo y jengibre, una onza menos cuarto por cada libra y se come después de las comidas. Sus provechos: excita el apetito y digiere los alimentos, calienta los riñones y aumenta la orina. (299)

[Take one pound of green [immature] walnuts and poke several holes in them with a skewer; then let them soak for three days. Remove them from the water and for each pound of nuts add three of honey with its froth skimmed off. After blanching the nuts, take them out of the water and return them to the honey and boil until a paste forms. Flavour with cinnamon, clove, and ginger, three quarters of an ounce for each pound. It is eaten after meals. Its benefits: it stimulates the appetite and aids in the digestion of food, it warms the kidneys and increases urine output.]

Martínez Montiño's recipe "Nueces en conserva" [Preserved walnuts] is similar in terms of puncturing the immature walnuts, soaking them, combining them with sweetener (he gives the option of either honey or sugar), and flavouring them with cinnamon and clove, but ginger is not included (483–5).[29]

Aldonza's catalogue also contains a series of savoury dishes that highlight specific vegetables and spices that often accompanied them. Historians have documented many of the Muslim's culinary contributions through agriculture.[30] What we find in the anonymous Hispano-Muslim cooking manual Kitāb al-tabīj is a preference for eggplant, fennel, and bottle squashes, followed by carrots, turnips, and lettuce, and then by cabbage, artichokes, and spinach. Other vegetables include celery, Swiss chard, and cucumber. Onion and garlic are widely used, particularly in the preparation of poultry dishes but also in lamb, mutton, beef, sheep, rabbit, and fish and occasionally in vegetables dishes, particularly eggplant. In a uniquely organized effort, Ibn Razīn lays out the manual's ten chapters in the introduction to his work. He explains that chapter 7 is dedicated to vegetables and is divided into ten sections: bottle squashes from the vine; eggplant; carrots; truffles; asparagus; artichokes; wild mushrooms; spinach, cardoons, lettuce, and similar things; vegetable garnishes, and taro (75–6). Unfortunately, only the first three and the last survive today.

Most, if not all, of these vegetables cut across socio-economic boundaries and were enjoyed by all echelons of society. The first dishes, "nabos sin tocino y con comino" [cumin turnips without lard], and "col murciana con alcaravez" [Murcia-style cabbage with caraway], are found in the anonymous Kitāb al-tabīj. The author first explains that a common meat and vegetable dish prepared with vinegar and saffron is known as terciados [hodgepodges]. "Todo plato que se cocina con carne, azafrán, vinagre y hortalizas, como los nabos, berenjenas, calabazas, zanahorias o cabezas de lechugas sin sus hojas, se llama terciado" [Any dish made with meat, saffron, vinegar, and vegetables such as turnips, eggplants, bottle squash, carrots, or heads of lettuce without its leafs, are called hodgepodges] (268). He then continues with simple vegetable recipes, all of which contain meat as well. The former Aldonza dish finds its match in one called "Hechura de nabo, también simple" [A turnip dish, also simple] (269) and the latter in "Receta de col blanca" [White cabbage recipe] (269).

What stands out when comparing these elite recipes with the common ones Aldonza describes is that in both cases and across centuries and social strata, the same spices are used, cumin with turnips and caraway with cabbage. In fact, in the manuscript, the author explains how cumin commonly accompanies dishes that have a heavy vinegar component while caraway is almost always used in cabbage dishes. Aldonza makes reference to this common combination of cumin and vinegar when she describes a casserole that she makes expertly: "cazuela con su agico y cominico, y saborcico de vinagre, esta hacía yo sin que me la vezasen" [a casserole with a little garlic, a pinch of cumin, and a hint of vinegar, I could make this without anyone having to show me] (178). In the manuscript, the author explains the health benefits of these spices.

El *comino* entra en los platos de vinagre ... por disolver las ventosidades y por su digestibilidad ... La *alcaravea* entra en los platos de col y de verduras para purificarlas y cuando hay col y espinacas en un plato o empanada, es precisa la alcaravea, porque bonifica el manjar, le da sabor y aleja los gases de las verduras. (115–16)

[Cumin is in vinegar dishes ... because it reduces wind and is digestible ... Caraway is in cabbage and vegetable dishes to purify them and when cabbage and spinach are in a dish or an empanada, caraway is necessary because it improves the delicacy, gives it flavour, and releases the vegetable gases.]

We know from Avenzoar's twelfth-century *Kitāb al-Aǧḏiya wal-adwiya* (*Tratado de los alimentos*) [Treatise on food] that cabbage was extremely popular in spite of its detrimental effects on one's health:

La gente toma col y hace elogios de ella, aunque es la peor de todas las verduras, pues genera atrabilis, sugestiones, lepra, repugnante sarna y epilepsia. No conozco ninguna verdura peor que ella, salvo la berenjena, con la que guarda un gran parecido. Es caliente y seca, y no se le reconoce ninguna propiedad beneficiosa con la única excepción de que, tanto si se come cruda como cocida, aclara la voz de una forma extraordinaria y maravillosa. Si la toma quien tenga ronquera, ésta le desaparece. Si se cuece y se prepara un emplasto con esta cocción y harina y se pone sobre los tumores, los hace madurar. (García Sánchez, *Kitāb al-agdiya* 84)

[People eat cabbage and extol its praises even though it is the worst of all vegetables as it creates black bile, susceptible minds, leprosy, revolting scabies, and epilepsy. I am not familiar with any vegetable that is worse than this one, with the exception of eggplant, which is fairly similar. It is warm and dry and has no recognized beneficial property with one exception, whether eaten raw or cooked it clears up one's throat in an extraordinary and marvellous way. If someone is hoarse and eats it, it disappears. If you cook it and make a poultice with cabbage and flour and put it on one's tumours, it makes them come to fruition.]

Similar detrimental properties describe the eggplant. "Todos los médicos concuerdan – y están en lo cierto – en que la berenjena, como alimento, es una hortaliza nada recomendable, aunque no tanto como la col" [All doctors concur – and they are right to do so – eggplant, as a food product, is not recommended, although it is not as bad as cabbage] (García Sánchez, Kitāb al-agdiya 85).

The rest of Aldonza's food memories mainly focus on stews and other casserole dishes and pay homage to one of the most important vegetables for both Jews and Muslims in spite of its alleged nutritional deficiency: the eggplant. As described in chapter 1, both Hispano-Muslim cooking manuals have an abundance of recipes for eggplant. For example, among the dozens of recipes in which eggplant is the primary ingredient are recipes for fried eggplant; sautéed with meat; stuffed with hen; prepared with sheep, hare, lamb, or cheese; baked; twice baked; and souffléed. Aldonza mentions three different dishes that feature eggplant: boronía [alboronia], caçuela de berengenas moxíes [twice baked eggplant casserole]; and caçuelas moriscas [Morisco-style stews]. Her memory of boronía is another tie between early modern food memories of the underprivileged and the preferences of the thirteenth-century Muslim elite. "Otro plato llamado al-būrānīya ('alboronia')" [Another dish called alboronia], is one of the more complex recipes of Ibn Razīn's manual. He describes a layered eggplant-meat dish and offers several variants on its preparation (140–1).

Although not as prolific in the early modern Castilian cookbooks, eggplant recipes appear in all of them. Similar to her caçuela de berengenas moxíes is Nola's "Cazuela mojí" [Twice- baked eggplant casserole] (316). He explains that after the vegetable is salted, dried, and fried, it is chopped and mixed with grated cheese, breadcrumbs, and spices that include coriander, caraway, pepper, cloves, and a little ginger. It is cooked again with egg batter, and then baked in a Dutch oven with an additional pepper-saffron-clove egg mixture until the mixture sets. It is then finished with a dab of honey and powdered spices. Martínez Montiño also includes "Cazuela mogí de berenjenas" [Twice- baked eggplant casserole] in his cookbook and insists on mixing honey and sugar together for the sweetener (245–6). Cervantes would include this same casserole in his play, *Los baños de Argel* [The baths of Algiers], in which a sacristan and a Jew appear on stage, the former holding the dish.

(Sale[n] el SACRISTÁN con una cazuela mojí, y tras él el JUDÍO).
JUDÍO: Cristiano honrado, así el Dío
   te vuelva a tu libre estado,
   que me vuelvas lo que es mío.
SACRISTÁN: No quiero, judío honrado;
   no quiero, honrado judío.
JUDÍO: Hoy es sábado, y no tengo
   qué comer, y me mantengo
   de aqueso que guisé ayer.
SACRISTÁN: Vuelve a guisar de comer.
JUDÍO: No, que a mi ley contravengo.
SACRISTÁN: Rescátame esta cazuela,
   y en dártela no haré poco,
   porque el olor me consuela.   (1672–84)

[(The sacristan enters holding a twice- baked eggplant casserole and behind him, the Jew)
JEW: Honourable Christian, now that God
   Has returned to you your freedom,
   Please return to me what is mine.
SACRISTAN: I refuse, honourable Jew;
   I refuse, honourable Jew.
JEW: Today is Saturday, and I have
   Nothing to eat and can only sustain myself
   With what I cooked yesterday.
SACRISTAN: Make yourself another one.
JEW: No, I cannot violate my law.
SACRISTAN: Take your casserole back
   And know that returning it to you is no small feat
   Because its aroma gives me comfort.]

In Cervantes' play, the reference to the Sabbath and Jewish law prohibiting work on that day is clear as the Jew explains why he cannot simply prepare another casserole. But beyond this, we see once again the cross-cultural shift of eating habits and food appreciation between Christians and Jews. The sacristan wants to feast on the Jewish casserole and indicates this through his sense of smell acknowledging that before he even tastes the eggplant, he indulges in the pleasure of its aroma. As the priest reluctantly returns the casserole to the Jew, not only eggplant itself, but also the traditional way it is prepared by Jews is acknowledged as a culinary contact point that unites the two cultures.

Similar to Aldonza's Morisco-style stews, Nola also includes recipes for "Berenjenas a la morisca" [Morisco-style eggplant] (285), and "Calabazas a la morisca" [Morisco-style bottle squashes] (287). Later, Martínez Montiño writes about "Morisco-style" poultry dishes as well.[31] More than any single cooking style or ingredient, these recipes acknowledge Muslim influences in Spanish cooking through their titles. Sometimes the references are vague. For example, spices common to Hispano-Muslim recipes – coriander, caraway, black pepper, clove, ginger, and saffron – abound in the early modern cookbooks. Other times, a recipe like Nola's "Berenjenas a la morisca" makes specific reference to Muslim food laws: "y sean muy bien sofreidas con buen tocino o con aceite que sea dulce, porque los moros no comen tocino" [and make sure they are thoroughly fried with good lard or in a sweet oil because Moors do not eat lard] (286). Early modern cookbooks outside the court also reference Morisco-style dishes. For example, in *Manual de mugeres* [Manual for women], the anonymous author creates "Olla morisca" [Morisco-style stew], a mutton and goat stew with garbanzos that is seasoned with cinnamon, clove, and a pinch of caraway (58–9).

While meat choices, particularly pork, instantly segregated social groups in the early modern period, an individual's taste for specific vegetables underscores common eating practices across social and ethnic divides. From the fictional primary sources of novels and plays in which the lower classes savour the same vegetable dishes as those recorded in the court manuals and cookbooks, we get a sense of some of the central tastes of Spanish cuisine. Aldonza's selective and seductive food memories do more than position the reader in her childhood kitchen. They offer us cultural memory, a window into early modern eating practices among the working classes. Her description of her grandmother's kitchen stands as the nexus between the food habits of Jewish, Muslim, and Christian ethnicities, between elite and underprivileged communities, and across centuries. By going back in time to the thirteenth century and turning the pages of the Hispano-Muslim cooking manuals, one can ground the early modern court recipes in culinary heritage and see clear links between numerous grain, vegetable, and sweet dishes that Muslims and Jews prepared and consumed and how elite Christians ate centuries later. In this way, cooking manuals and Delicado's picaresque novel serve as contact zones that testify both to established and shifting cultural eating habits. Additionally, legal documents illustrate food preparation and eating practices among minority groups that seek to segregate communities and simultaneously reveal a fuller picture of Spain's culinary history.

The author of the *Sent Soví*, Ruperto de Nola, or Martínez Montiño offer no direct reference to any of the Hispano-Muslim manuals and to date, no evidence has been found that either of these manuscripts was translated into Latin or any Romance language. Indeed, most food historians agree that it is impossible to establish any direct links between these works. However, health and nutrition manuals were most definitely translated from Arabic into Catalan and Spanish and thus, medieval understandings of food nutrition, as we will see in the following chapter, informed early modern writers of both prescriptive and fictional discourses. Moreover, in the court cookbooks and beyond, cook-authors acknowledge their indebtedness to Muslim and Jewish culinary influences in cooking methods, recipe titles, and direct references to ethnic food laws that affect how a dish is created. In the end, the combined discourses of fictional literature, Inquisitional texts, and cooking manuals and recipe books enable us to gain a greater understanding of how Jews, Muslims, and Christians defined themselves through the food they ate and of shared culinary tendencies from the Middle Ages through the early modern period.

Chapter Five

"Lantejas los viernes": Perceptions of Health and Christian Abstinence

Las lentejas ... el que las comiere ... está apto a ser leproso

[Lentils ... he who eats them ... is capable of becoming a leper]

Lobera de Ávila

In early modern Spain, lentils, and more generally legumes, are a paradox. They are perceived both as deeply spiritual food to be consumed on days of abstinence yet they are shunned as food fit only for peasants. They are dismissed as having no nutritional value for the healthy yet broths made from legumes are one of the first remedies for curing the ill and at times have aphrodisiac powers. Lope de Vega describes this pulse as "la triste y debil lenteja" [the poor, weak lentil] (388) in his ode to fruits and vegetables in *La Arcadia*, yet Covarrubias define them as embodying, "la virtud de la templança" [the virtue of temperance] (760). And the royal doctor Lobera de Ávila condemns them for provoking leprosy (133). What is it about these gentle brown legumes that figure so prominently to describe what Alonso Quijano eats each Friday? Using this description as a point of departure and investigating lentils' appearance in other early modern discourses, we come to understand that lentils first and foremost define social class, as the regular consumption of any kind of pulse was an indicator of poverty. Beyond their association with the poor, lentils held different meanings for doctors and medical advisors of the day. For some, they provided relief for certain ailments while others criticized their detrimental effects but all believed that they produced melancholy when eaten. Additionally, lentils, and other legumes, were common foodstuffs consumed on abstinence days in the church and together with what Alonso Quijano eats on Saturdays and Sundays, this meal exemplifies the notion of Christian sacrifice and commonly accepted eating practices in the early modern period. This chapter begins with lentils' common association with labourers and low social class and goes on to explore lentils from perspectives of health and religious identity as found in a variety of early modern texts.

Lentils are one of the oldest food products, first cultivated by man more than 10,000 years ago (Kaplan 277).[1] Along with the pea and the broad bean, they have been traced to central Asia and existed in Spain centuries before the rise of the Hapsburg empire. In the sixteenth and seventeenth centuries lentils are most definitely thought of as poor man's food and readers implicitly understood that Alonso Quijano's Friday diet, along with the scarcity of mutton in his weekly stew pot, was a clear indication of a waning social status for the humble hidalgo.

As discussed in chapter 2, all social classes had varying access to meat, fresh vegetables, bread, and wine, and the one-pot meal was the basis for a wide range of social classes throughout the different regions of Spain. For images of deeper levels of poverty, one must turn to literary representations, as cooking manuals attended to the diet of the elite and excluded recipes for the poor. Martínez Montiño does include a single recipe called "Sustancia de pobres" [Sustenance for the poor] but he explains that this poultry-mutton dish is not intended for those suffering from poverty but rather for those with impoverished health. As he describes how to season the dish, he clarifies that it is one of several recipes meant for the convalescent. "[L]a sazonarás de sal, y ha de ser muy poca, porque no hay mas mala cosa para los enfermos que hallar mucha sal en las viandas" [season it with salt but just a little as there is nothing worse for the ill than food with a lot of salt] (393). Furthermore, food available to the urban poor could widely vary from that available in rural communities. In the cities, food options for the poor could easily be reduced to "pan negro de cebada, cebollas, ajos, y eventualmente, un pequeño trozo de tocino" [dark, barley bread, onions, garlic, and eventually, a small piece of fat back] (Riera Melis, "Jerarquía" 94). Madame d'Aulnoy in her *Memoires de la cour d'Espagne: Relation du voyage d'Espagne* [Memories of the court of Spain: Account of the voyage to Spain] explains that often servants would get their food from public kitchens. "Hay cocinas públicas en casi todas las esquinas de las calles. Son grandes pucheros que cuecen sobre trébedes. Se va allí para adquirir toda clase de porquerías: habas, ajos, cebolletas y un poco de caldo, en el que mojan su pan" [There are public kitchens on almost every street corner that have big pots boiling away on trivets. They go there to get all sorts of terrible things: fava beans, garlic, green onions, and a little broth so they can dip their bread in it] (cited in Díez Borque, *La sociedad española y los viajeros* 101). In rural areas, onion and garlic, together with cabbage and turnips, were regularly eaten with bread made from various grains or possibly legumes. People who lived outside urban centres also maintained their own small vegetable gardens and, as Riera explains, even in the humblest of houses there were always bushels of grain, some cured meat, and wine but during the most difficult times in rural areas, peasants were forced to consume roots of wild plants, ferns, grasses, grape seeds, tree bark, walnut and almond shells, or even dust from slate ("'Panem nostrum'" 38) while in the cities, markets were supported by administrative institutions that could bring in grains and other products from afar ("Jerarquía social" 107).

Picaresque novels are filled with images of a poor person's diet in both urban and rural areas. From crumbs that Lazarillo is able to pilfer while under the tutelage of the priest of Maqueda to the over-developed embryos of the eggs Guzmán de Alfarache is served at a roadside tavern outside Seville representations of food for the impoverished come to life. One of the most well known scenes of exaggerated proportions of hunger and starvation comes from the pages of Quevedo's *El buscón* when Pablos is sent off to boarding school with his classmate Diego and lands in the hands of the miser, El Cabras.

> Comieron una comida eterna, sin principio ni fin. Trajeron caldo en unas escudillas de madera, tan claro, que en comer una dellas peligrara Narciso más que en la fuente. Noté con la ansia que los macilentos dedos se echaban a nado tras un garbanzo güérfano y solo que estaba en el suelo ... Venía un nabo aventurero a vueltas, y dijo el maestro en viéndole, "¿Nabo hay? No hay perdiz para mí que se le iguale ..." Repartió a cada uno tan poco carnero, que, entre lo que se les pegó a las uñas y se les quedó entre los dientes, pienso que se consumió todo, dejando descomulgadas las tripas de participantes. (104–5)

> [They ate an eternal meal, with no beginning and no end. They brought broth in wooden bowls, so clear, that to eat from one of them would have been more dangerous for Narcissus than the spring. I anxiously watched lean fingers swimming after one orphan garbanzo at the bottom of the bowl ... An adventurous turnip insisted on showing up and when the master saw it, he said, "There's a turnip? For me, no partridge can match it" ... He gave everyone such a small portion of mutton that between what

got caught under their nails and stuck between their teeth, I think it all got
used up, leaving the guts without anything, guilty by association.]

In this scene of exaggerated proportions, Quevedo uses the myth of
Narcissus to imply that little more than water filled their soup bowls. He
also includes a singular garbanzo and turnip, as representations of the
meagreness of the meal; they are contrasted with partridge, as much a
sign of affluence as pulses and turnips are of poverty. Mutton also forms
part of the students' diet, a fact corroborated by the dozens of mutton
recipes in Hernández de Maceras's university cookbook, but here
Quevedo wildly exaggerates how little the students ate to show that there
was not even enough meat on the bones to make it to their stomachs.

Lentils and other pulses make infrequent appearances on the stage
and when they do, they generally are in reference to poverty or abstinence.[2] In Tirso de Molina's hagiographic play *Santo y sastre* [Saints and
tailors], the main character, Saint Homobonus of Cremona, discusses
how to accommodate beggars who come knocking at his door when
he has nothing to give them. In response, Pendón, the comic relief of
the play, uses lentils and breadcrumbs as examples of how to stretch a
meal, a technique frequently found within medieval and early modern
cooking manuals.

HOMO: Pues dale pan.
PENDÓN: Si le hurtamos.
   ¿Eres hombre tú que dejas
   ni aun para guisar lentejas
   un migajón? ¿No tomamos
   cuenta al arca y sus rincones
   acabados de comer;
   pues por no hallar que roer
   aun no hay en casa ratones?   (2163–71)

[HOMO: Then give them bread.
PENDÓN: If we steal it.
   Are you not a man who would use up
   the last bits of bread for a lentil stew?
   Didn't we check
   the breadbox and its every corner
   after eating
   and found not even a crumb
   for a mouse in this house to gnaw on?]

Giving bread to beggars echoes the efforts of hospitals and convents that provided bread and soup to travellers and to the homeless. On his travels through Spain in the sixteenth century, Albert Jouvin notes that "en todos estos pueblos hay hospitales para recibir allí y alojar a los peregrinos pobres, a los que dan un trozo de pan y alguna sopa" [in all of these villages there are hospitals that receive and offer lodging to poor pilgrims to whom they give a piece of bread and some soup] (cited in García Mercadal 781). Those living in convents also ate their fair share of pulses as San Juan Bautista de la Concepción describes in his chapter "De los oficios mas communes" [On the most common offices] (1607). Here, he distinguishes between garbanzos and lentils as the former goes well with meat while the latter does not. "En no habiendo carne a prima noche, ponga su olla de legumbres, como esotros días, que si la trujeren, no cairá mal sobre una olla de coles o de garbanzos juntándolo todo; y si no fueren cosas compatibles, como lantejas y carne, puédese quedar para otro día la olla de las lantejas o darse a los pobres" [If there is no meat for the evening, make a stew of legumes, as with those other days; if you can add some meat, it would not taste bad combining all together in a cabbage or garbanzo stew; but if it were not compatible, like lentils and meat, you could make a lentil stew for another day or give it to the poor] (cited in Gázquez Ortiz, La mesa 99).

Another way to understand lentils' lowly position within society is to look at records from prison kitchens. Matilde Santamaría Arnaiz in her study La alimentación de los españoles bajo el reinado de los Austrias en el siglo XVII [Food of the Spaniards in the reign of the Austrians of the seventeenth century] notes that in the Libros de la Sala de Gobierno de los Alcaldes de Casa y Corte [Courtroom books from the judge of the royal house and court], there were clear instructions on what to feed the prisoners: "medio pan a cada uno y libra y media de baca entre dos" [a half bread for each one and a pound and a half of beef for two] (cited in Valles Rojo, La cocina 203). Later, details are written down for prison food served on abstinence days as well: "los días de pescado se de a los dichos pobres su caldo de garbanços y berdura o lentejas o nabos, según el tiempo y cada media libra de pescado abadejo con azeite y vinagre" [On fish days, give to said prisoners a broth of garbanzos and vegetables or lentils or turnips, depending on the season and [for] each a half pound of haddock fish with oil and vinegar] (cited in Valles Rojo, La cocina 203). Images of impoverished eating habits increase when turning to women's prisons. Here, they were given "un trozo de queso con pan negro y algunos nabos o berzas y solo de vez en cuando algo de carne" [a piece of cheese with dark bread and some turnips or cabbage and only once in a while some meat] (cited in Valles Rojo, *La cocina* 203). Beyond pulses being put in stews or soups, they were also ground into flour and used for making bread. Bread made from pulses stood in stark contrast to wheat bread, the most valued of all breads; indeed, it was considered inferior to all grain-based breads.

Legumes and Nutritional Privilege

Felipe Fernández Armesto reminds us that food has been a marker of social privilege since time began and that from the work at palaeolithic burial sites anthropologists can correlate levels of nutrition and signs of honour within the community (163). Greek, Arab, and later Spanish doctors such as Averroes and Maimonides affirmed the connections between health and diet in their medical writings. In early modern Spain, approaches to food consumption were based on the ancient notion of humourism, which put forth that in order to maintain a healthy constitution, an individual must sustain equilibrium among the body's four humours and a steady flow of spirits through the body's channels. Essentially, the human body consists of four basic substances, or humours: blood, yellow bile, black bile, and phlegm. Their balance indicates the health of an individual and, by extension, any illness or disease is a result of an excess or deficiency of one or more of these humors. In 450 BCE, Empedocles formulated the cosmogenic theory that the earth was made of air, fire, earth, and water and that between these elements existed a certain condition – air and fire: warmth; fire and earth: dryness; earth and water: cold; and water and air: moistness. To this scheme, Hippocrates (460–370 BC) attached four corresponding humours – air: blood; fire: bile; earth: black bile; and water: phlegm – thus, laying the foundation for the medical theory of humourism. Later Galen (129–c. 200 CE) added corresponding temperaments to each humour: air: sanguine; fire: choleric; earth: melancholic; and water: phlegmatic. And to those temperaments, he attached a series of characteristics (see table 5.1). Both Greeks and Romans, and later Arabs and Western Europeans that adopted and adapted this medical philosophy, believed that individuals were predisposed to each of the four humours and their corresponding element and that their temperament would fluctuate in function with diet and daily activity.

In Spain, the writings of medical doctors like Ibn Zuhr (also known by his Latinized name, Avenzoar) (b. 1091), Maimonides (b. 1105), and

Table 5.1 Example of how the four humours relate to other life forces

Element	Quality	Humor	Temperament	Season	Characteristic
Air	Moist-warm	Blood	Sanguine	Spring	Spontaneous, dreamer
Fire	Warm-dry	Yellow bile	Choleric	Summer	Ambitious, energetic, passionate
Earth	Dry-cold	Black bile	Melancholic	Fall	Creative, preoccupied with tragedy and death
Water	Cold-moist	Phlegm	Phlegmatic	Winter	Calm, compassionate

Arnau de Vilanova (b. 1238) were instrumental in illustrating how individual food items had clearly defined relations with the elements and their corresponding humour, quality, and temperament. In addition, one's humoural balance was affected by how food acted on the body; whether it nurtured the body slowly, quickly, or moderately; and to what degree it sustained the body or awakened the vital spirit. For example, if a certain food or way of preparing it were related to the brain, then that food would affect one's reason. Again, if either the food itself or the way it was prepared were related to the heart, then it would affect one's spirit. Or, if either the food or its preparation were identified and tied to the liver, then ingesting that food would affect one's desire. An individual's natural temperament, whether it be sanguine, choleric, melancholic, or phlegmatic, was always shifting based on external factors such as food intake.[3]

Ibn Zuhr penned several treatises on medicine and surgical practices of which three are extant today. Born in Seville and educated in Cordoba, Ibn Zuhr spent most of his professional career in Seville and is considered one of the most important physicians and clinicians of the Middle Ages. His writings contain the first full explanations of a variety of pathological conditions and therapy. One of his works, *Kitāb al-Aǧdiya wal-adwiya (Tratado de los alimentos)* [Treatise on food] (1147–63?), contains very specific information on different foods and their qualities. These beliefs and practices, which influenced Maimonides, Vilanova, and other medical writers through the early modern era, were particularly important for curing the ill. Like other doctors before him, he confirmed that wheat bread was the best of all breads and that the meat of the hen was the best poultry. He noted that fresh goat milk drunk on an empty stomach was excellent nourishment for the body and that olive

Table 5.2 The four humoral qualities and corresponding food items. From Ibn Zuhr's *Kitāb al-agdiya*, ed. García Sánchez.

Food category	Moist-warm	Warm-dry	Dry-cold	Cold-moist

Animal/
dairy
	Pigeon
	Milk-fed lamb
	Hare
		Turtledove
		Quail
		Thrush
		Eggs from
		  these birds
		Sheep
		Mountain goat
		Doe, gazelle, fallow
		  deer, roe deer
		Locust
			Beef
			Camel
			Cat
				Fresh cheese
				Butter
				Curds of milk
				Cottage
				  cheese

Vegetable	Borage Onion Turnip Carrot	Cabbage Garlic Artichoke	Hearts of palm Lentils	Lettuce – Chicory Squash Cucumber Melon –Watermelon Truffle
Fruit and nuts	Fig Must (from grapes) Raisins Almonds	Walnut Hazelnut Pistachio Pine nut Date	Acorn	Peach Apricot Grapefruit Vinegar
Bread	Wheat bread	Darnel bread Rice bread	Barley bread Millet bread Lentil bread Fava bean bread Sorghum bread Acorn bread	

oil was a perfectly balanced food between warm and cold, moist and dry (95). Beyond these specific recommendations, Ibn Zuhr categorized all foods and labelled them with a specific quality, which in turn corresponded to a certain humour, temperament, etc. (see table 5.2).

In the sixteenth-century dietary manuals on how and what to eat proliferate.[4] Following the ideas of Hippocrates (*Corpus hippocraticum* [The Hippocratic corpus], about 400 BCE), Polibus (*Sobre la naturaleza del hombre* [On the nature of man], 400 BCE), Galen (*De sanitate tuenda* [Galen's hygiene], also known as *Regimen sanitatis* [Rule of health] 129–200 CE), Haly Abbas (*Liber Pantegni* [Complete book of medical science] 994), Ibn Zuhr (1147–63?), Maimonides (*Guía de la buena salud* [Guide to good health] 1198), and Arnaldo de Vilanova (*Regimen de Salud* [Regimen of health] 1308), among others, authors of dietary manuals combined the traditions of ancient and medieval doctors to form the basis of sixteenth-century medical practices. The sheer quantity of health manuals that examine food's role in physical and spiritual health indicates how fashionable these texts were in the sixteenth century. Fray Bernardino de Laredo's *Metaphora medical* [Medical metaphor] (1522), Luis Lobera de Ávila's *Banquete de Nobles Caballeros* [Banquet of noble gentlemen] (1530) and subsequent revision *Vergel de sanidad* [Orchard of health] in 1542, Fernán Florez's translation of the Italian *El regimiento de toda la sanidad y de todas las cosas que se comen y beben* [Regiment of everything related to health and of what one eats and drinks] by Miguel de Savonarola (1541), Nicolás Monardes's edition of Juan de Aviñón's *Sevillana medicina* [Seville medicine] (1545), Pedro Jimeno's third part of *Dialogus de Re Medica* [Dialogue on medical matters] (1549), Francisco Núñez de Oria's *Aviso de sanidad* [Health news] (1569) with at least three subsequent editions, Pedro Mercado's *Diálogo de Filosofía natural y moral* [Dialogue on natural and moral philosophy] (1574), and Enrique Jorge Enríquez's *De regimine cibi atque potus* [On regiment of food and drink] (1594) are some of the texts circulating throughout the early modern period that treat the relationship between food and health.

When Don Quixote explains a knight's diet to Sancho, he implies that humble foods, like those usually eaten by servants and the working man, are also foods of the knights who show their valour through sacrifice: "su más ordinaria comida sería de viandas rústicas, tales como las que tú ahora me ofreces" [his usual fare would be made up of peasant food, just like what you are offering me now] (1.152). In response, Sancho also acknowledges that different classes eat different foods. But, nowhere in Cervantes is the relationship between food, health, and class so defined or satirized, than in Part 2 of *Don Quixote* when Sancho becomes governor of Barataria. Famished after a hard day of advising, Sancho enters the dining hall to a lot of fanfare, manifestation of his newly acquired power: music to welcome him, hand washing and a bib so he can wash before he enjoys his food, and a prayer to bless his meal. The room is filled with the duke's hired help: a steward, musicians, attendants, pages, a student, and, finally, the doctor, Pedro Recio de Agüero de Tirteafuera. The doctor's name alone, a pun on bad omens and "get lost," begins this extended humorous scene.[5] Using his whalebone wand, the doctor evaluates the dishes offered to Sancho, essentially eliminating anything that Sancho attempts to taste. Angered and frustrated, Sancho demands an explanation as to why the tantalizing dishes have been removed from the table. Pedro Recio explains:

> No se ha de comer, señor gobernador, sino como es uso y costumbre en las otras ínsulas donde hay gobernadores ... miro por su salud mucho más que por la mía, estudiando de noche y de día, y tanteando la complexión del gobernador, para acertar a curarle cuando cayere enfermo; y lo principal que hago es asistir a sus comidas y cenas. (2.387)

> [You should not eat, lord governor, except what is usual and customary on other isles where there are governors ... I look out for their (governors') health much more than my own, studying day and night and examining the governors' constitutions, to cure them when they fall ill; and the most important thing I do is attend to their lunches and dinners.]

Like Don Quixote before Sancho's arrival to Barataria, Pedro Recio tries to educate Sancho in the ways in which his cultural practices will reflect his status as governor. Pedro Recio's insistence on consuming certain foodstuffs while rejecting others draws on contemporary medical theories, like those stated above, to legitimize his claims.

The cultural historian Massimo Montanari cites Savonarola, author of *El regimiento de toda la sanidad y de todas las cosas que se comen y beben* [Regiment of everything related to health and of what one eats and drinks], who explains that "the rich should not partake of heavy soups, like those made from legumes or entrails, which were not very nutritious and difficult to digest; the poor instead were to avoid excessively select or refined foods which their course stomachs could not easily manage" (87). According to this theory of nutritional privilege, "the relationship between 'quality of person' and 'quality of food' was not a simple fact tied to the chances of wealth or need, but rather a basic and ontological postulate: to eat well or poorly was an intrinsic individual characteristic (and hopefully unalterable), just as was social class" (Montanari 87). Pedro Recio reiterates this idea and corroborates it with elitist notions of diet that required time ("estudiando de noche y de día") and attention ("tanteando la complexión del gobernador"). He continues his explanation:

> mandé quitar el plato de la fruta, por ser demasiadamente húmeda y el plato del otro manjar también le mandé quitar, por ser demasiadamente

caliente y tener muchas especies, que acrecientan la sed; y el que mucho bebe, mata y consume el húmedo radical, donde consiste la vida. (2.387)

[I ordered the plate of fruit be removed because it was too moist and the other food on the plate I also had removed for being too warm and having many spices that increase thirst; for he who drinks a lot, kills and consumes the root moisture wherein life exists.]

Sancho, anticipating a negative outcome to the doctor's proclamations, tries to reason with him asking which of the dishes he can eat. The doctor again denies him a variety of dishes: "plato de perdices asadas ... bien sazonadas ... conejos guisados ... ternera ... asada y en adobo [dishes of roast pheasant ... well seasoned ... stewed rabbit ... veal ... roasted and marinated] (387–8). He explains his decisions by overquoting Hippocrates and disdaining either the food's inherent nature or the preparation methods. These decisions, key to the humour of the entire dining episode at Barataria, draw on contemporary medical trends supported by the bio-psychological theory of the humours to satirize Sancho's stint as governor.[6] The duke and duchess, via their nutritionist trained in the Hippocratic school of medicine, use food as one of the many ways they attempt to destabilize Sancho's governorship, thus ridiculing the humble squire's aspirations of improving his station. The doctor's explanations were conveniently elitist and although the theories of nutritional privilege had been around for centuries, in the early modern period they "took on a new and unprecedented systematic rigor" (Montanari 88) and produced the type of social stratification that ruling classes embraced.

The following morning Sancho unhappily breaks his fast with meagre portions of preserves, a ration of bread, grapes, and "cuatro tragos de agua fría" [four sips of cold water] (2. 425). Again, the narrator recounts that Pedro Recio explains that his decisions are based on nutritional privilege: "los manjares pocos y delicados avivaban el ingenio, que era lo que más convenía a las personas constituidas en mandos y en oficios graves, donde se han de aprovechar no tanto de las fuerzas corporales como de las del entendimiento" [Light and few delicacies sharpen one's wit, which is what most agrees with people destined to command and in serious positions, where one does not resort so much to brute strength as to strength of mind] (425). Sancho, as it turns out, successfully navigates many of the challenges with which he is presented as governor, offering sound advice, judiciously resolving problems of his citizens, and establishing just tax laws, but in the end, it is his diet, and more specifically, his frustrations at the governor's table and his inability to enjoy a meal, that push him over the edge and lead him to renounce his position: "más quiero hartarme de gazpachos que estar sujeto a la miseria de un médico impertinente que me mate de hambre" [I would rather fill up on bread stews than be subject to the misery of this impertinent doctor who is trying to starve me to death] (444). He succumbs to the notion that each person is born into a social station and should remain there: "bien se está cada uno usando el oficio para que fue nacido" [everyone is well off practising the office for which he was born] (444).

However, the role of food in sustaining proper health also became fuel for those who opposed the notion of inherited nobility. If eating right, like receiving a solid education, fortified the development of proper habits, good morals, in short, noble behaviour, then perhaps scientific reasoning, and not birthright, could explain the "better" blood of the nobility. Certainly the exploration of one's actions defining a person's worth is at the heart of *Don Quixote*, whose protagonist affirms, "cada uno es hijo de sus obras" [everyone is a son of his own deeds] (1.97). And other writers also take up the idea that eating right affects the quality of one's blood. In *El buscón* Quevedo expresses this very idea in Book Two when Don Toribio explains to Pablos: "sin pan y carne, no se sustenta buena sangre, y por la misericordia de Dios, todos la tienen colorada, y no puede ser hijo de algo el que no tiene nada" [without meat and bread, no one has good blood and by the love of God, we all bleed red. You cannot be the son of someone if you have nothing" (82).[7]

Returning to Alonso Quijano's diet and given the medical conventions of the day, we learn that eating lentils regularly, which was a food that produced melancholy, would most certainly contribute to Don Quixote's mental imbalance. In his article "Renaissance Medical Psychology in *Don Quijote*," Daniel Heiple brought to light how Cervantes used contemporary medical theories to make Don Quixote's mental breakdown more viable. Lentils, together with the hot, dry air; lack of sleep; and loss of appetite and physical activity are causes established by centuries of medical theories that reasonably support how the knight's brain dried up. We know from Ibn Zuhr that lentils have a dry-cold quality. Arnau de Vilanova in his *Regimen de salud* also admonishes their consumption when he writes that "los legumbres nunca son buenos para los cuerpos templados mientras tuvieran sanidad, por lo cual conviene no comer de ellos, en particular si son secos" [legumes are never good for temperate, healthy bodies; as such it is not advisable to eat any of them, especially the dry ones] (cited in Cruz Cruz, *Dietética*

317). His advice manual continues declaring that peas, garbanzos, and fava beans are far superior to other legumes, i.e., lentils, and that if one must eat any of the pulses to combine them with ginger and saffron and cook them in almond milk (317). To further complicate the place of legumes in dietary health manuals, Vilanova also explains that garbanzo or pea juice cooked with white wine, spikenard, and saffron is very beneficial for cleansing the body: "Porque la tal bebida abre y limpia las venas capilares del hígado y las vías de la orina, y por el consiguiente, preserva de piedra y arenas" [Because such a drink opens and cleanses the liver's capillaries and the urinary tract, and as a result helps prevent stones both large and small] (318).

In the sixteenth century, Gabriel Alonso de Herrera, the father of modern agriculture, continues to support the theory that lentils have negative effects on the body: "da gruesso mantenimiento y de mala digestión, engendran sangre melancólica ... traen dolor de cabeza y hacen sonar sueños muy desvariados y espantosos; hacen ventosidades" [they lend themselves to a stout build and indigestion, they produce melancholy in the blood ... bring on headaches and make one dream delirious and horrific dreams; they create flatulence] (39). In the same way, the medical advisor of the Holy Roman Emperor and king of Spain Carlos I, Luis Lobera de Ávila, in his *Banquete de nobles caballeros* (1530) explains that lentils are good but "son de complixión melancólica" [have a melancholic constitution] (133). Turning to cooking manuals, Domingo Hernández de Maceras in his university cookbook, *Libro del arte de cocina* [Book on the art of cooking], also cautions the consumption of lentils. In his "De caldo de lentejas" [On lentil broth] recipe, he boils his lentils, and then adds sautéed onion and garlic as well as breadcrumbs as a thickener. He finishes the dish with standard spices, parsley and spearmint. But, at the end of the recipe Hernández de Maceras admonishes, "es buen caldo, sino que es melancólico, como dice Galeno, cap. 5." [it is a good broth but it is melancholic, as Galeno says in chap. 5] (234).

In spite of this tradition of the ill effects of lentils, Lobera de Ávila writes them up as specifically one of the first foods to give to someone who is ill. "Los manjares han de ser de buen nutrimento, de fácil y buena digestión. Al principio, de un caldo de lentejas con vinagre y agraz o algunas camuesas asadas o lechugas esparragadas y si la virtud estuviere flaca pasará a un caldo de pollo con agraz o vinagre" [Food should be nutritious and easily digested. In the beginning, prepare a lentil broth with vinegar and sour grape juice or some roasted apples or some lightly sautéed lettuce and if one's virtue is weak, you should try a chicken broth with sour grape juice or vinegar] (201). This recipe follows those found in Hispanic-Muslim cooking treatises that also include lentils for healing someone with a fever. The recipe "'Muzawara' provechosa para los calenturientos de tercianas y de fiebres agudas" ["Muzawara" good for those 48-hour fevers and acute fevers] is another lentil dish recommended for the ill that also contains squash, chard, or lettuce in addition to vinegar and spices (*Kitāb al-tabīj* 215).

Martínez Montiño is clearly aware of doctors' recommendations yet he is sceptical as he insists that his duty is to make dishes taste good and not to comment on whether it cures one or not.

> Lo han de ordenar los Medicos, porque en algunas mandan echar oro, y en otras raxitas de calabazas, y en otras garvanzos negros, y otras cosas conventientes para la enfermedad del enfermo, que no sean de mal gusto; y en algunas mandan echar tortugas, y pepitas de calabaza, y en esto no tengo que meterme, mas que sacar muy bien la sustancia. (391)

> [Doctors order it because in some prescriptions they include gold, in others squash shavings, and in others dark garbanzos, and other things pertinent to the disease of the sick person that do not taste bad. In some cases they prescribe eating turtle, and squash seeds, and I do not get involved with all this except for making the dish taste good.]

Although he does not specifically reference lentils, his examples include another pulse, the garbanzo. In other advice manuals, garbanzos enhance aphrodisiac qualities of food. Regarding hare meat, Ibn Zuhr explains that, "esta carne tiene virtudes afrodisíacas, sobre todo si se cuece con zumo de cebolla o con agua en la que se hayan puesto en remojo garbanzos" [this meat has a certain aphrodisiac quality especially when cooked with onion juice or with water in which garbanzos have been soaking] (57). Although not among the most appreciated food, lentils and other pulses are recognized by both writers and doctors as part of the common man's diet.

Lentils and Christian Dietary Practices

Beyond the medical texts warning of their ill effects and beyond their connection to poverty, lentils are definitively tied to abstinence and meals of religious sacrifice. Lentils and other legumes were not so much foods valued in and of themselves but rather in function with long-established Christian dietary proscriptions that formed the basis of a deep social identity and cultural bond. The *Diccionario de Autoridades* includes this Christian context in the definition of *potaje* [vegetable stew]: "Por antonomasia se llaman las legumbres guisadas para el mantenimiento de los días de abstinencia. También se llama así las mismas legumbres y semillas secas; y así se dice, que se ha hecho provisión de potajes para la Quaresma" [By antonomasia legumes cooked for sustenance on abstinence days are called this. Also, the legumes and dried seeds themselves are called this; and thus it is said that one has provisions for vegetable stew for Lent] (3.340). Many authors allude to the biblical story of Esau who sold his birthright to his twin brother Jacob in exchange for a bowl of lentils; these include Tirso de Molina in his allegorical play *El colmenero divino* [The divine beekeeper], and Lope de Vega in *La corona mayor* [The greatest crown]. Lentils also figure in Muslim and Jewish writing, thus exemplifying how this humble legume cut across ethnic divides. One way lentils are prepared in the Hispano-Muslim cooking manuals is with onions, cilantro, saffron, and vinegar. Eggs and figs are later added and the stew simmered until the lentils begin to dissolve (Ibn Razīn 280–1). In the Sephardic poem "Lamento de un judío pobre" [Lament of a poor Jew] lentils are presented as part of a stark, Jewish diet.

> Lechuga el domingo
> Migajas y agua el lunes.
> Puerros el martes.
> Las sobras de los puerros el miércoles.
> Lentejas secas el jueves
> Los restos de las lentejas el viernes.
> Mientras que en sabat lo más prudente es no cenar.
> Ni mucha carne, ni mucho vino.   (cited in Arbelos 149)

> [Lettuce on Sundays
> Bread and waters on Mondays
> Leeks on Tuesdays
> Leek leftovers on Wednesdays.
> Dry lentils on Thursdays
> The rest of the lentils on Fridays.
> While on the Sabbath the most prudent is not to eat at all
> Not much meat, not much wine.]

This diet, listed out by the days of the week, and the overlapping of lentils on Friday shows affinities with the opening of *Don Quixote* and again accentuates the importance of this humble legume across ethnicities and throughout the centuries.

For Christians, the concept of abstinence and fasting has existed since the early days of Christianity and has included to varying degrees Wednesdays, Fridays, and Saturdays throughout the year in addition to specific events of the liturgical calendar such as Lent, Advent, Ember Days, and Rogation Days.[8] In the early modern period in Spain, there were some 150 days of full or partial abstinence, with a clear distinction between the abstinence of Friday, no meat whatsoever, and that of Saturday, when people could eat other parts of birds and land animals that did not include its flesh. Reasons for abstention are complex but include penitence as one would renounce the pure pleasure of eating meat. Abstaining from meat would also aid in abstaining from sexual activity as scientific arguments put forth that meat consumption encouraged sexuality. Other possible reasons for abstinence were to avoid association with pagan imagery of animal sacrifice and to support the philosophy that vegetarianism inspired pacifism (Montanari 78–9). Although abstinence included both meat and other products derived from animals, as far back as the Middle Ages Spain benefited from bulls that granted first soldiers and then all Spaniards dispensation from refraining from eating meat from the extremities, intestines and organs, and animal byproducts such as cheese on partial abstinence days. For example, during the reign of the Catholic Monarchs, the Bull of the Holy Crusade, granted in 1478, 1479, 1481, 1482, 1485, 1494, 1503, and 1505 and continually renewed throughout the Hapsburg dynasty, included dietary dispensations (Fernández Llamazares 42–51).

Estando en el espresado territorio español (pero no fuera de él), pueden comer carnes por consejo de ambos médicos, spiritual y corporal, si lo exijiese la necesidad o la debil salud del cuerpo, ú otra cualquier causa, en los tiempos de ayuno de todo el año, aunque sean los de Cuaresma, y en los mismos por su arbitrio huevos y lacticinios. (Fernández Llamazares 42–51, 96)

[Being in said Spanish territory (but not outside it), they can eat meat on the advice of both their spiritual and corporal doctor, if need or weak health necessitates it or for any other reason during fast days throughout the year, even if it is Lent, and on these same days, on account of this adjudication, eggs and dairy products.]

This dispensation was originally written for anyone involved in holy warfare but was later extended to, "todos los vasallos del Rey Católico" [all the king's vassals] (Fernández Llamazares 115). Europeans who travelled through Spain commented on this unique situation. Madame D'Aulnoy writes about the exceptional practice in her journal: "Permite comer manteca y queso durante la Cuaresma y los viernes y los sábados de todo el año" [They are allowed to eat lard and cheese during Lent and on Fridays and Saturdays throughout the year] (cited in Díez Borque, *La vida española* 75).[9] Typically, on a full abstinence day like Friday, fish, eggs, and cheese were eaten, but when fish was not available, legumes were often served as the meat alternative for the day. With this in mind, the description of Alonso Quijano's weekend diet aligns perfectly with Christian eating practices of strict abstinence on Friday, partial abstinence on Saturday, and a celebratory meal on Sunday.

In fact, fish so defined abstinence days that people commonly divided the week between meat days and fish days. Coastal Spain enjoyed a wide variety of fish that varied from region to region and included hake, cod, sea bream, tuna, grouper, and sardines. Off the coast, dried, smoked, or pickled fish (mostly sardines, cod, herring, and salmon) was available throughout the year. Valles Rojo reports that in Castile turbot, lamprey, grouper, salmon, eel, and sole were the most valued fresh fish while cod, Conger eel, and hake were the most valued dried fish (*Cocina* 245). Although generally understood as an ecclesiastic imposition rather than a preferred dish, fish has no small presence among the cooking manuals of the early modern period. In both Nola's *Libro de guisados* [Book of cooking] and Hernández de Macera's *Libro de arte de cocina*, over 20 per cent of the recipes are for fish dishes.[10] Looking more closely at Nola, we realize that generally for each fish he included a recipe for an empanada and a stew and often times, a third recipe for grilled or boiled fish. Salmon, trout, barbel, shad, swordfish, sturgeon, dentex, palamida, Conger eel, moray eel, tuna, and grey mullet are all examples of this triple approach to preparing fish.

Eggs were readily available and regularly consumed by all members of society in an infinite number of ways. Not exclusively relegated to "fish days" as were fish and legumes, eggs were poached in soups, hard boiled in salads and empanadas, scrambled alone, or cooked together with virtually any meat or vegetable. They were used as a batter for meat, fish, and vegetables, and bread was dipped in eggs before being fried. They are essential to custards, cream-filled pastries, candied yolks, meringues, and cakes. They were also consumed raw in beverages or sauces. Medical advisors also believed that eggs formed good humours and were essential in curing what ailed you. In fact, at the beginning of Part 2 of *Don Quixote* the housekeeper explains that she should feed her master an unusual amount of eggs to help restore his health: "venía tal el triste, que no le conociera la madre que le parió: flaco, amarillo, los ojos hundidos en los últimos camaranchones del celebro; que para haberlo de volver algún tanto en sí, gasté más de seiscientos huevos, como lo sabe Dios y todo el mundo, y mis gallinas, que no me dejarán mentir" [this sad man arrived in such a state that even the mother who gave birth to him would not have recognized him; he was thin, yellowed, with eyes sunken way back into the recesses of his brain; to get him to return to his usual self, I used more than six hundred eggs, as God and everyone well know, and my chickens, they will prove I'm not lying] (2.85).

In 2006, the French chemist Hervé This systematically categorized the chemical possibilities of the egg and argued that when dealing with the yolk, the white, or the two together and simple transformative cooking processes, the possibilities for preparing the egg are endless. The earliest manuals both on the peninsula and throughout Europe contain literally hundreds of recipes that use eggs. In fact, Manuela Marín notes that eggs are more frequent in the cooking manuals of the West when compared to those of the East. "La frecuencia y las cantidades con que aparecen los huevos en la *Fuḍāla* son verdaderamente llamativas, por lo que se han considerado como una de las características más señaladas del recetario y, por extensión, del gusto gastronómico andalusí" [The frequency and quantity with which eggs appear in the *Fuḍālat* are really striking, and for this reason, they have been considered one of the most important characteristics of the recipe book and, by extension, of gastronomic taste of Al-Andalus] (Marín, *Relieves* 48). Some recipes call for up to thirty eggs (Marín, *Relieves* 48) and in both the *Fuḍālat al-ḥiwān* [The delicacies of the table] and in the *Kitāb al-tabīj* [Treatise on cooking] the egg's versatility defines the two texts.

One way in which the egg distinguishes itself early on in Spain is as a finishing device for savoury recipes. Often recipes include instructions for coating a dish with a whipped egg mix after the main ingredients have cooked. For example, in the poultry dish "Hechura 'Yilīdīya'-correosa" [Yilidiya creation, tough] after stewing the bird in a raisin juice-vinegar broth, the meat is finished with a mixture of whipped eggs, ground nuts, and breadcrumbs, covered, and baked over low heat (*Kitāb al-tabīj* 79). This use of egg batter as a finisher is also found in all the later, Christian cooking manuals.

In the seventh dialogue of *Ejercicios de lengua latina* [Latin language exercises] (1539), which treats university food, Juan Luis Vives highlights eggs as one of the more popular foods consumed on abstinence days. "En los días en los que no está permitido comer carne, en lugar de ésta tenemos huevos asados, fritos o cocidos, solos o mezclados con un pastel en la sartén con unas gotas, mejor que con un chorro, de vinagre o de aceite" [On days when eating meat is not allowed, in its place we have eggs, roasted, fried, or boiled, by themselves or mixed into a pie, in a frying pan with a sprinkle of, or even better, a good pour of vinegar or oil] (19).

Cheese, like bread and eggs, was enjoyed by rich and poor alike, and not exclusively associated with "fish days." Derived from cow, goat, and sheep milk depending on the region, and eaten both fresh and cured, it is one of the most referenced foods in *Don Quixote*, appearing over two dozen times in the novel (Valles Rojo, *Don Quijote* 10). Although recipes on how to make cheese do not form part of either the medieval or the early modern cooking manuals, recipes that include cheese certainly appear. Martínez Montiño includes dozens of recipes for soups, vegetable torts, and sweet and savoury pastries that require hard or soft cheese as an essential ingredient or grated cheese as a garnish. Likewise cheese appears on every seasonal banquet menu as a suggested finisher served with fruit.

Returning to the realm of pre New World pulses – lentils, garbanzos, and fava beans – lentils are considered the most humble. They rarely appear in the cooking manuals of Spain in spite of the fact that authors dedicate entire sections of their cookbooks to food for Lent/abstinence days. Ruperto de Nola's fourth chapter is titled "Tratado para guisar y aparejar las viandas en tiempo cuaresmal" [Treatise on cooking and finishing food during Lent] (345). Hernández de Maceras divides his cookbook into three main sections: "De los guisados de carnero" [On young mutton dishes] (195), "La comida de sábados" [Saturday meals] (221), and "Pescados y diferencias de huevos, y platos de vigilia, y potages" [Fish and different eggs, and dishes for abstinence days and stews] (229). Diego Granado dedicates several different chapters to Lenten foods: "De diversas viandas y guisados de pescado, platos y potajes cuaresmales" [On diverse food and fish stews, Lenten dishes and soups] (163), "Escudillas de pescado y otras viandas para días de Cuaresma" [Fish soups and other food for Lenten days] (255), "Para hacer pasteles de varios tipos de pescados y otras materias para días de ayuno" [For making various types of fish cakes and other things for fasting days] (280), "Tortas y tortadas y tortillones de pescados y otras cosas para días de Cuaresma" [Small, medium, and large fish pies and other things for Lent] (300), "De diversas maneras de tortas y costradas de frutas y legumbres para días de Cuaresma y cosas de leche a usanza de Italia" [On different types of fruit and legume torts and turnovers for Lenten days] (307), and "De cómo se han de hacer yelos (geles, gelos, gelatinas) y salsas de diversas maneras para días de carne y de Cuaresma" [On how to make gels, jellies, and gelatins and different types of sauces for meat days and Lenten days] (327). Together these chapters make up almost half of the 755 recipes.

Even those who do not formally divide their cookbooks into meat and non-meat days are very aware of the differences. In one of Martínez Montiño's recipes for cardoons he ends with a general tip: "Y advierte, que todos los platillos que tengo dicho, que se han de cocer con manteca de vacas, o buen aceite, se entiende que en dia de carne ha de ser tocino en lugar de la manteca, y caldo de carne en lugar de caldo de garbanzos" [And note that of all these dishes in which I have said to use beef tallow or good oil, it is understood that on meat days you can use fat back instead of tallow and beef broth instead of garbanzo broth] (300).

While cooks are clearly aware of the different foods for abstinence days, in the Christian court manuals lentils make only a rare appearance in the fourteenth century. A single recipe for lentils appears in the index to the Catalan cooking manuscript, Sent Soví though it is missing from the actual recipes. Santanach i Suñol explains "En las rúbricas del Sent soví, después de la leche de almendras, se menciona una receta de lentejas; la lectura del texto de esta preparación, conservada en el Llibre d'aparellar, permite constatar que se trata de una crema pastosa de lentejas, similar al pure de garbanzos o de guisantes que recomendaba el medico real" [In the Sent soví chapter outline, after almond milk a lentil recipe is mentioned; the text itself for this recipe, preserved in the Book of Food Preparation, confirms that it is a thick lentil soup, similar to a garbanzo or pea purée that the royal doctor recommends] (Libro de Sent Soví 35–6).

This legume is absent in the early modern works of Nola and Martínez Montiño, who include recipes for garbanzos and fava beans, though it does appear in Diego de Granado's Libro del arte de cozina [Book on the art of cooking]. As we know from chapter 1, the majority of Granado's recipes are translations or adaptations from the Italian Bartolomeo Scappi. Thus, the inclusion of "Para hacer escudilla de lentejas secas"

[Soup from dry lentils] (270) is more a reflection of Italian court cooking practices than Spanish ones. Lentils also appear in Hernández de Maceras's university cookbook, *Libro del arte de cocina*, exemplifying that lentils reached the kitchens of the elite student body – and here, only in a nominal way. In Hernández de Maceras's work, he states that lentils form part of the foods typically consumed during Lent and on days of abstinence: "Los potajes que ordinariamente se suelen dar en las Cuaresmas son los siguientes, arroz, natillas, espinacas, castañas, almidón, hormigo, turmas de tierra, borrajas, lechugas, garbanzos, espárragos, tallos de acelgas, calabaza romana, bretones, lentejas, zanahorias, berenjenas" [The dishes that are regularly served during Lent are the following: rice, custard, spinach, chestnuts, starch, porridge, truffles, borage, lettuce, garbanzos, asparagus, stalks of chard, Roman squash, Brussels sprouts, lentils, carrots, eggplant] (229). In this third section of his cookbook, dedicated to fish, eggs, and other Lenten food, he includes one recipe for lentils called "De caldo de lentejas" [On lentil broth] (234). As stated above, he adds sautéed onion and garlic for flavouring and bread to thicken the mixture. He then adds the appropriate spices, parsley and mint, but cautions his reader to take care as it will most certainly affect one's humoural balance.

Corroborating Hernández de Maceras's entry for abstinence foods, Vives describes what university students traditionally eat: bread and butter and seasonal fruit for breakfast, and vegetables and porridge with some meat for lunch. On non-meat days, lentils figure into the menu when fish is not an option. "[L]os días de vigilia, tomamos el suero de la leche en escudillas (obtenido al hacer la mantequilla) con algunos trozos pequeños de pan, algo de pescado fresco si hay alguno a precio tolerable en el mercado del pescado, de lo contrario, tomamos salazón bien macerado y después guisantes o garbanzos o lentejas o habas o altramuces" [On abstinence days, we have whey in bowls (obtained from making butter) with some breadcrumbs, some fresh fish if there is any at a reasonable fish market price, and if not, we eat salted fish, well soaked, and afterwards peas, garbanzos, lentils, fava beans or lupins] (18–19).

In Lope's 1621 comedia *Amor, pleito y desafío* [Love, argue, and challenge] when two servants lightly talk about the scarcity of food during the master's absence, they allude to Friday as bean day, but here, their reference is to garbanzos as opposed to Alonso Quijano's lentils: "los garbanzos, por los viernes/ hacen con dulce armonía/ bailes de a cuatro en el caldo" [garbanzos, as it is Friday/ dance with sweet harmony/ in groups of four in the broth] (Act 1). Here, pulses are not only referenced as a fish-day food but also defined in terms of their scarcity.

In comparison to lentils, garbanzos appear more frequently in the cookbooks and are more valued by the writers of the day. At first glance, garbanzos would seem to be on par with lentils as both pulses are often described together as a suitable alternative when no fish is available. In one garbanzo recipe, "Cómo se han de aderezar los garbanzos" [How to cook garbanzos] (236), Hernández de Maceras writes that the cooking process is the same for "De caldo de lentejas" [On lentil broth] in that it uses sautéed onion and garlic, bread, and spices, although here, he also includes eggs and other vegetables in the dish. In another recipe, for example, he adds garbanzos to one of his spinach dishes that also includes spices, garlic, and bread as a thickener (231). However, when examining the court cookbooks, we begin to understand that this legume was held in somewhat higher esteem than the lentil. Although Nola does not include it in his cookbook, in Martínez Montiño's manual, garbanzos appear in a handful of recipes. He includes garbanzos in his recipe "Cabeza de cabrito" [Head of kid] (219) and in "Como se aderezan las espinacas" [How to season spinach] (265). This latter recipe is similar to today's *espinacas a la catalana* [Catalan-style spinach] (without the garbanzos) in that it is a sautéed spinach dish with pine nuts and raisins. He even includes two sweet recipes for garbanzos: "Garbanzos dulces con membrillo" [Sweet garbanzos with quince] (249–50) and "Otros garbanzos dulces" [Other sweet garbanzos] (251). In both recipes sugar and cinnamon flavour the garbanzos. And, of course, garbanzos are the legume of choice for all *olla podrida* recipes. In fact, Diego de Granado distinguishes between light and dark garbanzos and suggests using both in his version of the stew.

In spite of this rich diversity of garbanzo recipes, the most common way that garbanzos are included in dishes is as a stock. Used as vegetable stock, garbanzos become a flavourful broth to a wide variety of vegetable and fish dishes such as "Olla de atún" [Tuna stew] (288), "Pastel de criadillas de tierra" [Truffle pie] (297), "Pastel de cardo" [Cardoon pie] (300–1), and "Cebollas rellenas" [Stuffed onions] (302). Martínez Montiño even includes garbanzo broth in a recipe for frog meatballs (319–20). This comes as no surprise as doctors of the day considered garbanzo stock to be much healthier than the legume itself. Even centuries earlier, Hispano-Muslim cooking manuals recognized the benefits of the broth as superior to that of the bean itself. The author of *Kitāb al-tabīj* writes, "el garbanzo en su cascara no tiene aplicación en las diversas clases de cocina, porque es un plato de la gente del campo y de los glotones; los que quieren con él aumentar sus fuerzas, solo toman su jugo y lo anaden a la carne y hacen con él un plato o una empanada" [the garbanzo in its shell has no place in different cooking styles because it is a dish meant for country folk or gluttons. Those who want to increase their strength should use just the broth and add it to meat and make a dish or an empanada] (117).

Of the three main pulses, fava beans were a cut above lentils and garbanzos, which, together with cabbage, leeks, onion and garlic, were considered beneath the elite. Riera Melis explains that fava beans "ocupaban un lugar destacado en la alimentación campesina y eclipsaban a las restantes legumbres" [had a prominent position in the peasant diet and eclipsed all the other legumes] ("Jerarquía social" 102). This privileged space among the peasantry is echoed in the court cooking manuals as it is the only legume to appear in all three court manuals of the early modern period (and prior to that as well). Nola's recipe "Haba real" [Royal fava beans] (373) is included in an appendix at the end of the cookbook with eight additional non-meat recipes. As an introduction to the appendix, Nola defends the value of Lenten foods: "aunque algunos digan que las viandas cuaresmales no son tan provechosas como las del carnal, a esto digo, que no es sino voluntad de personas; porque hay algunos señores que les contentan más unas viandas que otras" [even if some people say that Lenten food is not as good for you as meat dishes, to this I say, it depends on the person because some will like some foods more than other foods] (369). Martínez Montiño has three main fava bean recipes: "Potage de habas" [Fava bean stew] (240), "Otras diferentes" [Another different one] (241), "Habas en día de carne" [Fava beans for meat days] (241–2).

When Cervantes chose to define his character as one who regularly ate lentils for his Friday meal, he inscribed his main character with a humble social class, reinforced by nutritional theories that insisted that lentils were hard to digest and provoked excessive melancholy, a possible instigator of Alonso Quijano's mental breakdown. This small, round legume also represented the values of Christianity, as it served as a substitute for fish on abstinence days. Thus, with this passing legume reference, readers can more deeply understand Alonso Quijano's identity as a humble, Christian hidalgo and reflect on foods of restraint and sacrifice. It is not until the postwar years of Francoism in Spain that legumes once again take on such a strong sense of poverty, lack of nutritional privilege, and sacrifice. In spite of these ties to poverty and hardship, lentils continue to enjoy immense popularity in Spain. The country is one of the top fifteen producers of lentils in the world and in every town across Spain lentil soup or lentil salad appears as part of a "menu del día" [daily lunch special] in both high and low end restaurants.[11] The fact that this foodstuff, which is so tied to difficult economic times throughout Spain's history, is still ingrained as a definitive part of its culinary identity speaks to its ability to endure in spite of its clear associations with poverty, poor health, and the Catholic Church. At the opposite end of the food spectrum from the impoverished lentil, is *palomino* [squab], poultry reserved for the celebratory Sunday meal that will be more fully discussed in the following chapter.

Chapter Six

"Algún palomino de añadidura los domingos": The Theatrics of Food and Celebration

Ningún alimento de los que Dios puso en la tierra, [es] más apto para el sustento y nutrición del ser humano, que los diferentes tipos de aves

[No other food that God put on this earth (is) more suited to sustain and nurture human beings than different types of fowl]

Sorapán de Rieros

As a man of modest means, Alonso Quijano would reserve a domesticated fowl, specifically a *palomino* [squab] for the Sunday meal, an act that reflects the Christian custom of recognizing Sunday as a sacred day. The liturgical calendar, most noted by Advent, Christmas, Epiphany, Carnival, Lent, Easter, and patron saint days, was celebrated with feasts, and the Sunday meal is an extension of this deep-rooted connection between eating and religious ceremony. But beyond its connection to religious ritual, Alonso Quijano's Sunday dinner is also the first of many special meals served throughout the novel. In Part 1 and especially Part 2, characters gather to share a meal that reveals a genuine hospitality and often celebrates a special event. Don Quixote's meal with goat herders before his speech on the Golden Age, the wedding feast of Camacho and Quiteria, Sancho's famed governor's banquet, as well as countless spontaneous roadside meals all point to the importance of food as a social event and clear sign of both hospitality and celebration. Cervantes' novel marks the countless forms of discourse that not only signal an exceptional event with food, but more specifically, with poultry. It is no accident that Alonso Quijano eats squab as the main part of his Sunday meal. As we will see in other parts of *Don Quixote*, poultry takes on the same privileged significance. When knight and squire stop at an inn on the road to Barcelona, Sancho inquires about dinner to which the innkeeper confidently states that he can order whatever he desires: "que pidiese lo que quisiese: que *de las pajaricas del aire, de las aves de la tierra* y de los pescados del mar estaba proveída aquella venta" [that he should order whatever he wanted: that *from little birds in the sky to birds on the ground* and fish in the sea, his inn would provide] (2.484, emphasis mine).[1] The innkeeper's euphemism for having the best to offer shows that poultry is defined as a highly desired commodity. It is no wonder then that it appears on the tables of kings and in the fantasies of those who dream about magical lands of milk and honey. This chapter brings to light the significance of poultry as food for the privileged and a necessary part of celebratory meals before turning more generally to how food is used as a signifier of plenty and of deep-rooted desires for satisfying basic biological urges.

Poultry as a Signifier of Prestige

In Martínez Montiño's cookbook *Arte de cocina: pastelería, bizcochería y conservería* [The art of cooking, pie making, pastry making, and preserving], the cook describes a Christmas banquet for Felipe III that includes no less than three courses with twelve dishes in each course. For each course, half the options are poultry. In the first course he includes *pavos asados con su salsa;*[2] *pichones, y torreznos asados,*[3] platillo de arteletes de aves sobre sopas de natas; *perdices asadas con salsa de limones, capirotada con solomo, y salchichas, y perdices; pollas asadas* [roasted turkey with gravy; squab, with roasted pork fat, small dishes of cream soup with mint and ginger poultry roll; roast partridge with lemon sauce, casserole with pork, sausage, and partridge, roasted chicken] (14). Among the second course selections are *capones asados, anades asadas con salsa de membrillos, platillo de pollos con escarolas rellenas, empanadas inglesas,*[4] *zorzales asados sobre sopas doradas, platillo de aves à la Tudesca* [roast capons, roast duck with quince sauce, small dishes of chicken-stuffed escarole, English pasties, roast thrush in a golden soup, small dishes of various birds cooked German-style] (15). Finally, the third course includes *pollos rellenos con picatostes de ubres de ternera asados, gigotes de aves, platillo de pichones ahogados, empanadas de pabos en masa blanca, palomas toraces con salsa negra,* and *manjar blanco* [chickens with roast veal udder stuffing, minced poultry casserole, small dishes of stewed squab, turkey pie with white dough, wood pigeons with black sauce, and blancmange] (15–16).

From banquets to daily dining, poultry was ever present at the king's table. Sánchez Meco writes that "las carnes más preciadas por Felipe II fueron las aves, siguiendo un criterio muy difundido en la época por médicos y dietistas, quienes consideraban estos animales, como los idóneos para la alimentación humana" [Felipe II's most valued meat was poultry, which followed the well-known criteria for all doctors and nutritionists of the day who considered these animals to be the most suitable as food for humans] (132). Actually, one of the first and principal foods princes and princesses ate after being weaned was poultry. The medical team – Dr Valle, Dr Álvarez de Perea, Dr Sosa, and Dr. Guerrera – who attended the young prince Felipe (IV) in 1608 when he was just three years old, recommended the following diet:

> Mediodía: Tres platos. Uno de cocido y dos de asados de capon, perdigón o gazapo, y con cada uno de estos asados unas mollejuelas de cabrito. Se le permite uno de los dos asados. Cena: Un plato que puede ser "picadillo de polla muy tierna," "mollejuelas" o "huevos frescos." (cited in Simón Palmer, *La cocina* 21)

> [Mid-day meal: Three dishes. One of one-pot stew and two of roasted capon, partridge chick or young rabbit, and with each one of these roasts, sweetbreads made from kid. One of the two roasts is allowed. Dinner: A dish, possibly "tender chicken mincemeat," "gizzards," or "fresh eggs."]

This medical attention to poultry within the diet of future kings extended to other court members and those of high-ranking nobility and informed theories of nutritional privilege.

As mentioned in chapter 5, in the *Kitāb al-Aǧḏiya wal-adwiya (Tratado de los alimentos)* [Treatise on food] (1147–63?), the medieval physician Ibn Zuhr (Averzoar), like Galen and Dioscorides before him, confirms the role of poultry in a healthy diet and that the meat from a hen was the best poultry (95). But in the early modern period, the emphasis on poultry takes a new turn. Humanists like Platina in *De honesta voluptate et valetudine* [On right pleasure and good health], put forth that "peacocks and other edible birds … are more delicious than others and more suitable to the tables of kings and princes than the lowly and men of little property" (243). Here, Platina is clearly asserting poultry's preeminent position on the elite table. His stance creates an elitist diet and supports a theory of nutritional privilege among higher social classes.

This privileged space for certain types of poultry is seen time and again on the stage as well. In Tirso's *La elección por la virtud* [The choice of virtue], Sixto's father describes the rich and the poor through the food on their table in his own *beatus ille*:

> el que es de tu gusto esclavo
> estimara más que el pavo,
> el francolín y el faisán,
> pobre mesa y negro pan,
> añejo jamón, y al cabo
> dos cascos de una cebolla,
> que en la labradora mesa
> siempre que anda el hambre en folla
> son, en vez de la camuesa,
> mondadientes de la olla.   (Act 1)

> [he who has your enslaved taste
> enjoys more than turkey,
> francolin and pheasant,
> a poor meal with dark bread,
> old ham and in the end,
> two onion skins,
> that on the working man's table,
> where hunger always plays its part,
> instead of a golden apple, are
> toothpicks for the pot.]

Turkey, francolin, and pheasant are signifiers for elite taste and contrasted with the working man's palate that is accustomed to the flavours of bread and onions. Sancho, too, offers this same distinction when Don Quixote insists that he join him and the shepherds for the evening meal. To excuse himself from the formalities of the group, Sancho uses these same food images of bread, onion, and poultry: "mucho mejor me sabe lo que como en mi rincón, sin melindres ni respetos, aunque sea pan y cebolla, que los gallipavos de otras mesas donde me sea forzoso mascar despacio, beber poco, limpiarme a menudo, no estornudar ni toser si me viene gana, ni hacer otras cosas que la soledad y la libertad traen consigo" [whatever I eat in my own corner tastes so much better, without affectation or respect, even if it is bread and onions, than turkey at other tables where I would be forced to chew slowly, drink a little, wipe my mouth often, not sneeze or cough if I wanted to, nor do any of those things that solitude and freedom bring with them] (1.154).

Regarding theories of nutritional privilege, like Platina and Ibn Zuhr before him, the Spanish physician Lobera de Ávila describes the health benefits and risks of consuming poultry in his work *Banquetes de noble caballeros* [Banquet of noble gentlemen]. Citing from a wide range of authoritative sources, he explains that wild fowl produce an excess of anger while aquatic fowl are too moist. Meat from partridge, however, "es de maravillosa sustancia" [makes a marvellous stock] and the meat and broth from hen, and even more so from chicken, temper the humours and aid the stomach (77). Regarding pigeons and their squab, the older birds have a dry, warm disposition but the younger squab, like those Alonso Quijano ate in his Sunday meal, contain "supérflua humidad" [unnecessary moisture] that often leads to headaches (77). Perhaps the Sunday squab was served in an effort to restore the balance of Alonso Quijano's misaligned humours. Don Quixote may never have sallied forth had his diet contained more balanced food like chicken and less extreme food like squab or even lentils that unhinged his humours.

Returning to the king's table and according to kitchen records, Felipe IV's grandfather, the young teenager Prince Felipe (II), ate poultry every day. For example, the week of 3–10 August administrators from the kitchen in which the prince's meals were prepared bought hens every day, more than any other foodstuff with the exception of bread. Farm-raised squab was purchased with as much frequency as mutton, beef, and eggs; and capons, chickens, wild squab, partridge chicks, and geese also regularly appeared in the purchasing records for the prince's pantry (cited in Valles Rojo, *Cocina* 144).

Another way to understand the primary role of poultry in the diet of the adolescent prince is to examine how much was spent on different items. Seven months later, in March 1540, palace records show that the following was spent on food for the prince:

Gallinas tres, que costaron las dos a sesenta y cuatro mrs. cada[5]
Una y la otra por dos reales y medio que son: 179
Un capón que costó 2 reales y medio que son: 85
Dos palominos mansos por sesenta mrs.: 60
De carne para cocido y asado ocho libras a ocho mrs. la libra: 64

De pan para la mesa: 28
De pan para la cocina: 12
De pan para los perros y pájaros sesenta y tres mrs.: 63
Huevos para las torrijas y el tordo seis por nueve mrs.: 9
De almidón una libra: 24
De leche para potajes dos azumbres por treinta y seis mrs: 36
De aceite para el perro: 3
Otros gastos:
    De leña seis cargas, dos de acémilas y cuatro de asnos, que costaron todas
siete reales y medio que son: 255
Suman los gastos ordinarios de este día y otros gastos: 818 mrs.
    Los gastos de la despensa del príncipe N.S. del mes de marzo de 1540.
(cited in Valles Rojo, *La cocina* 146)

[Hens, three, of which two cost sixty four mrs. each
One at the other (price) of two and a half *reals* which totalled: 179
One capon that cost two and a half *reals* that totalled: 85
Two farm-raised squab for sixty mrs.: 60
For meat for *cocido* and roasts eight pounds at eight mrs. the pound: 64
For bread for the table: 28
For bread for the kitchen: 12
For bread for dogs and birds sixty-three mrs.: 63
Eggs for sweet fried bread and the thrush six for nine mrs.: 9
For starch one pound: 24
For milk for stews two *azumbres* for thirty six mrs.: 36[6]
For oil for the dog: 3
Other expenses:
    For firewood six loads, two mule (-sized) and four donkey (-sized) that
cost in total seven and a half *reals* that is: 255
The usual daily expenses and the other expenses add up to: 818 mrs.
The pantry expenses for H.M. the prince in the month of March, 1540.]

From these figures we can see that 324 of a total of 818 maravedis, or almost 40 per cent was spent on poultry and if just food costs are figured, then almost 60 per cent of the daily food allowance was spent on poultry alone!

Poultry's esteemed position was not just found at court. In early modern Spain birds were hunted and many farms had a pigeon loft that housed different birds for food throughout the winter. Nobility and villagers alike consumed a wide variety of fowl, including chicken, capon, goose, hen, duck, quail, and pheasant. Enrique de Villena includes twenty-nine different birds in his fifteenth-century *Arte cisoria* [The art of carving] and in both medieval and early modern cooking manuals, fowl is prominently featured.[7] Chicken, for example, was served at special banquets at court, and according to the accounts of a confraternity in Valladolid, at 70 per cent of the banquets for officials, chicken was served while beef was reserved for the poor (Rucquoi 298).[8]

Different types of farm-raised and, to a lesser extent, wild birds were also consumed among lower social classes both in rural and urban areas. Like the meat of quadrupeds explored in chapter 2, within poultry there is a definite culinary hierarchy. Among the farm-raised birds the preference from highest to lowest is as follows: "capón cebado, capón, polla cebada, polla, pavo, gallina, gallina cebada, pollo" [fattened capon, capon, fattened (female) chicken, (female) chicken, turkey, hen, fattened hen, (male) chicken], and among other birds: "perdices, francolín, perdigón, buchón, ansarón, ánsar, astarna, zorzal" [partridges, francolin, young partridge, pigeon, gosling, goose, grey partridge, thrush] (cited in Valles Rojo, *La cocina* 238). Beyond cooking manuals and court-related testimonies, the presence of domestic poultry and its central role on the privileged table appears time and again in multiple early modern discourses.

For example, in chapter 7 of *Menosprecio de corte y alabanza de aldea* [Contempt for court and praise for rural life] Antonio de Guevara writes about the virtues of country men and the vices of those at court. In doing so, he extols the excellent poultry found in the small towns.

> ¡Oh!, vida bienaventurada la del aldea, a do se comen las aves que son gruesas, son nuevas, son cebadas, son sanas, son tiernas, son manidas, son escogidas, y aun son castizas. El que mora en el aldea come palominos de verano, pichones caseros, tórtolas de jaula, palomas de encina, pollos de enero, patos de mayo, lavancos de río, lechones de medio mes, gazapos de julio, capones cebados, ansarones de pan, gallinas de cabe el gallo, liebres de dehesa, conejos de zarzal, perdigones de rastrojo, peñatas de lazo, codornices de reclamo, mirlas de vaya y zorzales de vendimia. (176–7)

> [Oh, happy village life, where they eat fowl that is fat, young, grain-fed, healthy, tender, full of flavour, well-selected, and even Castilian-bred. He who lives in a village eats wild squab in summer, farm-raised squab, collared doves, farm-raised collared doves, wood pigeons, chicken in January, duck in May, wild duck, suckling pig, young rabbit in July,

fattened capons, bread-fed goslings, hens next to the rooster, hare from the fields, rabbits from the briar patch, free-range partridge chicks, snared prey, decoy quail, blackbirds from the bush, and thrushes at harvest time.]

And, in the well-known travel journal of Madame d'Aulnoy, she asserts that, along with the one-pot meal, *cocido*, poultry in Spain is excellent: "Lo mejor que aquí se ofrece son los pichones, las gallinas y el cocido, que de veras lo considero excelente" [The best [Spain] has to offer are squab, hen, and *cocido*, that I consider to be truly outstanding] (203). It is clear then, that from both literary and non-literary texts, poultry was privileged food, formed a central part of the royal family's diet, and was repeatedly used by writers as a marker of the elite.

The Banquet as Spectacle

The presence of poultry is but one of the many indicators of social rank. In fact, more generally, food and celebratory banquets allow individuals to confirm their position within the social hierarchy. But, what exactly is a banquet? By definition it involves food, people, and spectacle. Covarrubias explains its meaning in the following way:

> vale tanto como un festín, convite y comida espléndida, abundante de manjares y rica en aparato. Tomó nombre de las bancas, o mesas sobre que se ponen las viandas, como llamamos mesa franca el dar de comer a cuantos quieren sentarse a la mesa, que sean de las calidades que se requieren; y hacer plato el admitir un señor a su mesa de ordinario, el número de caballeros competente; de manera que debajo destos nombres banco, mesa y plato, se entienda el convidar en la forma sobredicha. (162)

> [It is equal to a feast, a dinner party with splendid food, abundant in delicacies beautifully displayed. The name comes from benches or tables on which food was placed, in the same way we say *open table* when anyone who wants to sit at the table is fed, as long as he has the necessary social standing; and *to make a plate for* when a nobleman admits the appropriate number of gentlemen to his everyday table; so that from these names *bench*, *table* and *dish*, it is understood that one invites in the way explained above.]

Thus the table is the centre of the banquet that is as much defined by the dishes placed at its centre as it is by the people who are seated around

√ it. The table brings community together but also forces hierarchies, webs of inclusion and exclusion. Meals served on special occasions indicate the image people want to present of themselves. As Bourdieu put forth, the style of meal is "the systematic expression of a system of factors including, in addition to the indicators of the position occupied in the economic and cultural hierarchies, economic trajectory, social trajectory, and cultural trajectory" (72).

And nowhere is this positioning of prestige as prevalent as it is at court. This show of wealth and decorum took on unprecedented importance during the rule of Felipe IV and the Count-Duke of Olivares. In her study on Madrid as cultural capital in the early modern era, María José del Río Barredo reports that "La recepción y agasajo de los visitantes ilustres extranjeros fue uno de los objetos centrales de las etiquetas y cortesía en el Madrid de las décadas de 1620 y 1630. Lo había sido, desde luego, también con anterioridad, pero en estos años se convirtió en materia de Estado en el sentido liberal del término" [The receiving and welcoming of illustrious foreign visitors was one of the main tenets of etiquette and courtesy in the Madrid of the 1620s and 1630s. Previously, of course, it had also been that way, but during these years it became a public affair of the state in the most liberal sense of the word] (162). Del Río Barredo goes on to explain that beyond lodging and feeding foreign visitors to the state, the king would send his own personal attendants (or those of the queen for female guests) to attend to his guests (167).[9]

Directly related to court are many examples of these economic, social, and cultural trajectories. Typically, a nobleman would host an event for royalty to reassure his own place both at the table and among the power struggles playing out at court. Some of the outstanding banquets recorded from the Habsburg dynasty include the one that the President of the Court in Valladolid hosted for the arrival of the new king, Carlos I, in which "había mandado construir y edificar en medio de su casa una hermosa fuente sobre el suelo, de la cual salía vino por dos caños" [a beautiful fountain was ordered to be built and staged on the floor in the centre of the house from which wine poured forth from two spouts] (Vital 349). Generations later, in 1624, the Duke of Medina Sidonia organized a banquet that extended over days to honour Felipe IV as he travelled to southern Spain. For this occasion he ordered foodstuffs beyond his own land: "de diferentes partes, se embiaron a Doña Ana, diez y seys días, cinquenta cabritos y quatrocientas perdizes y conejos, mil gallinas, quinientos pollos, sin muchos capones y pabos cebados de leche. Del condado de S. Lúcar llevaron cien mil guevos" [from different parts over the course of sixteen days fifty kid and four hundred partridges and rabbits, a thousand hens, five hundred chickens, without many capons or milk-fed turkeys were sent to Doñana. A hundred thousand eggs were sent from San Lúcar county] (Espinosa and Bernal 11). Later towards the end of Felipe IV's career, Luis XIV's ambassador, the Duke of Agramont, held a banquet for the king's petition of the hand of María Teresa de Austria y Borbón, in which they served 500 meat dishes and 300 starters and desserts (Cubillo de Aragón).

For a more detailed look at early modern banquets, the reception of Lord Charles Howard, the Count of Nottingham, Admiral of England and ambassador for King James I to Spain, is an excellent example. Thomé Pinheiro da Veiga's account of the party that the Duke of Lerma threw on 7 June 1605, one of many for Lord Howard over those few weeks in summer, exemplifies how celebratory meals position both host and invited guests. Pinheiro da Veiga writes pages describing the multiple and intricate facets of this lavish banquet including the dishes, tablecloths, and tapestries that create the right ambiance:

En la otra habitación estaba la vajilla de oro y esmaltes, toda de piezas notables, que ocupaba la mesa y gradas de una pared hasta arriba, cosa admirable de ver; y en la otra había solamente vidrios y cristales engastados en oro, con pies, asas y tapas de oro y labores en toda su extensión, y los vidrios de colores, cosa nobilísima ... El banquete se dio en una galería grande, armada de brocados, como las demás de las cosas, donde pusieron 24 alacenas por medio de la casa para 80 personas, que comieron a la mesa con el Almirante, y estando con él en la sala muchos señores y títulos y muchas damas y señoras rebozadas, que todos entraron con asaz trabajo ... Estuvieron el rey y la reina viendo todo por una celosía que quedaba frente al extremo de la mesa, escondidos; y se afirma que sirvieron a la mesa 2.200 platos de cocina, y que fue de ver, además, los dulces secos, los frascos de conservas, y sobre todo la invención de empanadas de mil figuras de castillos y navíos, todo dorado y plateado. (64–5)

[In the other room was the dinner service made of gold and porcelain, all considerable pieces that sat on the table and terraced shelves that ran all the way up the wall; it was a remarkable thing to behold; and in another room, there were just glasses and crystal set in gold, with golden bases; handles and covers completely worked, and the coloured glass, it was magnificent ... The banquet was served in a huge gallery, filled with brocades and everything else, where twenty-four cupboards were placed around the house for eighty people who ate at the table with the admiral, and with him in the room were many gentleman and nobility and gentlewomen and ladies with their faces covered, and all fit but not without some difficulty ... The king and queen could see everything hidden behind latticework that was placed at the end of their table and it was confirmed that 2,200 dishes were served from the kitchen, and that it was quite a sight; in addition (were) the pastries, the jars of preserves, and above all, the empanadas creatively shaped into thousands of different castles and ships, all golden and silvery.]

At this banquet, royalty sat apart from other guests; they were central to, yet separate from, the feast. Those of rank, both men and women, joined the ambassador at the central dining table. Pinheiro de Veiga delights in describing the extravagant details that inform the spectacle. Beyond those objects already cited of gold dinner service, crystal glassware, room décor, and elaborately designed food displays, he also describes the music and other festivities that made up the event.

In figure 6.1 an engraving of the banquet that took place in Saint-Jean-de-Luz, France, to celebrate the nuptials of Louis XIV to María Teresa, princess of Spain, in 1660 includes images of elaborate platters, jewel-encrusted glassware, linens, tapestries, and musicians, that provide similar attention to detail as Pinheiro de Veiga's written account.

For the feast of Corpus Christi the following week, dinner was served to the esteemed guests at a monastery under the Duke of Lerma's patronage. The meal included the following:

Antes: ensalada, alcaparras, rábanos y espárragos; primer servicio, pasteles y ternera frita con huevos, pernil y pichones, pato albardado[10] y olla; segundo, perdiz, capones rellenos, otra olla y pierna de carnero, jigote, cabrito, ternera y cabezuelas; postres, peras cubiertas y rábanos, suplicaciones y aceitunas, otras peras y medios quesos. (83–4)

[(For) starters: salad, capers, radishes, and asparagus; first course (savoury) pies and fried veal with eggs, ham, and squab, bacon-wrapped duck and stew; second, partridge, stuffed capon, another stew, and leg of lamb, stewed meat, kid, calf and goat heads; desserts, covered pears and radishes, wafers and olives, more pears and half cheese wheels.]

Perhaps there were not 2,200 dishes served that evening, but from reading the menu, one gets a sense both of the excessiveness of the variety

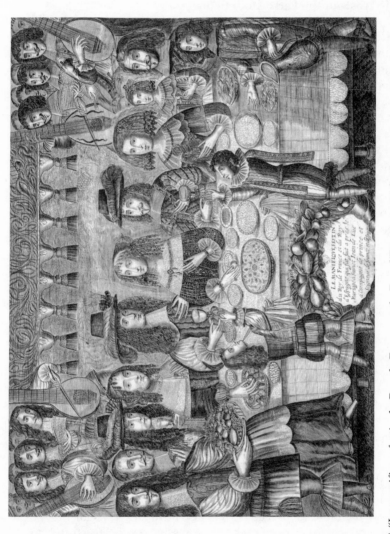

Figure 6.1 "Le manifique festin du Roy de France et du Roy d'Espagne qui fut fait après le mariage à Sainct Jean de Luc acompagné de prince et seigneur de France et d'Espagne." [The magnificent feast of the King of France and King of Spain that was celebrated after the marriage in Saint-Jean-de-Luz accompanied by the prince and lord of France and Spain] (17th c.). Image courtesy of the Département Estampes et photographie, Bibliothèque Nationale de France.

of dishes at each course and, once again, of the central role that poultry plays in the spectacle of the banquet.

Fantastic Feasts of the Early Modern Stage

Far from the realities of the king's lavish table, plays on the early modern stage often used poultry and, more generally, food in celebrations of a different kind to explore concepts of appetite, desire, and fantasy. The earliest examples are found in Lope de Rueda's *pasos* [interludes], in which food imagery is used to explore concepts of desire and taste through the creation of fantastic meals. Lope de Rueda was probably producing plays by 1540 and continued until his death in 1565 (Shergold 153). Among the works attributed to him are four plays, three pastoral colloquies, and four *autos* [allegorical plays] (González Ollé 11–12). However, he is best remembered for his *pasos* of which twenty-four are extant.

The *pasos* are characterized by their simplicity, minimal number of actors (usually two or three), and their practical function. Performed on stage between acts of a full-length production, they allowed for prop and costume change between acts, created the illusion of passing time, and lengthened the overall dramatic show (Listerman 133–4). Previously critics have treated Lope from a historical perspective, concentrating on his evolutionary role in the creation of the theatre and his role as a transitional figure who brought ideas from popular Italian theatre to Spain (Arróniz, Del Río, Johnson). Critics, particularly Carroll Johnson and Randall Listerman, have explored the vitality of Rueda's language, his theatricality, and the power of his character sketches.[11] In this chapter, I am engaging with Lope de Rueda's *pasos* to recover the historical, sexual, and social underpinnings of the use of food and food imagery in *La tierra de Jauja* [The land of Cockaigne], one of his most well-known interludes.

Although food images inform several of Lope de Rueda's plays, absent from the *pasos* are general associations of foods with hospitality, grace, bonding, compassion, and celebration. There is no spiritual significance to a food event. Instead food stimulates biological urges, promotes craving and lust, and as such is intrinsically tied to sexual desires and needs. In the *pasos* the presence or lack of food also instigates lies, violence, humiliation, and fear, basic responses to a repressive power structure.

Claude Lévi-Strauss, who maintained a structuralist approach towards foodways with emphasis on binary oppositions, for example, between the raw and the cooked, argued that, "the raw/cooked axis is characteristic of culture ... since cooking brings about the cultural transformation of the raw" (142). *La tierra de Jauja* reveals this very transformation from raw to cooked and also addresses the relationship between food and sex. Lévi-Strauss understands what Lope de Rueda did some 400 years earlier, that food acts encode social events.

The origin of the word *jauja* is uncertain, yet Corominas suggests that it derives from the name of a Peruvian city (344). It corresponds to a distorted, popular version of the mythology of Eden that took shape between the twelfth and the fourteenth centuries known as the land of Cockaigne. "The best cure for fear of hunger," the Italian culinary historian Massimo Montanari explains, "lay in dreams: dreams of tranquility and a full stomach, of abundance and overindulgence; a dream of the land of Cuccagna where the supply of food was inexhaustible and readily available" (94). He continues, "These utopian descriptions also included the suggestion of a free and happy sexuality as well as a dream of eternal youth, more directly connected to the ancient age of Saturn or the mythical Eden (95). However, the Catalan Bernart Metge understood this land in more dismal terms. For him it was a land of idleness: "There [on the island of Cockaigne], there was neither God nor nature, since there was neither order nor measure, nor anything rational" (cited in Camporesi 80). It was, then, a false paradise, a grotesque version of the biblical land of milk and honey that reflected a deteriorating food situation and an increasing difficulty to satisfy one's appetite.

In the *paso*, the two thieves, Honzigera and Panarizo, are worried about where they will find their next meal. Fortunately, they encounter the simpleton, Mendrugo, who, with a baked rice dish in hand, is on his way to visit his wife in jail. As explained more thoroughly in chapter 4, the exact origins of rice in Spain are unknown. Some speculate that it was introduced by the Byzantines in the sixth century and that later, in the eighth century, the Arabs introduced its large-scale production. In early modern Spain, rice was traditionally cooked in a broth. Ruperto de Nola's 1520 cookbook *Libre del coch* [Book on cookery] contains a recipe for "Arroz en cazuela al horno" [Baked rice casserole]:

> y cuando el arroz estuviere dentro en la cazuela echarles has tanta cantidad de caldo, como te pareciere que será menester para que se cueza no más, y cátalo que esté bueno de sal y bien grueso, y ponerlo a cocer en el horno, y un poco antes que se acabe de cocer sacarlo del horno y echarle algunas yemas de huevos enteras que sean frescos, sobre el arroz, y después tornar la cazuela al horno para que se acabe de cocer ... y este es buen arroz. (289)

[and when the rice is in the casserole dish, add the same amount of broth, as much as you think is needed to cook and no more, and taste it to make sure it has the right amount of salt and fat, and put it in the oven to cook, and right before it is done, remove it from the oven and add some whole egg yolks, make sure they are fresh, on top of the rice, and then put it back in the oven so that it finishes cooking ... and this is good rice.]

This recipe corresponds to the type of casserole Mendrugo is bringing to his wife.

In order to distract Mendrugo and consume his casserole, the two thieves create an elaborate tale of a land full of succulent delicacies described in visual, auditory, and aromatic terms. Honzigera and Panarizo alternate back and forth in their description:

HONZIGERA: Mira, en la tierra de Xauxa, hay un río de miel; y junto a él otro de leche; y entre río y río, hay una puente de mantequillas encadenada de requesones ... que están diciendo: "Coméme, coméme" ...

PANARIZO: troncos son de tozinos ... las hojas son hojuelas, y el fruto d'estos árboles son buñuelos y caen en aquel río de miel qu'ellos mismos están diciendo: "Maxcáme, maxcáme" ...

HONZIGERA: las calles están empedradas con yemas de huevos; y entre yema y yema, un pastel con lonjas de tozino ... Y assadas, qu'ellas mismas dizen: "Tragadme, tragadme" ...

PANARIZO: Hay unos assadores de trezientos passos de largo, con muchas gallinas y capones, perdizes, conejos, francolines ... Y junto a cada ave, un cochillo, que no es menester más de cortar; qu'ello mismo dize: "Engollíme, engollíme" ...

HONZIGERA: hay muchas caxas de confitura, mucho calabaçate, mucho diacitrón, muchos maçapanes, muchos confites ... Hay ragea y unas limetas de vino que él mismo s'está diziendo: "Bevéme, coméme, bevéme, coméme." (162–4)[12]

[HONZIGERA: Look, in the land of joy there is a river of honey and right next to it another of milk and between the two rivers there rises a butter fountain surrounded by lush farmer cheese that are calling out, "Eat me, eat me"...

PANARIZO: trunks of fat back ... with leaves of fried dough, and the fruit from these trees are cream puffs that drop into a river of honey and they themselves are calling out, "Chew me up, chew me up"...

HONZIGERA: the streets are paved with sweet egg yolks and between each one, a savoury pastry with strips of bacon ... And roasts, and they themselves are saying, "Swallow me, swallow me" ...

PANARIZO: There are cooking spits three hundred yards long, with tons of hens and capons, partridges, rabbits, and francolins ... And next to each bird, a sucking pig, that only needs to be sliced, that itself is saying, "Gobble me up, gobble me up."

HONZIGERA: There are many boxes of sweets, a lot of candied squash, a lot of citron, many marzipans, many sweets ... There are candies and bottles of wine that are calling out: "Drink me, eat me, drink me, eat me."]

The thieves' description begins with the raw, sensual foods of milk and honey, continues with prepared foods – butter, cheese and baked pastries – and then turns to a wide variety of cooked foods, eggs and bacon, the ever-privileged poultry (roasted hens and partridges), and rabbits. Orality is emphasized both by the spoken language and by the act of eating. "Eating, like talking, is patterned activity, and the daily menu may be made to yield an analogy with linguistic forms" (Wuthnow et al. 251). Here, the two are intrinsically linked together; story telling leads to eating. The thieves are able to achieve one oral act by producing the other; as they speak, they eat.

Orality is also emphasized by the relationship between food and sex. Martin Elkhort discusses the physiological relationship between the enjoyment of eating and the enjoyment of sex and explains that biological urges and bodily sustenance are frequently connected with sexual desire and lust (107).[13] Abstinence only heightens these needs. In *La tierra de Jauja*, Mendrugo is the nexus that links the two desires to consume.[14] He is bringing food to his wife in jail as she has been arrested for her practices as *alcahueta* [go between]. Her absence from the home suggests his unfulfilled sexual desires while his presence underscores her unfulfilled gastronomic needs. Honzigera begins the description of the land of Jauja with "un río de miel" [a river of honey] (162). Though not very nutritious, honey is psychologically pleasing and connotes erotic imagery. It is sweet, delicious, and pure. It does not need to be cooked, cultivated, or civilized. Honey is basic, primordial sustenance. It is raw pleasure, sex, animal instinct without human control, nature without culture.[15] For Honzigera and Panarizo, honey is their point of departure into a world of illusion and deception, one that advances from simple, raw pleasures into complex, "cooked" gluttony and debauchery that eventually deceives Mendrugo and leads to his defeat.

Not only does their selection of food begin with the raw and natural and end with the cooked and cultured, their verbs progress from the normal to the absurd, climaxing with gorging and gluttony. In this fantastic land, the raw food calls out, "Coméme, coméme" [Eat me, eat me] (162), the cream puffs, "Maxcáme, maxcáme" [Chew me up, chew me up] (163), the bacon and eggs, "Tragadme, tragadme" [Swallow me, swallow me] (163), and finally the poultry and sucking pig exclaim, "Engollíme, engollíme" [Gobble me up, gobble me up] (164). Their language then, begins with basic palatal gratification and culminates in lubricious gluttony. The sumptuous description ends with sweet desserts, and wine; only then does Mendrugo, previously absorbed in the opulent descriptions, realize that the two thieves have consumed his food as he has consumed their story. In exchange for such a vivid description, the two thieves satiate their appetites, but Mendrugo is left empty-handed to visit his wife, without means to fulfil either his wife's gastronomic or his own sexual appetite.

Another writer who continually uses food imagery to develop his plays is Juan Ruiz de Alarcón. In each of his twenty plays he included allusions to food, gastronomic metaphors, or plays on alimentary words. Perhaps this is not so unusual as metaphors such as "engaños que *alimenten* mi deseo" [deceptions that *feed* my desire] (*Las paredes oyen* [The walls have ears], act 1) or plays on words such as "Juan: 'Sancho amigo, *no convino*' / Sancho: '¿Sancho amigo y *no con-vino*? / Pues sin vino, ¿qué será?'" [Juan: Sancho, my friend, *he didn't agree.* Sancho: Your friend Sancho and *with no wine*? Come on, without wine, where would he be?] (*El semejante a sí mismo* [The like himself], act 1) seem common enough. However, many of Alarcón's works contain convivial scenes that develop both the play's action and the theme. Perhaps his most well known is *La verdad sospechosa* [Suspect truth] in which the main character, García, creates an elaborate banquet of the senses. When he unexpectedly runs into some of his acquaintances García needs little, if any, provocation to indulge in the most elaborate of fabrications. He charms his listeners by inventing a grandiose feast and fantastic scenario with his beloved. This famous banquet scene has been the source of a number of exciting articles, particularly James Burke's "Banquet of Sense."[16] Drawing from the medieval and Renaissance debates on the difference between man and beast, Burke argues that the hierarchy of the five senses – sight, sound, smell, taste, and touch – as presented in García's fabrication of his fantastic evening points to his over-stimulated imagination and exemplifies García as a "bestial" soul.

The Renaissance concept of spiritual and sensual pleasure is derived from Plato, who wrote that physical beauty is inferior to spiritual knowledge.

In attempting to reconcile Plato's ideas with Christianity, Marcilio Ficino privileges sight and sound while degrading the other senses.

> Since ... the mind, the sight, and the hearing are the only means by which we are able to enjoy beauty ... love is always limited to the pleasures of the mind, the eyes, and the ears ... Love is therefore limited to these three, but desire which arises from the other senses is called not love, but lust or madness. (*Commentary* 130)

However, he also recognizes that physiology and the intellect have equal importance. In a letter to Bembo, Ficino makes the convivial scene the place where both reach their maximum potential: "Only the meal [convivium] embraces all parts of man, for ... it restores the limbs, renews the humours, revives the mind, refreshes the senses and sustains and sharpens reason" (*De suffucientia* 739). For Ficino and other Renaissance intellectuals, physical functions and psychological states are interdependent; food affects the body while it also influences the workings of the mind. The banquet unifies both corporeal and spiritual elements and gives pleasure to the senses. But too much indulgence will lead to man's downfall. Ficino warns, "For whoever completely submerges himself in the darkness of the lower world will not be illumined by the rays from the higher" (*Meditations* 84).

Although Ficino allows for different interpretations on the role of the senses in man's search for a higher realm, in general, the banquet of sense is not regarded as a good thing because of its association with the gratification of the lower soul. García's speech is an opulent mixture of multiple senses which begins with a lush description of the evening:

> Entre las opacas sombras
> y opacidades espesas
> que el soto formaba de olmos
> y la noche de tinieblas,
> se ocultava una quadrada,
> limpia y olorosa mesa.   (665–70)

> [There in a river grove, deep and dark, amid
> The high and overshadowing elms was hid
> A secret clearing, black as the face of night,
> In which there stood a table, fragrant and bright.][17]

Here, sight, touch, and smell collaborate to captivate his friends' interest. In fact, throughout García's sumptuous description, the five senses blend together creating an eclectic stimulating description of the riverside festivity. García continues describing the opulent table with elaborately folded napkins and expensive silverware and crystal. He describes the intense beauty of his lady comparing her to precious stones, the spectacular fireworks that lit up the sky, and the enchanting music of clarinets, violas, flutes, guitars, and harps that softly floated through the night. Ficino also advocates a musical accompaniment to the banquet that can echo the celestial harmony and move the mind while the body is being renewed. While Ficino's writings in relation to the "banquet of the senses," particularly his commentary on Plato's symposium, are a dialogue with the classic sources, there is another tradition, inspired by Arabic writers, that also contributed to contemporary thought on the connection between food, the mental faculties, and a higher realm.

In discussing the relationship between food and magic in the Middle Ages and the Renaissance, Sarah Peterson points to the influence of Arabic cooking and the importance of fragrance. For many Muslims, the joys of this world and the next are corresponding planes of pleasure. For example, the tenth-century Arab poem "Meadows of Gold" records a history of the world that revels in the voluptuous meal that is part of the sensual paradise brought down to earth (Peterson 15). In the poem the fragrances of food take on special importance for enhancing the mental faculties, balancing the humours, and attuning one to celestial forces. Instead of the immoral gratification of the lower senses that separates man from the higher realm, for the Muslims, there exists a sense of continuity between the pleasures of eating in this world and the promised paradise to come (Peterson 12). Arabic cuisine was introduced into Europe as being at once sensual and luxurious, medicinal and divine. The senses, far from leading man astray or turning him into an animal, would help to heighten man's spiritual experience. The olfactory sense was the key. In Arabic theories, the medicinal properties of fragrance did not work directly upon the body but rather on the *spiritus*, or the breath, which was the entity that connected body and soul.

This notion of the *spiritus* was based on Galen's theory of the spirit, which, together with the Hippocratic theory of humours, accounts for the role of nutrition in both scientific literature and fiction. These theories, outlined in chapter 5, recommend a precise knowledge of the eater's temperament, the physical surroundings, and the constitution of the food to allow correct proportions to be determined in each case. For example, a person with a choleric temperament should be given cold and wet foods such as fruit, melon, and marrow; someone who is cold and wet be nature should favour hot, dry foods like unwatered wine, roasted meats, and bread. According to Galen, there are three kinds of spirits: natural, vital, and animal. The first, natural, is produced in the liver and spreads throughout the body to nourish it. In general this spirit is heavy and crude. The second type, vital, is lighter and sends vital warmth from the heart to the limbs via the arteries. Finally, the third, animal, is extremely refined and fluid. It originates in the brain and gives movement to the limbs by turning impulses from the brain into action through the nerves. Free from constraints of matter, although not totally immaterial, these corpuscles are volatile, vaporous, and mobile and circulate throughout the body. The filtering and distillation during digestion passes food products into the bloodstream and it is from the blood that, after successive refinements, the different spirits emanate.

García turns to the olfactory sense and stimulation of the spirits, after indulging in the sensual surroundings of the meal. Here, at the climax of his description, García returns to the smells:

El olfato no está ocioso
cuando el gusto se recrea,
que de espíritus süaves,
de pomos y cazolejas
y distilados sudores
de aromas, flores y yervas,
en el Soto de Madrid
se vió la región sabea.   (725–32)

[And as the tongue delighted in the taste
Of pleasure, the nose was no less busy. Graced
With soothing fragrances of potpourri
And perfume – flowers, herbs, and spicery
Distilled to sweet aromas – what had been
A grove became a heaven of muscadine.]

In this passage García points to an ancient tradition of inhaling aromatics. The practice of using aromatics, plants with fragrant properties, is recorded in the Koran. Arab chemists and magicians compounded oils for specific magical use (Rose 379). Scented flowers and herbs could camouflage unpleasant odours, promote hair growth, or increase sexual desire.[18] In short, inhaling volatile oils or aromatic substances could persuade an individual to respond in a certain way. The "pomos y cazolejas" [pomanders and cassolettes] that García describes were containers, typically made of ivory, silver, or gold with a perforated lid, that were used for diffusing aromatics. Introduced into Europe in the late sixteenth century, the former was in the shape of a ball, and suspended by a cord from the ceiling and the latter was a small box. Covarrubias explains that the pomander was typically placed over fire: "También se dize otro género de vaso, que, teniendo dentro de sí confeción de olores, se pone sobre el fuego para perfumar los aposentos, y éste se llama pomo" [There is another type of glass, that, when it has a mixture of aromas inside, is set over fire to perfume the rooms, and this is called a pomander] (876).

In the anonymous manuscript, *Manual de mugeres, en el cual se contienen muchas y diversas recetas muy buenas* [The manual for women in which is contained many, very good and diverse recipes], several recipes describe how to make aromatics for cassolettes. "Cazoleta de olor para perfumar" [Aromatic cassolette for giving off a perfume scent] typifies how these aromatics were blended. "Tomad tres onzas de menjuí, y onza y media de estoraque, y un adarme de algalia, y otro de ámbar; y si del algalia y ámbar quisiéredes poner más, será mejor. Y poned todas estas cosas en una cazuelica y ponedlas a cocer con poca lumbre" [Take three ounces of benzoin, and an ounce and a half of storax, and an adarme of civet, and another (adarme) of amber; and if you want to put in more civet and amber, it will be better. And put these things in a cooking-pot and put them to cook over a low fire] (53).[19]

García also alludes to the Sabean region, famous for its fragrant perfumes. And, as Francis Yates explains, Sabeans "were immersed in Hermetism, in both its philosophical and religious, and its magical aspects" (49). The *Picatrix*, for example, which is a comprehensive treatise on sympathetic magic, was written by an Arabic author under strong Sabean influence (Yates 49). These "aromas, flores y yervas" [aromas, flowers, and herbs] to which García alludes can only be ingredients that will further persuade his supposed beloved of his intentions and his now bewitched audience of his spectacular performance.

García's description of the grand buffet is a grand illusion, a figment of his vivid imagination, and an elaborate tale meant to impress his rivals at court. Much like the fantastic/phantasmic cook of his banquet, García has the power to persuade. He stimulates his listeners by producing opulent sights, sounds, and smells. Ironically, what is missing from his creative narrative is taste. He describes the quantity of dishes and how they were served, but the food's taste is all but absent from his fabrication.

Entre tanto, se sirvieron
treynta y dos platos de cena
....
Las frutas y las bevidas,
en fuentes y taças hechas
del cristal ...   (713–14; 717–19)

[And as they played, the waiters served the food –
Thirty two courses for the main meal
....
The fresh fruits, juices, wines, even the water
Were served in frosty crystal bowls and glasses ...]

The sights, sounds, and smells that he conjures up do not succeed in winning his love, who never does attend such a festivity; rather they enchant his listeners and win him the envy of his rivals. "Words related to the stomach," Michael Jeanneret writes, "awaken in language all sorts of dormant powers ... [G]randiose feasts and fantastic scenarios ... overturn the principles of moderation" (2). The banquet, then, like the theatre itself, is an illusion; what is real is the language that excites the palate and charms the ear. This connection between language and illusion becomes even clearer in Ruiz de Alarcón's *La cueva de Salamanca* [The cave of Salamanca].

This drama is based on the legend of the cave where the devil's magic was practised.[20] The play begins as the main character, Diego, runs into trouble with the authorities after pulling a foolish prank. To escape incarceration, he, along with his *gracioso* servant, Zamudio, and another friend, seek refuge in the house of the French magician Enrico. Shortly afterwards, the Marqués de Villena – a historical figure who, according to legend, practised magic in the caves of Toledo and Salamanca – arrives and promises to help the young students get out of trouble. The play continues with a series of spectacular magical acts – changing food into coal, a woman into a lion, a human into a bronze statue and back again. Paralleling Enrico's and the Marqués's magical activities are the love relationships of Diego and Doña Clara and of Zamudio and Lucía.

The play ends with a debate on the validity of magic, the king pardoning the foolish students for their mischief, and the lovers' promises of marriage to one another.

While "gastro-humour" seasons the entire play, I would like to focus on one particular scene when Zamudio, the servant, upon returning from Madrid, describes a woman he saw at the theatre in terms of the food that surrounded her.[21]

... en la comedia la vi
puesta en un aparador
....
Miraba yo desde el banco
en los platos relumbrantes
de almendra y pasa los antes,
los postres de manjar blanco.
Tal fiesta allí se celebra,
que halla cualquier convidado
platos de carne y pescado,
como en viernes de Ginebra.
Al salir se han de servir
los platos de la vïanda
que al entrar son de demanda,
y de vïanda al salir.
Vieras, mirando a estos platos,
mil mancebitos hambrientos
cual suelen mirar atentos
carne colgada los gatos.   (1007–8, 1013–28)

[At the play I saw her
at a sideboard
.....
I was looking from the bench
At the dazzling dishes
Of almonds and raisins as first course,
And blancmange for dessert.
There was such a celebration there
That any guest would find
Dishes of meat and fish
As if it were a Friday in Geneva.
Upon leaving the main course
Dishes are served,

The very ones everyone wants
Right as they enter
But are available only when they leave
You will see, staring at these dishes,
Thousands of hungry young men
Who, like felines, fix their gaze on
Racks of meat.]

Attending the theatre was more than just watching and listening to the play. As Zamudio points out, often the ladies who attended the show were of greater interest than the show itself. But instead of describing one particular woman, Doña Flor, in terms of her own beauty, he does so through the tantalizing food that surrounds her. His description appeals to taste and begins with the sweet hors d'oeuvres, almonds, and raisins, and dessert, blancmange, a popular sweet milk and poultry pudding usually flavoured with sugar and almonds. These sumptuous treats, like the woman's flirtations, are exciting but not totally fulfilling. The main dishes, *las vïandas*, are the real sustenance that the "mancebitos hambrientes" [hungry young men] hope to receive after the show ("que al entrar son de demanda/ y de vïanda al salir" [the very ones everyone wants right as they enter/ But are available only when they leave]).

Returning to Ficino's notion of indulging the senses and falling into "bestial love," these "mancebitos" are transformed into felines and the women into degrading racks of meat tantalizingly hanging over them. However, the young men's desires of consumption are left insatiate as the women, undecided about which suitor they should accept favours from, end up accepting from none.

Ellas no pueden sufrillo
....
y con tal gusto y espacio
siguen materia tan mala
que en regala o no regala
gastan todo el cartapacio.   (1029; 1037–40)

[They cannot take it
......
and with their taste and space
they see such bad products
that in merely thinking it over
they expend all their energy.]

As we have also seen in Lope de Rueda's interlude, using food desires to describe sexual desire is an easily understood metaphor. What is unusual, however, is that this scene occurs at the theatre, emphasizing even further that ingestion (of the food) and expression (of the theatre) are allied activities of taste and pleasure.

In the Renaissance there are hundreds of manuals and treatises that discuss food in terms of its effect on the physical and moral being.[22] Together, these works create a mythology of food that "expresses both a morality of pleasure and the demands of a refined culture, both a popular archetype and an erudite tradition" (Jeanneret 13). Erasmus was clearly intent on using rituals of meals to change manners and to make society more disciplined (Jeanneret 43). His aim was to control bodily pleasure and restrain sensuality. In *De civilitate morum puerilium* [A handbook on good manners for children] (1530) he argues that the observance of etiquette is an outward sign of inner distinction.[23] But these types of manuals would also promote affectation. Good conduct risks becoming a series of automatic gestures, an inauthentic system. Actors on the stage like those engaged in social dining experiences dealt in artificial forms adopting mannerisms and speeches to create works of art.

Another comic moment on the stage that deals with festivities and biological urges to satisfy both the stomach and the libido, is found in Cervantes' own version of *La cueva de Salamanca*. In his *entremés* [interlude], the cuckold Pancracio returns unexpectedly to his home where his wife, Leonarda, and servant, Cristina, have invited their lovers (the sacristan and the barber) to a dinner party. Another unexpected guest, a student from Salamanca (who Leonarda fondly refers to as *Salamanqueso*, thus highlighting the importance of food in the play), explains to Pancracio that he is a student of the cave of Salamanca and practises the dark arts. To satisfy Pancracio's curiosity, the student creates his own play within the play – once again focusing on acts of orality – and summons two devils (the respective lovers) and sets the stage for a grand banquet.

As the one-act play opens Cristina describes the contents of a laundry basket that the priest has discreetly sent to them:

una canasta de colar, llena de mil regalos y de cosas de comer, que no parece sino [u]no de los serones que da el rey el Jueves Santo a sus pobres; sino que la canasta es de Pascua, porque hay en ella empanadas, fiambreras, manjar blanco, y dos capones que aún no están acabados de pelar, y todo género de fruta de la que hay ahora; y, sobre todo, una bota de hasta una arroba de vino, de lo de una oreja,[24] que huele que traciende.

[a laundry basket, filled with hundreds of gifts and things to eat, it looks just like one of those large baskets the king gives to the poor on Holy Thursday, but it is really one of those Easter baskets, because inside there are savoury pies, cold cuts, blancmange, and two capons not yet fully plucked, and all kinds of seasonal fruit, and best of all, there's a one-gallon wine skin that has an excellent wine with a transcendent aroma.]

One of the key items in the basket, and in Ruiz de Alarcón's version of the play, is blancmange, a dish that appears in all early modern cooking manuals and was as popular in Spain then as paella is today.[25] It was associated with upper class dining, feasts, and special celebrations. Simón Palmer explains that it was eaten on special occasions: "se entrega como recompensa especial y en determinadas fiestas a algunas personalidades" [it was given as a special reward and on certain holidays to certain personalities] (*La cocina* 144). Into the early seventeenth century, the main ingredients for blancmange were hen breast, milk, and flour and it was generally thought of as a dessert or sweet snack, although it was also consumed to help improve the health of the convalescent. Over time, it lost poultry as a main ingredient and today it is served as a custard dessert.

In Martínez Montiño's manual the standard recipe for *manjar blanco* [blancmange] offers very specific instructions on how to boil and shred the hen breast, and on alternating milk and rice flour, carefully cooking the mixture before adding the sugar. His cooking instructions are very specific, "pon el cazo sobre unas trevedes con buena lumbre de tizon de carbon, y traelo a una mano con mucho cuydado, porque no se queme, ni se ahume, y quando comenzare a quajar batelo muy bien: tardará en cocerse tres quartos de hora, poco mas o menos" [put the pot on a trivet over strong charcoal embers, and stir it with one hand very carefully so that it doesn't burn or get infused with smoke and when it begins to thicken, stir vigorously; it should take approximately 45 minutes to cook] (228). Several additional recipes for blancmange include in *buñuelos* [cream puffs], over *picatostes* [fried bread], as *frutillas* [pastries], *cazolillas* [small custards], and *torta* [pie] (229–33).

Another indication that this poultry dish was seen as privileged food was how the government regulated it. In an effort to contain outward signs of the upwardly mobile in the late sixteenth century, the court instituted a series of statutes like one in 1592, in which blancmange, along with cream puffs, preserves, candied fruit, wafers, and other sweets, became illegal to sell on the street. "Las penas a los contraventores eran ejemplares: 100 azotes y dos años de destierro. En caso de que quien vendiera fuera un criado, a su amo le caerían dos años de destierro y 2.000 mrs." [The penalty for violators was exemplary: 100 lashes and two years of exile. And in cases in which servants were selling, the master would receive two years of exile and (a fine of) 2,000 maravedis] (cited in Alvar-Ezquerra 316).

The two capons that accompany the blancmange are additional markers of the festive occasion and also add humour by emphasizing the sexual tensions at play. When Leandra and Cristina want to know if the student can be trusted to keep their secret and help out with the preparations, they inquire if he knows how to skin a bird. "Desa manera, ¿quién duda sino que sabrá pelar no sólo capones, sino gansos y avutardas? Y, en esto del guardar secreto, ¿cómo le va?" [So, there's no doubt that you can strip clean not only capons but also geese and great bustards? And, keeping a secret? How are you at that?] Certain birds were euphemisms for types of men. In the case of *capón*, an effeminate man, quite possibly a reference to Leandra's husband, who is clearly not meeting his wife's needs. *Ganso* was slang for a simpleton, again, a passing reference to Pancracio who naively accepts as truth the tales that the student spins, and *avutarda,* for hardened criminal, bringing home the idea that the student can take care of any type of situation he might encounter.

As the *salamanqueso* sets the stage for consuming capons, blancmange and the rest of the goodies from the basket, like Zamudio and García and even earlier like Honzigera and Panarizo, he understands the intimate relationship between one act of orality and another. They all acknowledge this same power of food fantasy through fantastic fabrications. The student creates a play within a play, Zamudio is both in the play and at the play, García dazzles his listeners with his fictional food fantasy, and Honzigera and Panarizo create, through their words, an alternate space of desire. In doing so, all of the characters assert the legitimacy of natural instincts and restore the rights of the body and its impulses. Pleasures which are normally covert or repressed can be indulged, at least to a certain extent. In *La tierra de Jauja,* Honzigera y Panarizo are fully aware of the connection between creative expression and ingestion and, at least briefly, are able to convince their listener of a land of unrestrained access to food while they partake in their own unrestrained access to Mendrugo's baked rice dish. Zamudio, through comic relief, promotes a certain freedom or pleasure that, like the vision of women and food, offers a reprieve from society's conquest to tame the senses. García, through his ethereal banquet of the senses, taps into the connection between creative expression and ingestion as he, at least briefly, convinces his listeners of his superlative status at court through the invention of his banquet. And the student of Salamanca enhances his poetic illusions to secure gastronomic indulgences while others around him avoid punishment for their attempts at sexual fulfilment.

From Lope de Rueda to Ruiz de Alarcón and Cervantes, writers use food to reveal its function of fulfilling primary needs of food and sex and thus demonstrate the complexities between food and social systems. As a final note of interest, food points to the notion of consumption not only biologically, but also economically. There is a direct relationship between the consumption of food and the consumption of the text as a commodity. In the case of Lope de Rueda, his interludes, like cookbooks themselves, reveal a central connection between food and the written word. Elise-Noël McMahon reminds us in her article "*Gargantua, Pantagruel*, and Renaissance Cooking Tracts: Texts for Consumption" that "the discourse of cookery both produces and constrains a mixture ... the identity of the dish is determined by key ingredients, but that very determination opens the dish to variations potentially infinite" (193). She goes on to explain that there is no one fixed meaning in cookbooks, but rather, their value shifts as in a marketplace (194). In this way, the writing of recipes broke the absolute dependence of transmission of culinary knowledge through apprenticeship. As a writer, director, and actor for the stage, Lope de Rueda was able to control his work more than later playwrights who had to give up their text to directors and actors. The rapidly changing economic infrastructure forced distance between all involved in theatre. Lope's sustenance was this direct relation between poet and consumer, much like the cooking manuals that directly connected cooks, their dishes, and the consumer. In these moments of celebration, we see the workings of both culinary and literary arts and how they respond to appetite, desire, and fulfilment of fantasies. Whether it be on the stage, in the cooking manuals, or at the king's table, poultry ranks as one of the defining images of self-fulfilment within a celebratory event.

Chapter Seven

La sobremesa: Final Reflections on the Discourse of Food in Early Modern Spain

Shortly after the publication of Cervantes' novel *El ingenioso hidalgo don Quijote de la Mancha*, scholars began to debate how this masterpiece engages food matters and explain (and argue about) the meaning of foodstuffs and foodways found within its pages. The second line of the novel describes the protagonist through the food he eats, and with these words, Cervantes opens the door to understanding better Spain's culinary and, in a larger sense, cultural and social history. What "el señor Quijada o Quesada" ate reflects simply who he was socially and economically. As his persona changes from humble hidalgo to knight errant so too do his food choices and thus, mutton, *duelos y quebrantos*, and lentils never appear again in the novel while the *olla* and the *palomino* appear infrequently.

However, this novel alone does not tell the whole story. I write with a smile but also with firm conviction that all writers play with their food and that these actions reveal much more about Spain's culture and history than what is on the plate. Whether recording history, creating literature, or writing with another purpose, writers inform us about modes of production and distribution, food's relationship to health and human relationships, how food defines group identity, and how it provides communities with a medium of communication. In writing this book on representations of food imagery in both literary and non-literary texts, I am even more convinced of this truth. We see the playfulness most obviously in the fiction of literary artists like Cervantes, Quevedo, and many playwrights. The puns and carefully crafted food metaphors enrich readers' engagement with both the written and the performed texts.

For me, the complexity of food discourse in early modern Spain is most engaging when read in terms of the habitus of the very writers who are crafting these diverse texts. First is the issue of the cooking manuals themselves. Chapter 1, with its much-needed overview of pre-1700 cooking manuals in Spain, raises its own questions about the place of manuscripts and cookbooks in Spain's culinary history. Certainly these texts are essential as they focus on food and its preparation and presentation in ways that no other discourse provides. In this light, cooking manuals are essential to understanding Spanish culinary history. Yet, the works are problematic and potentially misleading. If studied without the context of other pieces of textual evidence, the cooking manuals can feed fantasies about culinary history. Written exclusively for contemporary and future cooks in the palace who prepare meals for the king, their audience (both the cook who consults the text and the monarch who enjoys the results of the culinary creations) is indeed limited. What then, can these manuals teach us about food practices of the overwhelming majority of the early modern population? Future studies must be particularly sensitive to this very issue. That said, reading these invaluable works in the context of other sources of evidence provides enormous insights into early modern food practices.

In addition to cooking manuscripts and books, the discourse of food in early modern Spain is made up of a myriad of voices and includes those of great works of fiction, travel logs, legal documents, and advice manuals. In turn, each of these voices is formed by a set of dispositions that have been learned, "inculcated" as Bourdieu would say, and inevitably reflects a series of social conditions that define how these values came to be. For this reason studying comparatively court cookbooks, village regulations, Inquisitional transcriptions, New World voyage logs, advice manuals directed toward women, and so on, provides scholars today with a fuller understanding of the social conditions that inform early modern Spain. According to Bourdieu, the habitus generates "practices and perceptions, works and appreciations, which concur with the conditions of existence of which the habitus is itself the product" (13). Consequently, examining closely the rich diversity of food discourse and digesting its significance has led to understanding the circumstances of their construction.

Not only do these literary and non-literary texts reveal food's role in the changing state of Spanish cultural and social history, but also, by examining representations of food in literary texts, we can understand its role in shaping early modern fiction itself. I mentioned earlier food metaphors that allow writers to develop their wit and sharp, social satire. We see multiple examples of food's comic role in the plays of

Lope, Calderón, and especially, Tirso de Molina, in which the *gracioso* (the comic relief figure) often adds gastro-humour to the text. As early as Lope de Rueda's *pasos*, food not only serves as a comic device but also as an actant that takes on an integral structural role in the one-act plays. This structural device is particularly evident in the case of the picaresque genre. Take, for example, Quevedo's *El buscón*. Here, meals shape the protagonist's character and life choices as Pablos grows into manhood. In book 1, food abuses both during carnival, when the crowd fires rotten food at Pablos, and at El Cabras's boarding school, when Pablos and his companions are literally starving, are moments of rude awakening for the picaresque hero. In book 2, as he settles into his life-style at the University of Alcalá, the reader understands that pilfering food, stealing from food vendors, and colluding with the housekeeper are regular actions that shape Pablos's future. Book 2 culminates in a feast of questionable meat pies and drunken debauchery among the unsavoury lowlife of Segovia that Pablos utterly rejects as he seeks to carve out his own space in the world. In book 3, as Pablos tries out his new lifestyle in the capital, food once again lends structure to the work. "Gentlemen" in search of food throughout the city, knowledge of the prison system and the rampant corruption exemplified through food bribery, and Pablos's attempt to pursue a woman of means through a picnic lunch he organizes in the Casa de Campo are additional ex-amples of how food imagery guides the reader through Pablos's literal and metaphoric journey. The novel closes in Seville where Pablos, over a shared meal and a lot of booze, is introduced to the criminal under-world and initiated into his newly found lifestyle.

Additionally, food imagery enlivens the pages of fiction with semiotic clues that reveal erotic desire, ethnic identity, cultural trends, and class hierarchy to name but a few of the salient topics explored in this study. From our postmodern perspective, readers also understand that food im-agery often destabilizes the text. In the meals and culinary conversations shared across *Don Quixote* it is Sancho who becomes the central char-acter while Don Quijote is absent or plays a secondary role. One need only think of Don Quijote and Sancho's journey in part II of the novel. At each culinary turn – the squires Sancho and Tomas Celial sharing a rab-bit empanada, the feast at Camacho's wedding, the governor's palace in Barataria, and the dialogue with an inn owner on the road to Barcelona – it is Sancho, not the errant knight, who is central to the plot development.

Returning to what we learn about food and society through literature, as the novel begins, Cervantes establishes his protagonist as belonging to a time, a place, and a social class through the food he eats on a day-to-day basis. We have learned that modest and traditional dishes reveal his humble status within the hidalgo hierarchy and remind readers of the political ramifications of food choices. These descriptions also reveal the diverse ethnicities that are so much a part of Spanish culture, the gender differences that surround food practices, the early modern understanding of medical practices, and the cultural norms of celebrations. With each phrase that describes how Alonso Quijano spent three quarters of his income, we form a deeper understanding about social constraints, national identity, and cultural heritage. We also understand how important both the medieval and early modern eras are to the development of Spain's gastronomy. Mutton as the preferred meat of choice has endured through today with the predilection for lamb at times of celebration. And while poultry no longer commands the same respect as food fit for royalty, it still holds its place as a healthy food option. Regarding plant-based foodstuffs, speculation still remains as to why some became the basis of Spanish cuisine: tomato, potato, pepper, eggplant, rice, lentils, garbanzos, parsley, and saffron, for example; while others never became part of the cuisine or faded from popularity: corn, peanuts, couscous, cilantro, and ginger.

In addition to enriching our understanding of how the representation of food influences the development of fiction, this monograph analyses and speculates on the changing sets of fields and dispositions that impacted, consciously or not, the writing of the authors studied. At the same time, I approach these texts acutely aware of my own role, motivations, and actions in the identification process.[1] My own set of fields and dispositions includes the fact that I am trained in literary studies and grounded in the humanities. As such, I have transferred analytic skills that I apply in the study of works of fiction to non-literary texts and in the process have drawn from the work of sociologists and anthropologists to get a fuller view of Spain's culinary heritage. As a twenty-first-century, American, female literary critic exploring works of primarily male, European writers from over 400 years ago, I am fully aware that I bring to this study a series of motivations and actions most likely not shared by those whose works I am studying. My interest in this project comes from a deep-rooted desire to explore fully food's connection to identity and to understand why certain foods were privileged while others disappeared from Spain's culinary heritage. In doing so, I have brought together New World contact points, laws prohibiting food sales and modes of preparation, religious mores, and perceptions of health in ways that were impossible to perceive as they were unfolding in early modern Spain. For example, by comparing Hispano-Muslim cooking manuals of the fourteenth century with a sixteenth-century picaresque novel, I can gather evidence that many of the same foodstuffs where consumed by people of diverse social standing. By comparing a manuscript that targets women who manage their own households, a university cookbook, and one written to cater to the tastes of the king, I can analyse how food practices in these very different spaces unfolded in ways that at times overlapped and at times ran their own course. And by comparing cooking manuals written between the thirteenth and the eighteenth centuries, I can document how specific foodstuffs were perceived and valued by society's most elite.

Work remains to be done in this burgeoning area of food representation in literary (and non-literary) texts in early modern Spain. The role of food in the lives of monastic men and women, in the staging of the *comedia*, as a motif of gastro-humor and its social significance, as it defines gender identity are a few of the areas that merit further examination. If nothing else, my hope is that this work will inspire other scholars to select, speculate, and analyse the myriad of ways writers play with their food.

Moving forward some 400 years and shifting continents, I would like to close this study with an anecdote that connects Cervantes and early modern food practices with the ever-changing world of gastronomy. José Ramón Andrés Puerta, the young Asturian-born and Bulli-trained chef who is owner of over a dozen restaurants from Washington DC to Los Angeles is a Quixotic figure. His visionary project of introducing Spanish cuisine to America and improving how Americans consider food is reminiscent of Cervantes' knight errant. In 2011, José Andrés was named the James Beard Foundation's Outstanding Chef, and in 2012, appeared among *TIME* magazine's most influential people. He thrives on simplicity and creativity, two essentials of Cervantes' work. In a TedTalk a few years back, he explained the importance of finding creativity in the simplest of places and not being afraid to move beyond one's comfort zone.

> In order to be creative, people of the world, we have to make sure we will not be afraid to look beyond the horizon, that we don't know what's behind. To take really that challenge of saying. "I'm going to move away from my comfort zone and I'm going to reach beyond what I don't know." This is really where we become creative. (2.46–3.16)

Consciously or not, his words recall the ethos of Cervantes and his ability to create inspirational and enduring works of art. What José Andrés, his predecessor Ferran Adrià, and a handful of other chefs have done with Spanish gastronomic heritage closely parallels the work of both Cervantes (in the realm of literature) and culinary masters of the early modern era. All keenly understand the importance of drawing from firmly established traditions as they look forward, renovate, and invent anew.

Appendix of Recipes

All selections in this appendix are discussed in previous chapters. Some highlight the uniqueness of the dish relative to all medieval and early modern cookbooks while others exemplify the culinary trends that continued through the centuries and across social, religious, and ethnic divides. If appropriate, an introductory comment precedes the recipe.

Kitāb al-tabīj fi l-Magrib wa-l-Andalus fi 'asr al-muwahhudin li-mu' allif mayhul (Tratado sobre cocina en el Magrib y al-Andalus en época almohade, de autor desconocido) [The book of cooking in Maghreb and Andalus in the era of Almohads, by an unknown author]. C. 1228–43.

1. RECETA DE FIDEOS [NOODLE RECIPE] (228–9)

This recipe indicates an early presence of pasta on the Iberian Peninsula (long before the travels of Marco Polo to Asia).

Esto se hace de masa y tiene tres clases: la alargada a modo de trigo, la redondeada a modo de grano de cilantro, que se llama en Bugía y su región *ḥamīṣ*, y la que se hace delgada con la delgadez del *kagīd* [hoja de papel] y es una comida de mujeres; la cuecen con calabaza, aromas y grasa; es una de los *qaṭāif*. La manera de cocer los fideos es como la de los macarrones.

[This is made from dough in three different ways: long like wheat, round like a coriander seed, which in Bugia and the surrounding region is called *ḥamīṣ*, and the thin type which has the thinness of *kagīd* (a sheet of paper). It is food for women, cooked with bottle squash, aromatics, and fat; it is one of the *qaṭāif* (shredded phyllo doughs). The way to cook noodles is similar to cooking macaroni.]

2. HECHURA DE LA COCCIÓN DE LOS MACARRONES [THE WAY TO COOK MACARONI] (229)

The author cooks the broth down leaving a rich pasta dish. A final note indicates that this same technique can be used just as easily for rice or noodles.

Se toma carne de las colas, de las piernas, del pecho, de la cintura y lo que haya de ellas que sea graso, se corta y se pone en la olla con sal, cebolla, pimienta, cilantro seco y aceite; se pone a un fuego moderado y se cuece hasta estar en sazón; luego se saca y se clarifica la salsa, se vuelve a la olla y se le añade mantequilla, grasa tierna y aceite dulce; cuando ha hervido, se ponen fideos finos en cantidad suficiente, se hierve y se agita suavemente y cuando se seca el agua y está a punto, se aparta del fuego y se deja un poco; se vierte en la fuente y se iguala hasta que se disuelva la grasa; luego se toma, si la quieres, cocida como está o frita y se alínea en la fuente, se maja algo de ello en los fideos y se espolvorea con canela y jengibre y se presenta; con esta receta se hacen el arroz y los fideos.

[Take meat from the tail, legs, breast, belly, and anything that is fatty, chop it up, and place it in a pot with salt, onion, pepper, coriander, and oil, on medium heat and cook until done. Remove it and clarify the sauce; then return it to the pot and add butter, a delicate fat, and sweet oil.[1] When that comes to a boil, add just the right amount of fine noodles, boil, and gently stir until the water is gone and it is perfect. Remove from the flame and rest. Turn it onto a platter, let it settle and the fat dissolve. Enjoy it as is or fried and arranged on the platter. Mash some of the meat into the noodles and sprinkle with cinnamon and ginger and serve it. This recipe can also be used for rice or noodles.]

3. TORTA CON CARNE DE CORDERO Y ESPINACAS, LECHE FRESCA Y MANTECA FRESCA [LAMB MEAT PIE WITH SPINACH, FRESH MILK, AND FRESH ANIMAL FAT] (227)

This is one of the few recipes that provides a name and a place of origin.

La hacía en Córdoba en las días de primavera el médico Abū-l-Hasan al-Bunānī, Dios se apiade de él y nos perdone a nosotros y a él. Se toma carne de cordero graso, se corta y se pone en la olla con sal, jugo de cebolla, pimienta, cilantro seco, alcaravea y aceite; se pone al fuego y cuando se acaba de hacer, se le pone la espinaca cortada y lavada en la cantidad suficiente, queso fresco amasado y manteca fresca; cuando ha terminado de hacerse, se saca la olla – del fuego – y se le vierte la manteca y habrá migas de pan de levadura moderada, sobre las que se pone su carne, y si le faltaba la carne de cordero, le hacía torta de espinacas y queso fresco, manteca fresca y las especias ya citadas y huevos en vez de carne.

[This dish was made in Cordoba in springtime by the doctor Abu al Hasan al-Bunani, may God take pity on him and forgive him and all of us. Take fatty lamb meat, cut it, and place it in a pot with salt, onion juice, black pepper, coriander, caraway, and oil. Put it on the fire and when it is done, add the right amount of spinach that has been chopped and washed, fresh cheese, and fresh animal fat. When it is done, remove the pot from the flame and pour off the animal fat and you should have large breadcrumbs made with moderately leavened bread over which you will pour the meat. If you have no lamb, you could make spinach and fresh cheese pies with the fresh animal fat and already cited spices and eggs instead of meat.]

4. PERDIZ JUDÍA [JEWISH PARTRIDGE] (102)

Se limpia la perdiz y se sazona con sal; luego se baten sus entrañas con almendra y piñones y se añade a esto *almorí* macerado, aceite, un poco de zumo de cilantro, pimienta, canela, canela de la China, espliego, cinco huevos y lo que baste de carne; se hierven dos huevos y se rellena con esto el relleno de la perdiz, se le recubre con los huevos hervidos y que esté el relleno entre la piel y la carne y algo de él en el interior de la perdiz; entonces se coge una olla nueva y se ponen en ella cuarto cucharadas de aceite, media de *almorí* macerado y dos de sal. Mete en ello la perdiz y ponla al fuego, después de reforzar su cubierta con pasta y re-muévela seguido hasta que se iguale, y cuando se seque la salsa, descu-bre su tapadera y échale media cucharada de vinagre, brotes de cidra y de menta y casca sobre ella dos o tres huevos; luego pon sobre ella una cazuela de barro y una olla de cobre, llena de brasas encendidas hasta que se tueste, y luego a su alrededor, hasta que se tueste el otro lado, y se fría todo; luego ponla en una fuente y pon a su alrededor el relleno y adórnala con las yemas con que has adornado la olla y espolvoréalo con pimienta y canela, después con azúcar y preséntalo, si Dios quiere.

[Clean the partridge and season it with salt. Then pound together the entrails with almonds and pine-nuts and add crushed *almorí*,[2] oil, a little cilantro juice, black pepper, cinnamon, Chinese cinnamon, lavender, five eggs, and any additional meat that may be necessary. Boil two eggs. Stuff the bird with the stuffing mixture by spreading it between the flesh and the skin, and with what remains, insert into the cavity along with the two boiled eggs. In a new pot add four tablespoons of oil, half (a tablespoon) of *almorí*, and two of salt. Put the bird in the pot and place it over the flame after you have covered it with dough and evened it out by shaking the pot. When the sauce has been reduced, open the cover and add a half-tablespoon of vinegar, citron and mint shoots, and, finish with two or three eggs broken over the top. Put a clay cover on top and a copper pot filled with burning embers until it browns and then move the embers all around browning all sides. Let cool and serve on a platter garnished with hard-boiled egg yolks and sprinkled with black pepper, cinnamon, and finally, with sugar, and present the dish, God willing.]

5. PLATO JUDÍO DE BERENJENAS RELLENAS CON CARNE [EGGPLANT STUFFED WITH MEAT, JEWISH STYLE] (266–7)

Se escaldan las berenjenas y se les sacan sus semillas y se las deja enteras; se toma carne de pierna de cordero, se pica con sal, pimienta, canela, canela de la China y espliego, se bate con la clara de ocho huevos y se separan seis yemas; con ese relleno se rellenan las berenjenas; luego se toman tres ollas y se ponen en una de ellas cuatro cucharadas de aceite, zumo de cebolla, especias, aromas y una cucharada de agua olorosa de rosas, piñones, un brote de cidra, otro de menta y lo suficiente de sal y agua; se hierve ligeramente y se le echa la mitad de las berenjenas rellenas y pone en una olla segunda una cucharada de vinagre, cebolla picada, especias y aromas, una rama de tomillo, otra de brezo, hoja de cidra, dos ramos de hinojo, una cucharada de aceite, almendra, garbanzos remojados y cosa de medio dírhem[3] de azafrán molido y tres ajos cortados; se empapa en agua suficiente hasta que hierva varias veces y se echa en ella el resto de las berenjenas rellenas y se pone en la tercera olla cucharada y media de vinagre fuerte, cebolla majada, almendra, piñones, un brote de brezo y hojas de cidra; se rocía con agua de rosas y se espolvorea con aromas y se adorna la segunda con yemas cortadas, brezo cortado y se espolvorea con aromas; se corta sobre la tercera un huevo cocido con brezo, se espolvorea con pimienta y se presenta.

[Scald the eggplant, remove seeds, and leave them whole. Take meat from a leg of lamb and mince it with salt, pepper, cinnamon, Chinese cinnamon, and lavender. Separate eight eggs, whip the egg whites, and reserve six yolks. Fill the eggplant with this filling. Then take three pots and in one of them put four tablespoons of oil, onion juice, spices, aromatic herbs, and a tablespoon of fragrant rose water, pine nuts, a sprig of citron, one of mint, and enough water and salt. Simmer and place half the stuffed eggplant in the pot. In the second pot place a tablespoon of vinegar, minced onion, spices and aromatic herbs, a sprig of thyme, one of heather, a citron leaf, two sprigs of fennel, a tablespoon of oil, almonds, soaked garbanzos, and about a half a dram of ground saffron and three chopped cloves of garlic. Add enough water to cover it all and bring to a boil several times. Add the remaining stuffed eggplant. In the third pot, add a tablespoon and a half of strong vinegar, mashed onion, almonds, pine nuts, a sprig of heather, and citron leaves. Rub in rose water and sprinkle with aromatic herbs. Garnish the second pot with slices of egg yolk, chopped heather, and sprinkle with aromatic herbs. Sprinkle over the third pot a chopped boiled egg and heather, sprinkle with black pepper, and serve.]

6. RECETA DE COL BLANCA [WHITE CABBAGE RECIPE] (269)

Se toma carne joven, gorda y se corta en una olla con sal, cebolla, pimienta, cilantro seco, alcaravea y aceite; se pone a un fuego moderado y cuando está casi en sazón, se toma repollo gordo de col, se tira su exterior y se toma su corazón y lo cercano a él, se le limpia de sus hojas, se mete el cuchillo entre os ojos y se tira el resto de las hojas hasta que quede blanco como el nabo; se pela y se corta en pedazos proporcionados y se echa en la olla, después de escaldarlos, como se ha indicado. Cuando se ha terminado, se saca al rescoldo y se exprime sobre él algo de zumo de cilantro y el que quiera este plato terciado, le añade vinagre y azafrán.

[Take young, fatty meat and cut it up (and place it) in a pot with salt, onion, black pepper, coriander, caraway, and oil. Put it on a moderate fire and when it is nearly done, take a cabbage filled with flowers, throw away the outside and take the heart and surrounding parts, and remove its leaves. Stick a knife between the "eyes" and throw away the rest of the leaves until it remains white like the turnip. Peel it and cut it up into even-sized pieces and place them in the pot, after boiling them, as has been indicated. When they are done, remove them from the flame to the embers and squeeze some cilantro juice over them. If you want this dish *terciado*, add vinegar and saffron.][4]

7. EMPANADA DE "RAGUĪFES" EN SARTÉN [NAPOLEAN-STYLE EMPANADA IN A FRYING PAN] (144)

This recipe resembles a Napoleon with alternating layers of thin dough and sweet cream. These layers are then covered with a thicker crust, soaked in a condensed milk mixture, and later sprinkled with cinnamon and sugar.

Se amasan dos libras de harina de trigo y se hace con ellas un pan muy delgado, se cuece un poco en el horno, se toma vaso y medio de leche y se agitan en ella ocho huevos batidos con algo de harina; se cuece al fuego y se toma otra sartén nueva y una libra de crema y se pone algo de ella en el fondo de la sartén y algo de leche y se le coloca encima un pan delgado, según esta receta, hasta que se acabe el pan delgado y la crema; luego se pone encima de la sartén un pan grueso que la cubra toda; luego envíalo al horno y cuando se ha cocido algo, envía por él y rocíalo con el resto de la leche hasta que se termine y la embeba toda; luego se vuelve al horno hasta completarse su cocción, luego se envía por ella y se pone en una fuente y se rompe la sartén suavemente para que salga entero; luego se corta con un cuchillo en dos pedazos separados, se espolvorea con azúcar y se presenta, si Dios quiere.

[Knead two pounds of wheat flour and with this make a very thin bread, bake it a little in the oven. Shake together a cup and a half of milk and eight eggs that have been beaten with some flour and cook over the fire. In a new pan, with a pound of cream, put some in the bottom of the pan together with some of the milk mixture and place on top (of the liquid) a thin piece of bread, according to this recipe, until all the cream and thin bread are used up. Then, put on top of the pan a thick piece of bread that covers it all and place it in the oven and when it is partially cooked, remove it, and pour on the rest of the milk until it is all gone and the dish is completely soaked. Put it back in the oven until it has finished cooking. Take it out and put it on a platter and gently break the pan so that the dish comes out whole. Then, cut it into two separate halves, dust with sugar, and serve, God willing.]

8. DULCE DE AZÚCAR [SUGAR SWEETNESS] (274)

Se toma una libra de azúcar molido y de harina candeal majada hasta que se haga como la harina de sémola, un tercio de libra; se le añade huevos y se bate con ello; entonces se pone la sartén a un fuego ligero con una libra de aceite dulce y cuando éste hierve, se vierten en él estas migas y el azúcar batido con huevos; se remueve al fuego ligero hasta que se ligue y se enfríe; se espolvorea con azúcar, espliego y canela.

[Combine one pound of ground sugar with one third of a pound of white flour that has been pounded until it looks like semolina. Add eggs and beat everything together. Then heat one pound of sweet oil in a frying pan on low heat and when it is boiling, drop the breadcrumb-egg-sugar batter into the oil and shake over a low flame until it binds together. Let cool and sprinkle with sugar, spikenard, and cinnamon.]

9. PASTA DE NUEZ VERDE [GREEN WALNUT PASTE] (299)

Another recipe for preserved walnuts appears in Martínez Montiño's cookbook (483–5). The two are similar in terms of puncturing the immature walnuts, soaking them, combining with sweetener (Martínez Montiño gives the option of either honey or sugar), and flavouring them with cinnamon and clove but in the other recipe ginger has disappeared.

Se toma una libra de nuez verde y se agujerea mucho con un pincho de hierro, luego se macera en agua tres días; se saca del agua y se toma para cada libra tres de miel limpia de su espuma, después de cocerse un poco las nueces; se sacan del agua y se vuelven a la miel y se cuecen hasta que tomen forma de pasta; se aromatiza con canela, clavo y jengibre, una onza menos cuarto por cada libra y se come después de las comidas. Sus provechos: excita el apetito y digiere los alimentos, calienta los riñones y aumenta la orina.

[Take one pound of green (immature) walnuts and poke several holes in them with a skewer and then let them soak for three days. Remove them from the water and for each pound of nuts add three of honey with its froth skimmed off. After blanching the nuts, take them out of the water and return them to the honey and boil until a paste forms. Flavour with cinnamon, clove, and ginger, three quarters of an ounce for each pound. It is eaten after meals. Its benefits: it stimulates the appetite and aids in the digestion of food, it warms the kidneys, and increases urine output.]

Ibn Razīn Tuyīǧbī. *Fuḍālat-al-Hiwan Fi Tayyibat al-Ta'am Wa-l-Alwan (Relieves de la mesa acerca de las delicias de la comida y los* *diferentes platos*) [The delicacies of the table and the finest of foods and dishes] C. 2nd half of 13th century.

1. RECETA DE PAN DE PANIZO [RECIPE FOR MILLET BREAD] (79)

Se coge harina de panizo y se pone en la artesa. Se le pone sal y se amasa muy bien con poco agua, porque no le conviene que sea mucha. Después se hacen obleas gruesas para llevar al horno, y finas para el anafe y la placa. Sobre la superficie de las obleas se pone sésamo, anises y granos de hinojo. Se cuecen deprisa porque, si no, se estropean.

Esta es, de todas las clases de pan de trigo, la que más aprecian los andalusíes, y la consumen en abundancia en la época de la cosecha del panizo.

[Take millet flour and place it in the kneading trough. Add salt and knead well with a little water, because it is preferable to use little water. Then make thick wafers for baking in the oven, and fine wafers for the portable oven or the griddle. On top of the wafers add sesame, anise, and fennel seed. Cook them quickly because, if you don't, they will break apart.

This is, of all types of wheat bread, the one that the Andaluces like best and abundantly consume during the millet harvest season.]

2. CONFECCIÓN DEL ALCUZCUZ [MAKING COUSCOUS] (130–1)

Similar recipes for both making couscous and then using it in other dishes are found in the 1611 cookbook by Martínez Montiño (360–4).

Se coge sémola fresca y se pone en la artesa. Se rocía con agua en la que se ha disuelto un poco de sal y se remueve con las puntas de los dedos para que la absorba. Luego se frota entre las palmas de las manos con cuidado para que tome la forma de cabezas de hormiga. Se sacude en un cedazo fino para que pierda toda la harina que tenga y se deja reposar tapada.

Se cocina de este modo:

Se coge carne de ternera grasa y de buena calidad y huesos grandes de lo mismo. Se ponen en una olla grande con sal, aceite, pimienta, cilantro seco y una pocas cebollas partidas. Se cubre con agua abundante y se pone al fuego. Cuando la carne comienza a estar tierna, se le ponen las verduras del tiempo que se tengan a mano, como col, nabos, zanahorias, lechuga, hinojo, habas verdes, calabaza vinatera y berenjenas. Cuando la carne y las verduras están a punto, se coge la olla dispuesta para hacer el alcuzcuz, que está agujereada por abajo, y se llena de alcuzcuz con cuidado. Se pone sobre la olla grande en la que está la carne con las verduras y se une a ella con una tira de masa para que no se escape el vapor. Se tapa la olla del alcuzcuz con una servilleta gruesa para que contenga el vapor y se cueza adecuadamente. Se sabe que está hecho por la fuerza del vapor que sube por la boca de la olla y porque, cuando se golpea al alcuzcuz con la mano, se oye un ruido. Cuando está hecho, se pone en la artesa y se frota con las manos con grasa de buena calidad, canela, almáciga y espicanardo, hasta que los granos quedan sueltos. Se pone en un cuenco, sin llenarlo del todo, dejando sitio para lo que ha de echarse encima. Después se comprueba si el caldo de la carne es suficiente o no. Si es escaso, se añade agua a la olla y se deja hasta que dé un hervor; cuando empieza a hervir, se retira del fuego y se deja que se afirme su cocción. Después se vierte moderadamente sobre el alcuzcuz, primero en el centro y luego por los lados. Se deja un rato tapado hasta que absorba el caldo. Se prueba con el dedo si lo ha absorbido y, si no, se añade más caldo, en cantidad razonable. Se sacan los huesos y se colocan verticalmente en medio del cuenco y, a su alrededor, la carne y las verduras. Se espolvorea con canela, pimienta y jengibre. Se come y que aproveche, si Dios Altísimo quiere.

Quien quiera hacerlo con carne de ovino y de gallina, puede hacerlo del mismo modo; por la potestad y fortaleza de Dios.

[Take fresh semolina and put it in the kneading trough. Sprinkle with water that has some salt added to it and stir it with your fingertips so that the water gets absorbed. Then carefully rub (it) between your palms so that it forms the size of ant heads. Sift through a sieve so that all the remaining flour comes out and let it rest, covered.

Cook it this way:

Select fatty veal of good quality and big bones of the same animal. Place it all in a pot with salt, oil, black pepper, coriander, and chopped onion. Cover everything with a lot of water and place over the flame. When the meat begins to become tender, add seasonal vegetables that you have on hand like cabbage, turnips, carrots, lettuce, fennel, fresh fava beans, bottle squashes, and eggplant. When the meat and vegetables are cooked just right, pick up the couscous pot with the holes on the bottom, and fill it carefully with couscous. Put it over the big pot with the meat and vegetables and join the two together with a strip of dough so no steam escapes. Cover the couscous pot with a thick napkin to hold in the steam and to cook it right. You know that it is done when the steam forces its way through the top of the pot and also when you hit the couscous with your hand, you will hear a noise. When it is done, place in the kneading trough and rub with a good quality fat between your hands, with cinnamon, mastic, and spikenard until the grains are loose. Place in a bowl, without filling it up so you have space for what comes on top. Then see if there is enough stock or not. If there is not enough, add more water to the pot and bring it to a boil; when it begins boiling, take it off the fire and check to see if it has cooked enough. After pouring a moderate amount over the couscous, first in the centre and then on the sides, let it stand, covered, for a while so that the stock gets absorbed. Use your finger to test the absorption; if it is not enough, add more stock, a reasonable amount at a time. Remove the bones and stand them up in the centre of the bowl and, around them, the meat and vegetables. Sprinkle with cinnamon, black pepper, and ginger. Eat and enjoy, if God Almighty is willing.

Whoever wants to make this with mutton or hen, can do it in the same way, by the authority and power of God.]

3. PLATO QUE SE LLAMA AL-ǦAMALĪ [DISH CALLED AL-ǦAMALĪ] (139–40)

The only part of this recipe copied here is the meatball section. Meatballs are generally served as part of other meat dishes. In this case, the dish is a type of stew made up of beef, tripe, garbanzos, almonds, fennel, garlic, and many different spices.

Se coge carne de morcillo, se limpia de nervios y se machaca muy bien en un almirez de madera. Se le pone sal, pimienta, jengibre, canela, espicanardo, clavo y claras de huevo y se amasa hasta que la carne se mezcla bien con las especias. Con esto se hacen albóndigas.

[Select a piece of shank, remove any vein or connective tissue and pound it well in a wooden mortar. Add salt, black pepper, ginger, cinnamon, spikenard, clove, and egg whites and knead it until the meat and spices are well mixed together. This is the way you make meatballs.]

4. OTRO PLATO LLAMADO AL-BŪRĀNĪYA ("ALBORONÍA") [ANOTHER DISH CALLED ALBORONIA] (140–1)

This is one of the more complex recipes of Ibn Razīn's manual. He creates a layered eggplant-meat dish and offers several variants on its preparation.

Se coge la carne mencionada [partes buenas de carne de vacuno] y se hace como antes, limpiándola y cociendo los callos con agua caliente hasta que blanquean, poniéndole las especias, yemas de huevo, albóndigas, etcétera, y llevándola luego al fuego. Después se cogen berenjenas grandes y se parten en rodajas redondas de tamaño mediano, ni muy finas ni muy gruesas. Se ponen en una tabla, unas sobre otras, y se les echa sal entre ellas, poniéndoles un peso encima para que suelten el jugo oscuro que tienen y pierdan el amargor; luego se lavan con agua clara y se ponen a escurrir. Se fríen en una sartén con mucho aceite hasta que se doran, cuidando de que no se rompan. Cuando está hecha la carne, se encostra la olla con huevos suficientes, como se ha visto anteriormente; se retira el fuego de debajo, dejándola reposar un rato. Cuando está encostrado y su grasa se ha coagulado, se pone en una fuente un lecho de hojas de cidro frescas y, sobre ellas, la mitad de las berenjenas. Se pone encima la carne, y sobre ella, el resto de las berenjenas. Se adorna la fuente con yemas de huevo [cocidas], albóndigas, huevos [cocidos] partidos y tallos de menta. Se le espolvorea canela y jengibre. Se come y que aproveche, si Dios Altísimo quiere.

También puede hacerse, si se quiere, cogiendo las berenjenas y pelándolas. Luego se cortan y se ponen en una olla con agua y sal. Se llevan al fuego hasta que están casi hechas; entonces se sacan y se lavan con agua clara caliente y se dejan escurrir. Después se coge carne y se machaca en un almirez, poniéndole especias como las de las albóndigas y claras de huevo. Se hace con ello una masa que quede bien trabada. Luego se coge una sartén y se pone al fuego con aceite. Cuando el aceite está caliente, se echan las berenjenas y se les da la vuelta con cuidado, sacándolas antes de que estén fritas del todo. Se coge la carne machacada y se cubren con ella. Se untan las manos con aceite y se aplana hasta que todo quede bien liso y se cubran todas las berenjenas. Se vuelve a poner en la sartén y se fríe con cuidado, dándole la vuelta para que se dore. Se saca y se le hace lo mismo con las berenjenas solas, que se ponen luego encima de la carne.

Si se quiere, se cogen las berenjenas, después de cocerlas, lavarlas y machacarlas en el almirez hasta que se haga una masa como la del tuétano, y se mezclan muy bien con la carne machacada con todas las especias. Después se untan las mano con aceite y se hacen con esto obleas redondas finas. Se fríen y se hace con ello lo que se ha dicho al principio con las berenjenas; has de tenerlo en cuenta.

Se puede hacer este plato, de la misma manera, con carne de ovino o de gallina. También se puede poner la carne en la cazuela, sobre una capa de berenjenas y otras dos más, una en medio y otra por encima;

se cubre [con agua] después de poner las berenjenas y se lleva al horno hasta que cuaje o se cocina en la casa poniendo encima otra cazuela con fuego hasta que cuaja y se dora su superficie. Es bueno, si se quiere, trasladarlo a una fuente; tenlo en cuenta.

Quien lo desee, puede coger las berenjenas, partirlas en dos mitades y vaciarlas; se rellenan con carne machacada y especiada que tenga claras de huevo. Después se rebozan con harina de adárgama, se fríen en aceite fino hasta que están a punto y sabrosas y con esto se hace la albornía.

[Take the aforementioned meat (good cuts of beef) and make it as before, cleaning it and cooking the tripe in hot water until it turns white, add spices, egg yolks, meatballs, etc. and put it on the fire. Then take big eggplants and slice them in medium-sized rounds, not too thin and not too thick. Spread them on a table, in layers, salting each layer and putting a weight on top so the dark juice is released and it loses its bitterness; then rinse with clear water and drain them. Fry in a frying pan with a lot of oil until they brown, being careful not to break them up. When the meat is ready, form a crust in the pot with the right amount of eggs, as you have seen before; remove from the flame and let rest. When the crust has formed and the fat has coagulated, put a bed of fresh citrus leaves on a platter, and on top, half of the eggplant. Place the meat on top and on top of that, the rest of the eggplant. Garnish the platter with hard egg yolks, meatballs, slices of boiled eggs, and shoots of mint. Sprinkle with cinnamon and ginger. Eat and enjoy, if Almighty God is willing.

If you want, you can also make them by taking the eggplant and peeling it. Then cut it up and put it in a pot with water and salt. Place the pot on the flame, cook until they are almost done; then remove them and rinse with clear water and let dry. Then take meat and grind it in a mortar, adding spices like the ones used with the meatballs, and egg whites. Make a mixture that is thoroughly mixed together. Then put oil in a frying pan and heat. When the oil is hot, cook the eggplants, carefully turning them and taking them out before they are completely fried. Take the ground meat and cover them with it. Grease your hands with oil and spread the mixture so it is flat and covers the entire eggplant. Return to the frying pan and carefully fry, turning it to brown. Remove it and do the same with the rest of the eggplant and put them on top of the meat.

If you want, take the eggplant, and after cooking, rinsing, and grinding in a mortar until it is the consistency of marrow, thoroughly mix with the ground meat and all the spices. Then grease your hands with oil and make delicate round wafers. Fry and then follow the directions for eggplant above; keep it all in mind.

You can make this dish, in the same way, with meat from sheep or hen. You can also place the meat in a pot over a layer of eggplant and repeat the layering twice, one in the middle and one on top; cover (with water) after arranging the eggplant, and put it in the oven until it solidifies or cook it at home putting another pot with a flame on top until it solidifies and the crust is golden brown. It is good, and if you like, transfer it to another platter; keep this in mind.

Whoever wants to can take eggplants, slice them in half, and remove the inside; fill them with ground meat that has spices and egg whites added to it. Then, dust with flour, and fry in good oil until they are cooked just right and flavourful and this is how you make *alboronia*.]

5. SOBRE LAS LENTEJAS [ON LENTILS] (280–1)

Lentils appear in Jewish, Muslim, and Christian writing, thus exemplifying how this humble legume cuts across ethnic divides. One way lentils are prepared in the Hispano-Muslim cooking manuals is with onions, cilantro, saffron, and vinegar. Eggs and figs are later added and the stew simmered until the lentils begin to dissolve.

Se lavan las lentejas y se cuecen en una olla con agua clara, aceite, pimienta, cilantro y cebollas partidas. Cuando están a punto, se les echa sal, un poco de azafrán y vinagre. Se les cascan tres huevos y se deja un poco sobre el fuego; después se retira. Se pueden cocinar sin cebolla o con colocasia hervida y partida. Se cocinan también con sicomoros disueltos con ellas, a fuego flojo; cuando las lentejas empiezan a cuajarse, se les añade manteca de buena calidad o aceite fino, en la cantidad que admitan, hasta que están a punto y han absorbido el aceite. Entonces se retiran del fuego y se les espolvorea pimienta.

[Wash the lentils and boil them in a pot with clear water, oil, black pepper, cilantro, and chopped onion. When it is cooked just right, add salt, a little saffron, and vinegar. Crack three eggs into the pot and let cook a little; then remove from the flame. You can make this without onion or with boiled, chopped taro. It can also be made with figs cooked in with the lentils very slowly; when the lentils begin to boil, add a good-quality tallow or fine oil, as much as you want until they are cooked just right and all the oil absorbed. Then remove from the flame and sprinkle with black pepper.]   ·

Libre de Sent Sovi [Libro de sent soví, Book of Sent Soví] 1st half of 14th c.

1. CELIANDRE [CORIANDER] (88)

Si vols fer celiandre així com mostalla – e dóna's ab polls en ast o ab perdi- us a malalt – pren lo gra del celiandre preparat e ametlles perades, cany- ella, gingebre, clavell, e sucre blanc; e pica-ho tot fortment, e destrempa- ho ab agror e ab dolçor. E val més ab vi de magranes agredolces.

[If you are going to make coriander the same way you make mustard – and serve it with roasted chicken or partridge for a sick person – take the grain of the prepared coriander, peeled almonds, cinnamon, ginger, clove, and white sugar and thoroughly grind it all together, and mix it with verjuice and sweetener. It is better with the wine of bittersweet pomegranates.]

2. SALSA VERD [GREEN SAUCE] (82)

Si vols fer salsa verd, hages fulla de juivert e, lo tendre, llava'l e eixuga'l al sol o sens sol. E pica'l molt ab canyella e gingebre e clavells, pebre e avellanes torrades. Amesura-ho de cascú e tasta-ho, e si veus que la una cosa sap més que l'altra, trempa-ho per egual. E destrempa-ho ab vi- nagre; e lo vinagre parega-hi mes. E pot-hi hom metre pa torrat banyat ab vinagre. Mit-hi mel o sucre a hom delicat o a malalt.

[If you are going to make green sauce, get parsley leaves and wash the tender parts and dry them in the sun or without sun. And thor- oughly grind them with cinnamon, ginger, and clove, black pepper, and toasted hazelnuts. Put in just the right amount of everything, taste, and if you think that an ingredient is too strong, correct the others with equal measure. And add vinegar so that it is noticeable. And you can add bread soaked in vinegar. Add honey or sugar if it is for someone who is weak or sick.]

3. SALSA DE BOLETS [MUSHROOM SAUCE] (76)

Si vols fer salsa a bolets perbullits e premuts e sosengats ab oli, fes aital salsa: pren ceba, juivert, vinagre, espècies, e destrempa-ho ab vinagre e un poco d'aigua. Fes peces d'ells, que els sosengues, o en dóna ab sosenga, e puis mit-los en sa salsa o els dóna cuits en brases ab sal e oli.

[If you are going to make a sauce with boiled, pressed mushrooms sautéed in oil, prepare it thus: take onion, parsley, vinegar, and spices, grind them all together and mix them with vinegar and a little water. Mince the mushrooms, sauté them or add them to the sauté and then add them to the sauce and serve them boiled or braised with salt and oil.]

4. SOLS [VINEGAR MARINADE] (84)

Si vols fer sols a què et vulles, a carn o a peix, pren de la carn o del peix fruit e fets-ne trossos, e gita'ls en vinagre; e dessús gita primerament farigola.

E si vols lo sols cald, hages pebre e safrà e vinagre, e del brou de la carn o del peix, e ceba tallada; e destrempa-ho tot e gita-ho dessús.

[If you are going to make a vinegar marinade for whatever, either meat or fish, take the meat or fried fish and cut it into pieces; put them in the vinegar but before doing so, sprinkle entirely with thyme. And if you prefer a warm marinade, combine black pepper, saffron, and vinegar and some of the meat or fish broth and chopped onion and mix all together and pour on top].

Manual de mugeres en el cual se contienen muchas y diversas recetas muy buenas [The manual for women in which is contained many, very good and diverse recipes]. 1475–1525.

1. REÇEUTA PARA HAZER UN OBISPO DE·PUERCO [RECIPE FOR SEASONING A BISHOP BLOOD SAUSAGE] (81)

Dos libras de puerco que sea de lomo y aya estado un día en adobo con la tripa. Lavadas después y picadas con una dozena de huevos cozidos y con una libra de manteca. Y después de picado, echallo en una almofia y juntar con ello una dozena de huevos crudos, y quarta y media de clavos,[5] y canela molida, y un poco de pimienta, y encorporarlo todo muy bien. Y después encorporado, y puesta la sal que fuere menester, henchir la tripa dello y poner a trenchos las hiemas de huevos cozidas que quisieren.

[Two pounds of pork that is from the back and that has been marinating for one day with the tripe. After washing (the meat) chop it up with a dozen boiled eggs and a pound of lard. And after chopping it, put it in a bowl and add a dozen raw eggs, and six pinches of cloves, and ground cinnamon, and a little black pepper, and mix it well. And once it is mixed, and the necessary salt added, fill the tripe with it and insert in intervals however many cooked egg yolks you might want.]

2. REÇEUTA PARA CAÇUELA DE ARROZ [RICE CASSEROLE RECIPE] (84)

This recipe is found in many cookbooks from the earliest ones through the seventeenth century. The flexibility in choice of meat is common to recipes found in both the Fuḍālat and Kitāb al-tabīj. For another option, see Ruperto de Nola's recipe "Arroz en cazeula al horno" [Baked rice casserole] (289).

Pondréis en una caçuela arroz y queso rallado, que sea muy bueno, y sal; y rebolbello todo muy bien. Y luego pondréis con ello el caldo que os pareçerá que basta, será el caldo de carne gruessa. Y pondréis ençima la carne que quisiéredes, e cozerá en el horno. Y quando esté casi cozida, sacadla y poné ençima de todo tajadas de queso fresco, y hiemas de huevos y espeçias. Y luego torne al horno y acabe de cozer. Y como sea cozida, haréis platos o escudillas dellos, qual más quisiéredes.

[Put rice and grated cheese, of very good quality, and salt in a pot; and stir it all well. And then put in as much broth as you think is enough, it should be stock from fatty meat. And put on top the meat of your choosing, and cook it in the oven. And when it is nearly cooked, take it out and put slices of fresh cheese on top, and egg yolks and spices. And then put it back in the oven and finish cooking. And when it is cooked, serve it on plates or in bowls, whichever you prefer.]

3. REÇEUTA DE UN MANJAR DICHO VIAFORA [RECIPE FOR A DISH CALLED *viafora*] (84–5)

The editor of Manual de mugeres, Alicia Martínez Crespo, notes that although the meaning of viafora is unknown, it could be related to the many tafaya dishes that appear in Hispanic-Muslim treatises (84n276).

Almendras medio tostadas, majadas y destempladas con caldo grueso de gallina o carnero. Colada aquella leche y puesta en una olla, poner con ella carne de carnero que sea de pierna no muy assada, picada muy menuda, y un poco de açúcar, y canela y muy poco de gengibre. Y cueza meneándola siempre hasta que se ponga espeso. Y como sea cozido, haréis escudillas dello con açúcar y canela por çima.

[(Prepare) almonds half-toasted, crushed, and thinned with thick chicken or mutton stock. Once this milk is strained and placed in a pot, add mutton; it should be from the leg and not thoroughly cooked, shredded very fine, and a little sugar, and cinnamon, and very little ginger. And cook it, stirring constantly, until it becomes thick. And when it has cooked, serve it in bowls with sugar and cinnamon on top.]

4. OLLA MORISCA [MORISCO-STYLE STEW] (58–9)

Tomá una olla y poné al suelo della una escudilla boca abaxo. Y echo dentro diez e ocho onças de sevo de cabrón o de carnero que sea de la riñonada, y una dozena o más de cebollas cortadas en quartos. Y ponedla al fuego, sea el fuego de carbón, y cueza una ora o más. Hazé pedaços tres libras de cabrón, que sea de lomo e del pecho, y otras tres de carnero. Y hechas pedaços, echaréislo todo junto en la olla y cozerá hasta que esté descozida. Pondréis con ellos unos pocos de garbanzos remojados y la sal que fuere menester. Y como sea cozida, poné en ella muchas especias de clavos, e canella y un poco de alcaravea. Y esto haréis quando lo queráis gustar.

[Take a pot and put a bowl upside down in the bottom. Put in eighteen ounces of goat or sheep tallow that comes from the loin, and a dozen or more onions, cut into quarters. And put it over the fire, made from charcoal, and cook it an hour or more. Cut up three pounds of goat meat, which is from the back and the chest, and another three of mutton. And after they are cut up, throw it all together in the pot and cook until the meat falls apart. Add some soaked garbanzos and the necessary amount of salt. And when it is cooked, put in a lot of spice of cloves, and cinnamon, and a little caraway. And you will make this when you want to please.]

Nola, Ruperto de. *Libro de guisados* [**Book of cookery**]. **1525.**

1. LECHE MAL COCIDA [BADLY BOILED MILK] (298)

This recipe first appears in the anonymous Sent Soví (110) although the two recipes have little more that their title in common. In Nola's recipe, there is no milk; rather, ground almonds and breadcrumbs are quickly sautéed together with beaten eggs to give a visual result of something that resembles curdled milk but that tastes delicious.

Majar almendras blancas con un migajón de pan: y desque sea bien majado pasarlo has por estameña; y desque sea todo pasado ponlo en una olla limpia; y ponlo al fuego: y cuando haya hervido quítalo del fuego; y toma algunas yemas de huevos batidos; y échalos en la olla meneándolo unas cuantas veces, y después hacer escudillas; y si pusieres el migajón de pan en remojo en agua rosada no puede ser sino mejor; aunque basta lo otro: la agua rosada siempre es buena en muchos manjares.

[Grind white almonds with some breadcrumbs. Once it is well ground, strain through a strainer and once it is all strained, place in a clean pot and put it over a flame. Bring it to a boil and remove from the flame. Then beat some egg yolks and place them in the pot, constantly stirring and then place in bowls. And if the breadcrumbs were soaked in rose water, it couldn't be better, although the other way is fine too: rose water is always good in many dishes.]

2. XINXANELLA A LA VENECIANA [VENETIAN JUJUBE] (320–1)

The recipe for Venetian jujubes is actually a broth with pasta. The pasta is made with cheese, fine breadcrumbs, eggs, saffron, and other herbs, pressed through a large grater that forms the dough into gnocchi-sized shapes that are then served in a broth. Xinxanella is a variant of guinja, synonym of azufaifa or jujube, the red, tear-drop shaped fruit of the jujube tree.

Tomar queso que sea grueso; y rallar una buena almuesta de ello;[6] y pan rallado que sea un panecillo de tres blancas y tres maravedís de salsa fina y un maravedí de azafrán y ocho huevos; y todo esto sea bien mezclado, y amasado todo junto; y desque todo sea bien majado tomar el rallo del queso, vuelto del revés; y poner esta pasta sobre él y desque el caldo estuviere muy hirviendo y bien gordo tú harás pasar aquella pasta por los agujeros del rallo sobre la olla, de manera que lo que pasare vaya dentro la olla y desque todo sea pasado dejarlo cocer como fideos o como morteruelo; y cuando fuere cocido hacer escudillas, pero que sean ralas, mezcladas con un poco de caldo, porque no sea tan espeso como los fideos, empero que el caldo sea bien grueso; y si fuere caldo de vaca muy grueso, será muy mejor vianda, y de las mejores del mundo; y con las cantidades que arriba dije se pueden hacer cerca de ocho escudillas.

[Take a hard cheese and grate a cupped handful of it. Take breadcrumbs from "three-penny" bread,[7] and three maravedis worth of
fine herbs and one maravedi of saffron[8] and eight eggs and mix it all
together well and knead it. And when it is all mashed together, take
the cheese grater turned upside down and put the dough on it. And
when the stock has come to a rolling boil and has a good fat content,
push the dough through the holes in the grater over the pot so that
whatever goes through falls into the pot, and when you are finished
let it all cook like noodles or *morteruelo* (a liver-breadcrumb spread).
And when it is cooked place it in bowls, but sparsely, mixed with a
little stock, so that it is not as thick as noodles but with a fatty stock.
If it is fatty beef stock, it will be a much better dish, even among the
best in the whole world. With the quantity I have specified above, you
can serve eight.]

3. POTAJE DE FIDEOS [NOODLE STEW] (289–90)

Limpiar los fideos de la suciedad que tuvieren y desque estén bien
limpios poner una olla muy limpia al fuego con caldo de gallinas o de
carnero bueno y gordo, y que esté bueno de sal, y cuando comenzare
de hervir el caldo, echar en la olla los fideos con un pedazo de azúcar;
y desque sean más de medio cocidos echar en la olla, con el caldo de
las gallinas o de carnero, leche de cabras o de ovejas, o en lugar de ello,
leche de almendras, que ésta nunca puede faltar, y cuezga bien todo
junto y desque sean cocidos los fideos apartar la olla del fuego y dejarla
reposar un poco y hacer escudillas, echando azúcar y canela sobre ellas; mas como tengo dicho en el capítulo del arroz muchos hay que con
potajes de esta calidad que se guisan con caldo de carne dicen que no se
debe echar azúcar ni leche, mas esto está en el apetito de cada uno; y en
la verdad, con fideos o con arroz guisado con caldo de carne, mejor es
echar sobre las escudillas queso rallado que sea muy bueno.

[Remove any dirt the noodles might have and when they are clean,
place them in a very clean pot over a fire with stock from hen or from
good, fatty mutton, and make sure the salt is good, and when the stock
begins to boil, add the noodles to the pot with a lump of sugar, and
when it is more than half cooked, add to the hen or mutton stock, goat
or sheep milk, or in its place, almond milk that is always tasty. Boil
everything together and when the noodles are cooked, take the pot off
the flame and let it rest a little before serving in bowls sprinkling it with
cinnamon and sugar. As I have stated in the chapter on rice, there are

many who say that stews of this quality that are prepared with meat stock should not have sugar or milk added to them, yet this is up to each person's taste and truth be told, noodles or rice prepared with beef stock are better when served in a dish with grated cheese on top; it is very good.]

4. CAZUELA MOJÍ[9] [TWICE BAKED EGGPLANT CASSEROLE] (316)

Tomar las berenjenas no muy grandes ni muy pequeñas, sino medianas; y abrirlas por medio y echarlas a cocer con su sal, y desque estén bien cocidas escurrirlas con un paño que sea basto; y después picarlas mucho, y echarlas en una sartén o cazo y échale buena cosa de aceite; y tomar pan y rallarlo y tostado echárselo allí dentro y echarle queso añejo rallado; y desque esté buen rato traído sobre la lumbre, tener molido culantro seco, y alcaravea y pimienta y clavos; y un poquito de gingibre; y traerlo sobre la lumbre y échale allí unos huevos; y traerlo sobre la lumbre hasta que esté duro; y después tomar una cazuela, y echarle un poquito de aceite; y asentarlo en ella; y batir unos huevos con pimienta y azafrán y clavos, y del mismo pan tostado que lleva dentro la cazuela y de queso rallado, y hacerlo espeso y asentarlo encima a manera de haz y ponerle sus yemas, y cuajarlo en el horno con una cuajadera, que es cobertera de hierro con brasa encima; y desque esté cuajada, quitarla de la lumbre y echarle un [sic] escudilla de miel que sea muy buena por encima y su pólvora duque.[10] Esta misma cazuela se puede hacer de acelgas o de zanahorias.

[Take medium-sized eggplants, not too big or too small, and cut them in half, salt them, and let them sweat, and when they are done, wipe them off with a course cloth and then mince them. Place them in a frying pan or a casserole pot with a good amount of oil. Grate bread, toast it, and then add it, and add aged grated cheese. Once it has simmered a while, add ground coriander, caraway, black pepper, and clove, and a little ginger, and let it simmer. Then add some eggs and let them cook until it has set. In another pot, add a little oil, enough to cover the bottom, and beat eggs with black pepper, saffron, and clove, and add the bread-cheese mixture to thicken it and shape it into a bundle. Add yolks and cook in the oven until set with an "egg-setting" lid, which is an iron lid with embers on top. Once it is set, remove it from the heat and drizzle it with a bowl of excellent honey and some Duke's powder. This same dish can be made with Swiss chard or carrots.]

5. EMPANADAS DE AZÚCAR FINO [POWDERED SUGAR TURNOVERS] (322)

Has de tomar una libra de almendras mondadas y majarlas en seco sin echarles ninguna agua ni caldo de manera que tornen muy aceitosas; porque cuanto más aceitosas fueren serán muy mejores; y después tomar libra y media de azúcar blanco bien polvorizado y mezclarlo bien con las almendras, y desque todo sea bien mezclado y majado, si fuese muy duro ablandarlo con una poca de agua rosada y desque esté un poco ablandada la masa polvorizar sobre ella un poco de gingibre a tu discreción, bien molido; y después tomar masa que sea de harina, y amasarla con buenos huevos y aceite dulce que sea fino, y desta masa hacer unas tortillas o empanadillas o rosquillas y henchirlas de la dicha masa, y después pornás una cazuela al fuego con muy buen aceite dulce, y cuando herviere echarle dentro de aquellas empanadillas y cuezgan hasta que tornen amarillas de color de oro; y cuando las quitares del fuego echarles encima miel derretida, y sobre la miel azúcar y canela.

[Take a pound of shelled almonds and grind them dry, without any water or stock, until they become oily, because the oilier they are, the better. Next, take a pound and a half of fine white sugar and mix it with the almonds so that it is well mixed and ground up. If it [the mixture] is very hard, soften it with a little rose water and once the mixture is a little soft, sprinkle over it a little ginger, finely ground, to taste. Then, take a flour dough and knead in some good eggs and a sweet oil, with a delicate flavour, and with this dough make tortillas or turnovers or little rings and fill them with the said filling. Next, heat a pot with good, sweet oil and when it is boiling, put in the turnovers and cook until they turn golden in colour. When you remove them from the flame, cover them with melted honey and over the honey, sugar and cinnamon.]

Granado, Diego. *Libro del arte de cozina* [Book on the art of cooking]. 1599.

1. OLLA PODRIDA [HODGEPODGE STEW] (82–3)

Toma dos libras de garganta de cerdo salada, y 4 libras de pernil desalado, dos hocicos, dos orejas y 4 pies de puerco partidos y recién sacados de un día, 4 libras de jabalí, joven y fresco, 2 libras de salchichones buenos, y limpio todo, hágase cocer con agua sin sal: en otro caldero de cobre cuézcanse también con agua y sal 6 libras de carnero y 6 libras de riñonada de ternera y 6 libras de vaca gorda y 2 capones y 2 gallinas y 4 pichones caseros gordos y de todas las dichas cosas las que estuvieren primero cocidas váyanse sacando del caldo antes que se deshagan y consérvense en un tarro de barro y en otro tarro de barro o de cobre con el caldo de la sobredicha carne, cuézcanse dos cuartos de liebre trasera cortados a pedazos, tres perdices, dos faisanes, dos ánades gruesas, salvajes y frescas, veinte tordos, veinte codornices y tres francolines y estando todo cocido, mézclense los dichos caldos y cuélense por cedazo advirtiendo que no sean muy salados. Ténganse aparejados garbanzos negros y blancos que hayan estado en remojo, cabezas de ajos enteras, cebollas partidas, castañas mondadas, judihuelas y fríjoles hervidos, y todo se haga cocer juntamente con el caldo y cuando estas legumbres estarán casi cocidas pónganse repollos, berzas y nabos y rellenar de menudillos y salchichas y cuando todo estará cocido antes tieso que deshecho, hágase de todo una gran mezcla e incorpórese, gústese muy a menudo en respecto a la sal y añádase una poca de pimienta y canela y después ténganse aparejados platos y escudillas grandes y póngase de las diferentes partes de toda esta composición sobre los platos sin caldo y tómese de todas las aves ya partidas en cuatro cuartos y de las carnes gruesas, y las saladas cortadas a tajadas y las aves menudas déjense enteras, y repártanse en los platos equitativamente junto con la composición, y sobre éstas póngase de la otra composición, la del relleno cortado y de esta manera háganse tres suelos y téngase una cucharada del caldo más gordo y póngase por encima, y cúbrase con otro plato, y déjese media hora en lugar caliente, y sírvase finalmente caliente con especias dulces. Puédense después de hervidas asar algunas de las dichas aves.

[Take two pounds of salted pork neck and four pounds of desalted ham, two jowls, two ears, and four split pig's feet all less than a day old, four pounds of young, fresh boar, two pounds of good sausage and all of these well cleaned; bring to a boil in unsalted water. In another copper pot, bring to a boil in salted water, six pounds of young mutton, six pounds of veal loin, six pounds of beef fat, two capons, two hens, and four young, fat squab. While all these ingredients are cooking, take out the first pieces of meat as they finish cooking but before the meat falls apart and reserve them in a clay pot. In another clay or copper pot with the broth of the aforementioned meat, boil two hindquarters of hare cut into pieces, three partridges, two pheasants, two ducks fat, fresh, and wild, twenty starlings, twenty quail, and three francolins. When everything has cooked, mix the said stocks together and strain through a sieve being careful that none of them is too salty. Mix together light and dark garbanzo beans that have been soaking, whole heads of garlic, onion halves, shelled chestnuts, green beans, and boiled beans, and cook it all together in the stock and when the vegetables and beans are almost done, add two types of cabbage and turnips and stuffing made of giblets and sausage. When everything is tender but not yet falling apart, mix everything together and blend well. Check the flavour often for salt and add a little black pepper and cinnamon. Next, have plates and big bowls ready and arrange all the different parts of this mixture on the plates without any stock. Then place the fowl that have already been cut into four quarters, the fatty meat and the salty meat that have been cut into slices, and leave the wild fowl whole. Divide equally among the plates together with the mixture that includes the sliced stuffing, and in this way make three layers and add a tablespoon of the strongest broth and spoon it over the top. Cover with another plate and let sit in a warm spot for a half an hour. Serve warm with sweet spices. After boiling the meat you can roast some of the said fowl.]

2. PARA HACER PLATOS DE LECHUGA CON CALDO DE CARNE DE DIVERSAS MANERAS [TO MAKE SEVERAL DIFFERENT LETTUCE DISHES WITH BEEF BROTH] (107–8)

Tómense de las lechugas las partes más blancas y lávense con muchas aguas, y póngase a cocer en agua que hierva, sáquense del agua y píquense sobre una mesa o partidas en 4 partes, háganse cocer con caldo gordo de carne, y con agraz entero y a la postre un manojito de hierbas, y no queriendo hierbas póngase huevos batidos y con un poco de caldo frío, añadiéndole pimienta, canela y azafrán y así como se acabaren de echar los huevos, désele luego una vuelta con la cuchara para que no se cuajen y sírvase caliente. De la misma manera se puede hacer la endívia que llaman también escarola blanca. Si quisieres rellenar la lechuga guarda el orden que hemos dado para las berzas a la Milanesa sin olvidar el agraz. Con las dichas lechugas se pueden poner a cocer rellenos de hígado, papada de puerco y tajadas de pernil y pollos rellenos y pichones de media pluma (tiernos) y cuando estuviere cocido, sírvase caliente todo con su caldo.

[Take the whitest part of the lettuce and rinse it many times with a lot of water. Put it in boiling water, take it out, and chop it up on a table or divide into four pieces. Cook in a fatty meat stock with whole unripe grapes and, to finish, a handful of herbs. If you do not want herbs, add beaten eggs and, with a little cold stock, add black pepper, cinnamon, saffron, and once you add the eggs, stir with a spoon so that it does not set, and serve warm. In the same way you can prepare endives that are also called white escarole. If you want to stuff the lettuce, maintain the order we have given for "cabbage Milanese style" and do not forget the unripe grapes. With said lettuce, you can cook stuffed with liver, pork cheek, and slices of ham, and stuffed chicken, and squab with medium-length feathers (tender), and when it is cooked, serve warm in its broth.]

Martínez Montiño, Francisco. *Arte de cocina, pastelería, vizcochería y conservería* **[The art of cooking, pie making, pastry making, and preserving]. 1611.**

1. ENSALADA DE ACENORIAS [CARROT SALAD] (98)

Las acenorias para ensalada, se han de buscar de las negras, lavarlas; y mondarlas de las barbillas, y cortarles el pezon, y la colilla, y meterlas en una olla, las colas por abaxo, y que estén muy apretadas; y poner la olla en el rescoldo, y echarla lumbre alrededor, y por encima, y se asarán muy bien. Luego sacarlas, y mondarles unas cascaritas que tienen muy delgadas, y sazonarlas de sal, y sirvelas con aceyte, y vinagre, y caliente; y si las quisieres echar azucar, podrás. La olla ha de estár boca abaxo. Hanse de poner estas acenorias adonde están las borrajas, y hazlas raxitas. (98)

[Carrots for salad; one should use the dark ones, wash them, scrub off the fine threads of roots, chop off the top and bottom, and place them in a pot, end down and packed together. Put the pot in embers so it is surrounded by them; stoke them and the carrots will roast well. Then remove them, peel off their fine outer layer, and season with salt. Serve them warm with oil and vinegar. If you like, you can sprinkle them with sugar. The pot should be face down. Serve on a bed of borage and cut into small pieces.]

2. OTRA MANERA DE CARNERO VERDE [ANOTHER WAY OF (MAKING) GREEN MUTTON STEW] (80–1)

Pondrás a cocer el carnero como está dicho, cortando el carnero á pedacitos tamaños como nueces, y echalo á cocer con agua, y sal, y un pedazo de tocino gordo y una cebolla entera: y quando el tocino, y la cebolla esté cocido, sacalo al tablero, y echale cantidad de verdura, peregil, yervabuena, y cilantro verde, y picalo todo junto asi caliente como está, y despues que esté bien picado, y el carnero bien cocido, echa la verdura, y el tocino picado dentro de la olla: y si vieres que tiene mucho caldo, saca un poco antes de echar la verdura, y sazona con todas especias, y echale un poco de agraz si fuere tiempo, y cueza dos, ó tres hervores: luego batirás tres ó quatro yemas de huevos desatadas con un poco de vinagre, y sacarás toda la flor del platillo con la verdura, y quajarlohas con las yemas de huevos, y sirvelo sobre revanadillas de pan. Luego echale toda aquella flor por encima: y si hubieres de hacer muchos platos juntos, no los quajes con huevos, sino toma una poca de buena manteca de puerco, y calientala bien, y echa dentro un poquito de harina, y friela un poco, de manera que no se ponga negra, no mas de quanto haga unas ampollitas blancas, y echala en el potage, y pondrás un poquito de azafran, y un poco de agrio, y viene á quedar muy bueno: y quando lo sirvieras, echale de la flor por encima.

[You can start cooking the mutton as is stated, by cutting the mutton into walnut-sized pieces, and bring it to a boil with water, salt, a piece of fat back, and a whole onion. When the onion and fat back are done, take them out and put them on a cutting board and add a good amount of herbs, parsley, mint, and cilantro, and chop it all up while still warm. After it is well chopped, and the mutton well cooked, add the herbs and the minced fat back to the pot: if you see that there is too much stock, take a little out before adding the herbs, and season with all spices, and add a little verjuice if there is time, and boil two or three times; then beat three or four egg yolks mixed with a little vinegar, and you will take the whole thing out along with the vegetables and set them with the egg yolks and serve it on a bed of sliced bread. Then put the whole thing on top; and if you were making a lot of dishes at once, do not set them with the eggs but rather with some good lard, and heat it up well, and mix in a little flour and fry it up so that it does not burn, only until it forms little white bubbles, and pour it into the stew and add a little saffron, and a little verjuice, and it is going to be delicious: and when you serve it, garnish it with a flower on top.]

3. SALPICÓN DE BACA [BEEF SALPICON][11] (36)

Pues que tratamos de salpicon, quiero avisar, que quando te pidieren salpicon de baca, que procures tener un poco de buen tocino de pernil, cocido, y picado, y mezclado con la baca, y luego su pimienta, sal, y vinagre, y su cebolla picada, mezclada con la carne, y unas ruedas de cebolla, para adornar el plato, es muy bueno, y tiene buen gusto.

[When dealing with salpicon, I must advise that when asked to prepare a beef salpicon, you add a small amount of good pork fat that has been cooked and diced and mixed with the beef. Later, add salt, pepper, vinegar, and minced onion to the meat and some onion wheels to garnish the dish. It is very good and very tasty.]

4. COMO SE ADEREZAN LAS ESPINACAS [HOW TO SEASON SPINACH] (265)

This recipe is similar to today's espinacas a la catalana [Catalan-style spinach], without the garbanzos.

Las espinacas, lo mas ordinario es guisarlas dulces, enjutas con pasas, y piñones, cociendolas primero, y picarlas, y esprimirlas del agua, y ahogarlas con un poco de buen aceyte, y cebolla, y sazonar con todas especias, y sal, y un poco de agrio, y luego echarles su dulce de miel, o azúcar, y sus pasas, o piñones, y algunas veces garvanzos, y estas no has de llevar asi caldo, porque han de ir muy enjutas.

[The most common way to make spinach is to cook it as a sweet dish, sprinkled with raisins and pine nuts. First, cook the spinach, chop it up and squeeze out the extra water. Pour a lot of olive oil over the dish, add onion and season with spices, and salt, and a little verjuice, and then add honey as a sweetener, or sugar, and its raisins, pine nuts, and sometimes garbanzos. And this spinach dish should have no stock, because it should not be a watery dish.]

5. POTAGE DE HABAS [FAVA BEAN STEW] (240)

Las habas en día de pescado las buscarás que sean muy tiernas, y las mondarás y pondrás aceyte que sea bueno en una cazuela de barro, o en una olla, y ponla sobre brasas: y quando esté caliente echar las habas dentro, y tendrás lechugas lavadas, y deshojadas y las torcerás en las manos, y las harás lo mas menudo que pudieres, sin llegar cuchillo a ellas, y esprimelas del agua, y las irás echando con las habas, y váyanse ahogando habas, y lechugas. Ellas irán echando agua de sí, que casi bastará para servir de caldo: echale de todas especias, y verdura cilantro verde mas que de las otras, y sazona de sal, y ponles un poquito de agua caliente, y un poco de vinagre, y cuezan hasta que estén blandas: echale unos huevos crudos para que salgan escalfados con las habas; y sirve las habas, y los huevos todo junto en la misma cazuela. A estas habas se suele echar un poco de eneldo, mas algunos señores no gustan de él.

[Beans, on a fish day get the ones that are very tender, and grind them up and put good oil in a clay pot or in a stew pot and place it over the embers. When it is heated, put in the beans. And wash lettuce, separate the leaves, tear them in your hands and make them as small as you can without bringing a blade to them. Squeeze out the water and add to the beans, and coat the beans and lettuce with oil. They will extract their own water, perhaps enough for the stock. Add all your spices and herbs, cilantro more than others, and season with salt. Add a little warm water and a little vinegar and cook until everything is soft. Add in raw eggs that will come out poached with the beans. Serve the beans and the eggs together in the same pot. It is common to add dill to this dish although some masters do not like it.]

6. MANJAR BLANCO [BLANCMANGE] (227–9)

Quiero poner aquí algunas potagerías de legumbres: y esto hago (como tengo dicho) para los mancebos, y mugeres, que sirven a algunos señores, y no saben estas cosas, aunque parecen muy faciles. El manjar blanco, para una pechuga, la sacarás de una gallina, acabada de matar, y tendrás la olla cociendo, y echala dentro: y cueza hasta que esté casi acabada de cocer: luego deshilala muy menuda, y ponla en un cazo, y echale medio quartillo de leche, y batela con el cucharon, de manera que no se corte, luego echale una libra de harina de arroz, y hechale otro poquito de leche, y batelo muy bien; luego vele hechando leche, y trayendolo a una mano hasta que tenga cinco quartillos, y echa una libra de azucar, y si le echares cinco quarterones será mejor: echarle un poco de sal blanca, cantidad de un panecillo de los de Madrid, y pon el cazo sobre unas trevedes con buena lumbre de tizon de carbon, y traelo a una mano con mucho cuydado, porque no se queme, ni se ahume, y quando comenzare a quajar batelo muy bien: tardará en cocerse tres quartos de hora, poco mas o menos. Para ver si está cocido, toma un poco en la punta de un cuchillo, y dexalo enfriar un poco, y llegalo a la mano, sino se pegare estará cocido. Advierte, que si haces muchas pechugas juntas, como si fuesen seis, no pueden llevar tanta leche, que a seis pechugas bastarán siete azumbres de leche, si no fuesen muy buenas las pechugas, aun sería mucha leche, porque trabajan mas las pechugas, y se deshacen mas, y no pueden llevar tanta leche, porque saldria el manjar blanco blando. Otro manjar blanco se hace con mas leche, y mas azúcar, mas yo me atengo a este.

[I want to write down here some bean stews and I'm going to do this (as I have said) for apprentices, and women, who serve lords and do not know these things even though they seem so easy. Blancmange; take a breast of a hen, recently slaughtered, and place it in a pot of boiling water. Cook it until it is almost completely cooked through. Then, finely shred it and place it in a pot. Add a half a pint of milk and beat with a large spoon so that the milk doesn't curdle. Then add a pound of rice flour and a little more milk and beat well. Then, continue adding milk, stirring with one hand, until there are five pints. Add one pound of sugar, and if you add a pound and a quarter, even better. Add a little salt, about the amount [you put in] Madrid rolls, and place the pot on a trivet with strong charcoal embers. Stir it with one hand very carefully so that it doesn't burn or get infused with smoke. When it begins to thicken, stir vigorously. It will take approximately 45 minutes. To see if it is done, put a little on the tip of the spoon, let cool, and when you touch it, if it doesn't stick, it is done. Be advised that if you cook a lot of breasts at once, for example, six, you cannot add as much (corresponding) milk. For six breasts, seven *azumbres* of milk is enough.[12] But if the breasts are not that good, even that would be a lot of milk, because the breasts need to cook longer, fall apart more, and cannot use as much milk because the blancmange would end up bland. Another blancmange uses more milk and more sugar but I prefer this one.]

Hernández de Maceras, Domingo. *Libro del arte de Cocina* **[Book on the art of cooking] 1607.**

1. DE ENSALADAS [ON SALADS] (183)

Tomen todas verduras bien picadas, y échenles alcaparras, y lávalas bien y échalas en un barreño, y échales aceite mucho, vinagre poco, haz de ellas tus platos, y luego ponle por encima, a cada un plato lonjas de tocino del pernil y de lenguas y truchas, o salmón, yemas de huevos y tajadas de diacitrón, maná, azúcar y granada, flor de borrajas porque parece bien.

[Mince all vegetables and add capers, wash them and put them in a bowl, and add a lot of oil, a little vinegar, and plate them up. To each add a slice of fat back, tongue, trout or salmon, egg yolk, citron, manna, sugar, pomegranate, borage blossoms because they look good.]

2. CÓMO SE HA DE RELLENAR UNA LECHUGA
[HOW TO STUFF LETTUCE] (211–12)

Ha de ser la lechuga atadera, y se le han de quitar las hojas malas de encima, y luego quitando las primeras, han de quedar dos hileras de ellas, y se le ha de quitar el cogollo a raíz de las hojas, y se picará una libra de carnero de la pierna muy bien picado, con tocino gordo, y perejil, y hierbabuena, y cuatro maravedís de especias, con su sazón de sal: y unos agraces, y un par de huevos, y se le pueden echar: unas ruedas de cañas de vaca también son buenas, y después que lo tengas muy bien sazonado, métalo dentro de la lechuga, y átala muy bien con un cordel, y échala a cocer con grasa, y en cosa holgada, y no cocerá hora entera: y después de cocida, se pondrá en una fuente hecha ruedas, sirviéndola con limones agrios, o agraz, es plato muy regalado: y de la misma manera se puede rellenar un repollo Murciano, y con el mismo aderezo.

[With lettuce that will be tied up, remove the ugly, outer leaves, and then after removing the first layer, there should be two rows of lettuce. You should remove the centre of the leaves. Mince a pound of young mutton leg with heavy lard, parsley, spearmint, four maravedis worth of spices, and the right amount of salt. Add verjuice and a couple of eggs and you could also add some beef bone marrow, which is very tasty. After it is all well seasoned, stuff the lettuce leaves and tie them up well with string. Cook them in heated up fat in a spacious pot. They will be done in less than an hour. After cooking, place on a platter in the shape of a circle and serve with bitter lemons or verjuice. It is a nice looking dish. You can also make it with cabbage from Murcia and with the same seasoning.]

3. CÓMO SE HA DE RELLENAR UNA LECHUGA
[HOW TO STUFF LETTUCE] (237)

This recipe is for a sweet dish.

Hanse de cocer unas borrajas, perejil, y hierbabuena en agua y sal, y en estando cocidas, pícalas, y échalas en un cazo con una poca de manteca de ganado, o aceite, para que se ablanden y échales piñones, pasas, y azúcar, y dos o tres huevos, y una poca de canela, y azafrán, y mételo

todo en la lechuga, y átala, y ponla a cocer. Servirásla con azúcar y
canela: y lo mismo se puede hacer del repollo.

[You need to cook borage, parsley, and spearmint in water and salt,
and once cooked, chop them up and put them in a pot with a little beef
tallow, or oil, to soften them, and add pine nuts, raisins, and sugar, and
two or three eggs, and a little cinnamon and saffron, and fill lettuce
with this mixture, tie it, and boil it. Serve it with cinnamon and sugar:
you can do the same with cabbage.]

4. CÓMO SE HAN DE HACER MANOS REBOZADAS
[HOW TO MAKE DEEP-FRIED KNUCKLES] (224)

Después de cocidas las manos, se les quitarán los huesos, y se han de
dejar helar, y se echará una poca de harina en un cazo con especias,
y sal, y cuatro, o cinco huevos conforme la cantidad de las manos, y
no ha de quedar muy espeso: y luego se mojará cada media mano,
en el batido, y se freirá, y se harán unas torrijas para poner debajo, y
se servirán con azúcar, y canela por encima. También se puede cocer
un poco de miel con especias, y vinagre, o agraz: y se le echará por
encima, y con su azúcar y canela: y ha de ser agridulce: y con esta
misma salsa se puede dar el cabrito rebozado, y cualquier género de
rebozado, como manos de ternera, de puerco, y de cabrito, y otras
cualesquiera manos.

[After boiling the knuckles, remove the bones, and let them congeal,
and add a little flour in the pot with spices, and salt, and four or five
eggs depending on the amount of knuckles, and it should not be very
thick. And then dip half of each knuckle in the batter and fry them, and
make some fried sweet bread to put underneath, and serve topped with
cinnamon and sugar. You can also cook with a little honey and spices
and vinegar or verjuice: and you can top with cinnamon and sugar and
it will be sweet and sour: and you can use this same topping to serve
over deep-fried goat or any type of deep frying, such as beef, pork, or
kid knuckles or any other knuckle.]

5. DE ZANAHORIAS RELLENAS [ON STUFFED CARROTS] (266)

Toma las zanahorias que sean gordas, y lisas, y límpialas muy bien,
y córtalas a trozos, pequeños, y sácales el corazón, sin que se quiebre
el trozo, y échalas a cocer en agua caliente, y en estando muy tiernas,

sácalas, y escúrreles el agua, y en azúcar, almendras, y nueces muy majado, amásalo con agua de azahar, y échale un poco de pimienta, clavos y canela todo muy bien mezclado, y rellena las zanahorias con ello: y luego bate los huevos que quisieres, y envuélvelas en ellos, y échalas a freír, y vuélvelas a los huevos, hasta que se acaben: y luego enmélalas, y échale su azúcar, y canela por encima.

[Choose carrots that are thick and smooth and wash them well and cut them into small pieces and remove the centre without breaking the piece and cook them in warm water. Once they are tender, remove them and drain out the water and in a mixture of sugar, ground almonds, and ground walnuts, bind it together with orange blossom water, and add a little black pepper, clove, and cinnamon that is thoroughly mixed together and stuff the carrots with it. And then beat as many eggs as you want and dip them in them and fry them, and repeat with the egg wash until finished. Then cover the carrots with honey and sprinkle with cinnamon and sugar.]

6. CÓMO SE HA DE HACER OTRO GUISADO LLAMADO ALBUJÁVANAS [HOW TO MAKE ANOTHER DISH CALLED ALBUJAVANAS] (197)

This is a recipe for minced lamb patties served with an egg-vinegar golden sauce. It takes its name from its Arabic origins but includes lard in its ingredients. This addition of pork fat exemplifies how dishes adapted over time to the regional, cultural norms.

Hase de tomar el carnero de la pierna, dos o tres libras, con forme los convidados, para cada uno media libra de carne, y hase de tomar la carne y picarla muy bien con tocino gordo, perejil, y hierbabuena: y después de picada con todo esto se ha de echar en una cazuela, y tomar cuatro, o seis maravedís de especias, y para cada libra un huevo, y se han de tomar estos huevos, y las especias, y sal molida, y vinagre, y echarlo todo en la carne: y hase de amasar muy bien, y después que estuviere amasado, se ha de tomar un cuarterón de carne, y ponerla en la mano, y hacer una torta: y se ha de tener una cazuela untada, y ponerlas en ella: y se ha de hacer en cada una un agujero en el medio que quede, y se ha luego de poner la cazuela a la lumbre, con poca lumbre debajo, y encima; y desde que estuvieren cocidas, batirse han un par de huevos con un poco de vinagre, y haráse un caldillo espeso, y luego se pongan en los platos, y se le ha de echar el caldillo por encima, y servirse han a la mesa.

[Take two or three pounds of mutton leg, depending on the number of guests, a half pound for each one, mince it well with heavy lard, parsley, and spearmint. After mincing all together, place in a casserole pot and add four or six maravedis worth of spices and for each pound, one egg. Take these eggs, spices, ground salt, and vinegar and mix it into the meat and knead it all very well and once it is kneaded, take a quarter pound in your hand and make a patty and place it in the greased casserole pot. Make a whole in the middle of each one that is left. Put the casserole pot over the flame, and have the fire both above and below the pot. Once it is cooked, beat a couple of eggs with a little vinegar and make a thick dressing. Place the patties on the plates and drizzle the sauce on top and serve them at the table.]

7. CÓMO SE HAN DE ADEREZAR LOS GARBANZOS [HOW TO COOK GARBANZOS] (236)

Los garbanzos para se cocer bien presto, se echarán en agua tibia, y se picará cebolla, y ajos, frito todo con aceite: y se le echará, seis huevos se echarán: luego se molerán seis maravedís de especias, y garbanzos, y un poco de pan: y se le echará todo para que se espesen: y se sazonarán bien de sal, con sus verduras, y un poco de vinagre.

[To cook garbanzos quickly, put them in warm water. Chop onion and garlic and fry them in oil and add it. Add six eggs and grind together six maravedis worth of spices and garbanzos and a little bread. Add it all to thicken it. Season well with salt, herbs, and a little vinegar.]

8. DE OTRO PLATO DE ESPINACAS, PARA SERVIRLAS EN ESCUDILLAS [ANOTHER SPINACH DISH, TO BE SERVED IN A BOWL] (231)

Echaranse a cocer unos pocos de garbanzos, hasta estén muy bien cocidos, y tomarán las espinacas, y échales más garbanzos, y se majarán especias, con unos ajos, y un migajón de pan, desatándolo con el caldo de la olla, y se le echará para que espesen y su aceite lo que fuere menester. Éstas son para dar en escudillas, y no se les eche dulce, sino un poco de agrio.

[Cook some garbanzos and when they are well cooked, take some spinach and add it to the garbanzos. Mash together spices with garlic and breadcrumbs, dissolving it with the stock from the pot, and pour it in to thicken. Add as much oil as necessary. This dish should be served in bowls and do not add any sweetener, but rather a little verjuice.]

Altamiras, Juan de. *Nuevo arte de cocina* [New art of cooking] 1747.

1. FIDEOS GRUESOS [THICK NOODLES] (73)

Rallarás pan, y queso a proporción, a seis partes de pan una de queso; echarás de todas especies, azúcar, y canela, huevos crudos correspondientes; harás pasta de esto, no muy dura, la amasarás con caldo de carne: hecho esto pondrás una perola con el caldo que te quedó a hervir con fuego lento, cogerás una espumadera de agujeros crecidos, pondrás la pasta en la espumadera, y con un cucharón la irás apretando, que caiga sobre el caldo, que estará hirviendo, déjalos cocer, y quedarán como cabos de cuchara: cocidos los echarás en los platos, y sírvelos con azúcar, y canela por encima.

[Grate some bread and cheese in the proportion of six parts of bread to one part of cheese. Blend together spices, sugar, cinnamon, and the corresponding amount of raw egg. Make a dough with this but not too hard. Knead it with meat broth. Once this is done, put stock in a saucepan and boil on a low flame. Take a skimmer with large holes and place the dough on the skimmer and with a large spoon, push the dough through so that it falls into the stock that is boiling. Let it cook and they will come out looking like the end of a spoon [like spaetzle]. Once cooked, place them on plates and serve with cinnamon and sugar on top.]

2. ABADEJO CON TOMATE [HADDOCK WITH TOMATOES] (87)

Cortarás las raciones, lávalas bien; luego las cocerás, espumándolas, ponlas a escurrir en una tabla; freirás cebolla, y tomates con abundancia; compondrás las raciones en una vasija ancha, cubre la primera superficie de ella con las raciones, sobre que echarás la cebolla, y tomate, perejil, y pimienta, ajos machacados, y de esta suerte irás prosiguiendo con las otras raciones, que de nuevo echarás, hasta llenar la vasija; echarás un poco de agua, cuanto baste a bañarlas, que den un par de hervores, lo sazonarás de sal: este no necesita de otra especie, por cuanto, suple el tomate; es así muy gustoso y cómo conservarás los tomates todo el año, verás más adelante.

[Cut into portions and wash well. Then cook them, scoop them out, and place them on a table to drain. Fry onions and a lot of tomatoes; place the portions in a wide pot and cover the bottom with the portions. Place on top the onion, tomato, parsley, black pepper, and mashed garlic and proceed this way with the other portions that you will place in the pot until it is full. Pour a little water over it, enough to bathe the pieces and have it bubble some, season with salt. This dish needs no other spice in so far as the tomato provides it all. It is very tasty and later on you will see how to preserve tomato for the entire year.]

3. CRIADILLAS DE TIERRA [TRUFFLES] (115)

Esta es una hierba muy regalada, críase como las patatas, debajo de la tierra, las mondarás, y las pondrás echar en remojo en pedazos: escáldalas, ponlas a cocer, y cocidas que sean, pon aparte el caldo con que se cocieron; vacíalas en una cazuela, échalas aceite con ajos fritos, componiendo una salsilla de caldo que apartaste, con todas especies, deja que dé un hervor, y si te queda algo del mismo caldo, lo compondrás como de carne, y será tan bueno, que dudarás si es de carne, o pescado. Las patatas se componen del mismo modo; y si comes muchas te advierto, estarás de tan buen aire, y tan favorable, que con el aire que soples puedes componer embarcación para ir al Papa, si no es que sea tan fuerte, que por romper las velas sea necesario su reparo, que no se hace a costa de patacas.

[This is a valued vegetable, grown like potatoes, underground; peel them and let them soak in pieces. Rinse and cook and once cooked, reserve the stock in which they were cooked. Put them into a pot, with oil and fried garlic and make a little sauce from the stock that you set aside, with all spices; bring to a boil, and if there is some stock remaining, use it like beef stock; it will be so tasty you won't know if it is from beef or fish. Potatoes are made the same way; and if you eat a lot, I must warn you that you will have such good and favourable air, that with the wind you blow, you can set sail to see the pope unless it's so strong that you rip your sails and have to mend them, in which case I hope you don't use potatoes.]

Mata, Juan de la. *Arte de repostería en que se contiene todo género de hacer dulces secos, y en líquido, bizcochos, turrones, natas, bebidas heladas de todos géneros, rosolís y mistelas, con una breve instrucción para conocer las frutas y servirlas crudas* **[The art of confectionary baking in which is found how to make all types of dry and liquid sweets, sponge cakes, turron, creams, all types of iced drinks, liquors and punches, and with brief instructions on recognizing and serving raw fruit] 1747.**

1. SALSA DE TOMATES A LA ESPAÑOLA [SPANISH-STYLE TOMATO SAUCE] (165)

Después de assados tres, ó quatro tomates, y limpios de su pellegito, se picarán encima de una mesa lo mas menudo, que ser pueda: puestos en su salsera, se les añadirá un poco de perejil, cebolla, y ajo, asimismo picado, con un poco de sal, pimienta, aceyte, y vinagre, que todo bien mezclado, é incorporado, se podrá servir.

[After roasting three or four tomatoes, their peel removed, chop them on a table as finely as possible. Put them in a saucepan and add a little parsley, onion, and garlic, all minced, with a little salt, black pepper, oil, and vinegar. Once it is all thoroughly blended and mixed together, it is ready to serve.]

2. OTRA MANERA [ANOTHER WAY] (165)

Asados, limpios, y picados los tomates, del modo dicho, se mezclarán con un poco de ajo, cominos, orégano, sal y pimienta, asimismo molido, y se desleirá todo con un poco de caldo de la olla, y quatro gotas de vinagre, con lo que se servirá caliente.

Executanse diferentes modos de estas salsas, según el gusto de cada uno, que por muy comunes, se omiten.

[Roasted, without peel, and minced, as already explained, mix with a little garlic, cumin, oregano, salt and pepper, all ground together, and pour in a little stock from the pot and four drops of vinegar, and serve warm.

There are many ways to make these sauces, depending on the taste of the individual. Since there are so many, they have been omitted.]

Notes

Prelims

1 For more on Spain's gastronomic revolution, see Luján (110–11); for developments in England, see Thirsk, and for developments in England and France, see Mennell.

2 Since their work, the field of food studies has exploded and it would be impossible to list all the significant contributions to the field of study. That said, Roland Barthes's work on food as a sign of society encoded by a certain "grammar" was also highly influential. Jack Goody examines the political economy of food at both the micro (household) and macro (state) levels. In his study on sugar, Sidney Mintz demonstrates how this single food item acts as a metaphor for social relations between producers and consumers. For an excellent source of the study of food across history and in the social sciences, see Murcott, Belasco, and Jackson.

3 For an overview of Bourdieu's theory of taste and society, see Bennett's introduction (Bourdieu).

4 Marín has changed our understanding of Hispano-Muslim cooking in Spain with her critical edition of Ibn Razín's cooking manual and numerous articles on food practices in Al-Andalus. Santanach i Suñol writes on the early Catalan contributions to Spain's gastronomy and Castro Martínez, on Moorish influences. Juan Cruz Cruz focuses more on the scientific techniques and nutritional philosophy as seen through the early modern recipe manuals of Martino da Como and Ruperto de Nola while María de los Ángeles Pérez Samper looks at cooking and eating practices in the seventeenth-century university setting. For comprehensive studies on Spanish food history, see Luján and Perucho, and Martínez Llopis (*Historia de la gastronomía española*). In addition to these studies, L. Jacinto

García (*Carlos V*) and Gregorio Sánchez Meco focus on food history during the reigns of Carlos V and Felipe II, respectively. Both study the novelties and trends of the time period as seen at the royal table and in nobles' houses. Both look at the popular culinary practices in modest homes and in the church. Jacinto García (*Carlos V*) also discusses the early influences of New World foodstuffs in Spain. Both include recipes and, in this way, invite the reader to recreate historic dishes and menus. Another notable historian, Santiago Gómez Laguna, often contextualizes Spanish culinary developments in a larger European context.

5 There are hundreds of scholars who have published comprehensive works, collected essays, and monographs that contextualize food production, preparation, and consumption within a literary context. Gian-Carlo Biasin (1993) analyses food representation in the modern Italian novel, Denise Gigante (2005) traces the concept of taste in its literary representations (primarily in English literature), Catherine Gautschi-Lanz (2006) writes about dinners and diners in nineteenth-century French literature, Nancy Gutierrez (2003) looks at eating disorders in early modern English literature; Chris Meads (2001) studies banquets in Elizabethan drama. These are just a few of the important publications within different European contexts.

6 In addition to Mennell and Montanari for more on the relationship between language and taste, see Ferguson.

7 All citations are from Luis Murillo's edition.

8 Unless otherwise indicated, all translations are my own.

9 Michael Hoey coined the term "discourse colony" to describe and analyze texts that are generally not read from start to finish but rather approached as a work containing individual units that share a common function but without a semantically important order. Besides cookbooks, other examples of discourse colonies are hymnals, newspapers, and conference proceedings. For more information, see 234–5n1.

1 *El Ante*: The Rise of Cooking Manuals in Spain

1 In Michael Hoey's seminal work *Textual Interaction: An Introduction to Written Discourse Analysis,* he distinguishes nine characteristics of discourse colonies: meaning is not derived from sequence; adjacent units do not form continuous prose; a framing context exists; the work is anonymous or there is no single author; one component may be used without another; components may be reused in subsequent works; components may be added, removed, or altered; many of the components serve the

same function; and there exists an alphabetic, numeric, or temporal sequencing (77–89).

2   There exist several other culinary manuscripts dating to the late Middle Ages. Joan Santanach references *Llibre de totes maneres de potatges de menjar* [The book of every kind of dish], *Llibre de totes maneres de confits* [The book of all kinds of candied fruit] and *Llibre de aparellar de menjar* [The book of food preparation] still an unpublished manuscript (2112) at the University of Barcelona. The first and the third contain a substantial number of recipes from the *Sent Soví*. In his introduction to Josep Lladonosa's *La cocina medieval* [Medieval cuisine] Martínez Llopis mentions three other medieval manuals of interest. *Llibre de coch de la canonja de Tarragona* [Book of cooking from the canon of Tarragona] (1331?), published in Barcelona in 1935, contains a series of food norms following the liturgical calendar for the religious order at the Seo de Tarragona. Francesc Eiximenis also wrote on dietary habits of the Catalan in *Terç del crestià* [The third part of the Christian] in 1384, which appeared as part of his multivolume work *Lo crestià* [The Christian]. Jaime Roig, physician to Alfonso V and Juan II of Aragón, published *Llibre de les dones, mes verament dit des consells* [Book of women, more truly understood as advice] in the fifteenth century (12).

3   Many of the titles translated into English are commonly accepted. The textual translations, except where noted, are my own.

4   Ibn Razīn's full name is: Abū l-Hasan 'Alī ibn Muḥammad ibn Abī l-Qāsim ibn Muḥammad ibn Abī Bakr ibn Razīn al-Tuyīğbī al-Andalusí.

5   This manuscript was also edited in Rabat (1981), Beirut (1984), and Fez (1997).

6   For more on contemporary Arabic traditions of the East, see Rodinson, Arberry, and Perry's *Medieval Arab Cookery*, or Ibn al-Karīm's *A Baghdad Cookery Book*.

7   The manuscript is in the National Library of Paris (7009). For an English translation of the work, see Martinelli.

8   Huici Miranda first published this piece in article form in 1961–2 in *Revista del Instituto de Estudios Islámicos* [Journal of Islamic Studies] before it was published as a book through the Instituto Egipcio de Madrid in 1965. Finally, in 1966 the city of Valencia sponsored the publication of the work under the title *Traducción española de un manuscrito anónimo del siglo XIII sobre la cocina hispano-magribí* [Spanish translation of an anonymous thirteenth-century manuscript on Hispanic-Magreb cooking].

9   Beyond the Trea editions of these cooking manuscripts, see García Sánchez, "La alimentación popular urbana en al-Andalus" and Bolens. For more general information on food in Al-Andalus, see García Sánchez's

edition of *Kitab al-Agdiya (Tratado de los Alimentos)* [Treatise on food] and Waines. For the early diffusion of food items from the Middle East to Europe, see Watson and Riera Melis, "Jerarquía social."

10 *Mudéjar* is the term used to describe a Muslim living in Christian Spain in the Middle Ages.

11 My count differs slightly from that of the editor on p. 28.

12 Waines also comments on the unusual measure of "disposable" earthenware pots: "These somewhat drastic measures were probably not always adopted, as pots could be adequately cleaned, under proper supervision of the domestics, with hot water and bran. Nevertheless, such circumstances explain the opening expression found in not a few recipes to 'take a new pot'" (727).

13 Bernard Rosenberger writes on the versatility of grains in precolonial North Africa. See "Diversité."

14 For more on the importance of spices in Hispano-Muslim cooking, see García Sánchez, "Especias y condimentos." In this article she includes graphs of use of spices in the two cooking manuals and in agricultural treatises, as well as their properties according to dietary and medical treatises.

15 *Aletría* comes from the Arabic *itrīya*, a type of noodle primarily used for sweet dishes. I have translated it here as angel hair pasta because the recipe for making *aletría* explains that one forms the noodle by making it as fine as possible (Marín, *Relieves* 135).

16 For more on the curious history of cilantro and parsley, see Marín (*Relieves* 39n59).

17 Bernard Rosenberger argues that the complier of the *Kitāb al-tabīj* is from the area of Cordoba-Seville and cites several recipes to support this position ("Usos del azúcar" 101).

18 *Almojábanas* also appear in Ruperto de Nola's cookbook (1520) and are still found in Spain today but do not usually include cheese. However, cheese is a common ingredient in *almojábanas* in Puerto Rico.

19 For more on the connections between medieval Muslim and Christian cooking manuals, see Marín, "From Al-Andalus to Spain: Arab Traces in Spanish Cooking," especially pp. 46–51.

20 In 2008, Barcino-Tamesis published an English translation of Santananch's edition entitled *The Book of Sent Soví. Medieval Recipes from Catalonia.*

21 Santanach's investigation into wills and inventories shows that nobility and clergy alike owned copies of this text (*Libro* 24).

22 The use of almonds and almond milk is a good example of how overlaps in ingredients do not necessarily reflect a direct influence from one cooking manual to the next. Almonds and almond milk are found in cooking

manuals throughout medieval Europe. For example, the fourteenth-century German text *Daz buoch von guoter spise* [The book of good food] (c. 1345–54) has several recipes but bears no direct influence on or from the *Sent Soví* or any of the Spanish cooking manuals.

23 For a comparison of how sugar is used in *Kitāb al-tabīj* and *Sent Soví*, see Rosenberger who states that in the former sugar appears in 14.3 per cent of the recipes and in the latter, 16.5 per cent ("Usos del azúcar" 107).

24 Six mushroom recipes appear in the oldest European cooking manual, Apicius's *De re cocquinaria* [On cooking] (1st–3rd c. CE). Three are also found in the fourteenth-century Italian manuscript *Anónimo toscano*, and one in the fourteenth-century Italian manuscript *Anónimo venenciano*. However, mushroom recipes do not appear in the French *Vivendier* (15th c.) and do not come into English cooking until late in the sixteenth century (Thirsk 41). One hundred years after the appearance of *Sent Soví* two recipes appear in Martino da Como's *Liber de arte coquinaria* (1450). For these recipes, see Cruz Cruz (*La cocina mediterránea* 153).

25 In the article "Chivalric Identity in Enrique de Villena's *Arte cisoria*," Miguel-Prendes argues that the treatise was a manifestation of Villena's desire to exert his influence in the political arena (2003). Since Russell Brown's edition in 1984, Pedro M. Cátedra has published a three-volume edition of Villena's complete works. For editions prior to Brown, see his edition, 41n72.

26 In his introduction, Brown notes that almost one third of the manuscript is dedicated to the character of the carver (20).

27 For an English translation of the manuscript, see *Manual de mugeres... The Manual de Mujeres*.

28 These three unedited manuscripts are housed in the Biblioteca Nacional de Madrid. For more information, see *Manual de mujeres* (14n14). Another well-known women's manual from thirteenth-century France is *Le ménagier de Paris* [The good wife's guide]. In this work the older husband instructs his young bride on the moral standards and practical responsibilities of a proper wife so that she might dutifully serve her future husband once he passes away. See Greco and Rose.

29 For a summary of the history of dietary manuals, see Cruz Cruz, *Dietética medieval* (14–25) and for those in the fifteenth and sixteenth centuries, see Luján (*Historia* 104–6). In terms of texts dedicated to hygiene in Spain, little work has been done on the early modern era. However, excellent studies that examine the social, moral, and gender implications of hygiene focus more on the nineteenth century. See, for example, Charnon-Deutsch and for French literature, see Corbin.

30 For detailed information on the history of Villanova's work and more background information on dietary manuals in Spain, see García-Ballester and McVaugh.

31 The numbers in parentheses indicate how many recipes are found in each category. The +1 sign indicates an exception. In the case of medical remedies, an additional recipe is included entitled "Betum para soldar bidrio" [Bitumen for soldering glass]. Martínez Crespo speculates that the bitumen "cures" a problem or that the verb *soldar*, related to *cicatrizar* [to scar], might explain why it appears here (*Manual de mugeres* 40n38). In the case of the other two, the additional recipes are listed in the index under "Tabla de lavatorios, polvos y otras cosas para los dientes y ençias contenidas en este libro" [Index of washes, powders, and other remedies for the teeth and gums found in this book].

32 *Tafaya* is essentially a slow-cooked lamb dish seasoned with coriander, pepper, and onion but also has many variations. For example a *tafaya blanca* [white tafaya] is made with almonds and coriander while a *tafaya verde* [green tafaya] is made with cilantro and mint. In the anonymous *Kitab*, the author explains that *tafaya* "es uno de los más nobles alimentos y de los más equilibrados en quimo y el más adaptado a todo temperamento" [is one of the finest foods and one of the most balanced during chyme (phase of digestion when food turns to thick liquid), and that best adapts for all temperaments] (121).

33 As it is common to include exact quantities in health-related recipes and no specific quantities or flexible quantities in food recipes, further research should study the relationship between food recipes that include specific quantities and health-related explanations that often come at the end of a recipe.

34 For more on when Nola wrote his cookbook and the scant biographical information that remains today, see Cruz Cruz, *La cocina mediterránea* (15–24).

35 The Catalan version was also republished six times in Barcelona in 1520, 1535, 1539, 1560, 1568, and 1578. The Castilian versions were printed in Toledo 1525; Logroño, 1529; Toledo 1529, two others from unknown cities in 1538 and 1543, Toledo in 1544; Medina del Campo in 1549; Valladolid in 1556; Zaragoza in 1562 and 1568; and Toledo in 1577. It was not republished again until 1929 in Madrid (Val xxiin 30). For a comparison between the first three editions (1520, 1525, and 1529), see Peyrebonne.

36 Aguilera Pleguezuelo suggests that Nola, by not including his last name in the Catalan edition – the author is simply, Mestre Roberto – was possibly trying to hide his Morisco identity (111).

37 All citations of *Libro de Coch* are from the Cruz Cruz edition (*La cocina mediterránea*), translations are my own.

38 *Culantro* and *cilantro* are often used interchangeably even though they are two different plants. For more information, see 248n10.

39 All citations of *Libro del arte de cozina* are from the Benet i Pinós edition, translations are my own.

40 Xavier Benet I Pinós, in his edition of Granado's work, surmises that Granado is from Valencia "pues los términos dialectales valencianos abundan en el escrito y con los pescados es corriente la denominación catalana según los términos corrientes de las playas valencianas" [because words from the Valencian dialect abound in his writing and with respect to fish, the Catalan designation of terms typical of Valencian shores is common] (9). Nicolás Antonio (1617–84) in his *Bibliotheca Hispana Nova* (1672) recorded his second last name, Maldonado, but with no biographical details (Val xviii).

41 For more on Granado's plagiarism, see Gómez Laguna ("Sobre Diego Granado" 21–3).

42 There are two significant sections of Granado's work that do not come from either Nola or Scappi. I suspect that these sections also originated from the work of other authors but the sources have yet to be identified. Val surmises that Granado was familiar with many manuscripts that are no longer extant but that were probably commonly used in convents and estates (xxiii–xxiv).

43 All translations for Scappi's cookbook are from Terence Scully's translation and critical edition. All citations will contain both the original page numbers followed by those corresponding pages from Scully.

44 Jeanne Allard cites 587 of 762 recipes in Granado's cookbook that come from Scappi. While exact numbers vary from one critic to another, all confirm the intense borrowing that occurred. The Val edition contains 762 while Benet i Pinós has only 755. This discrepancy is explained by the fact that the latter combined two recipes into one on several occasions so that the same recipes are in each but labelled differently.

45 Differing from the Spanish gastronomic historians Martínez Llopís, Xavier Domingo, and Néstor Luján who cite Granado as a pillar of culinary history, Gómez Laguna believes that Granado's work did not directly influence Spain's culinary history except for the fact that it inspired Martínez Montiño to write the definitive cookbook that influenced Spanish cooking for centuries ("Sobre Diego Granado").

46 According to records in *WorldCat*, Martínez Montiño's cookbook was published throughout Spain, ten times in the seventeenth century, ten times in

the eighteenth century, and six times in the nineteenth century until 1823. It was published again in 1982 when Tusquets printed a facsimile version and again in Valencia, 1994 and 1997. Recently three new facsimiles have surfaced: Valladolid, 2006; Seville, 2008; and Madrid, 2009.

47 Inés Eléxpuru writes about the Arab influences seen in both Granado and Martínez Montiño. She has found that Martínez Montiño includes more Hispanic-Muslim cooking in his work than Granado does (132).

48 Although Granado does have recipes for almost all of these, there is no reference to the sweet potato in the earlier work. In fact, in his prologue, Martínez Montiño is the first to mention this New World find in a cooking manual.

49 Later, in the note to his reader, Hernández de Maceras mentions forty years of kitchen work at the university (178).

50 In her introduction to the cookbook, Pérez Samper also notes that *Libro del arte de cocina* is a work that reaches a wider social stratum (65). While Gómez Laguna also acknowledges the shift in social class, he argues that the work holds little importance for Spain's gastronomic history; no additional editions were reprinted. He also criticizes the book for being disorganized and with little to offer beyond the recipes themselves ("Domingo Hernández").

51 Some food items are difficult to translate. *Albérchiga*, for example, from the Mozarabic pronunciation of the Latin *persicum*, is a peach variety and has no other equivalent in English.

52 *Lamprear* is a two-part cooking method that consists of cooking the fish or other food item, and then returning it to the pot with wine or vinegar, honey and sugar, and a fine herb mixture. It is then either brought to a boil and reduced or slowly simmered until done.

53 For these titles and others, see Simón Palmer *Libros antiguos* and *Bibliografía*. For secondary sources on chocolate and tobacco, see Norton.

54 For more on what Spaniards drank in the early modern period, see Herrero García.

55 For more on *Llibre de totes maneres de confits*, see Santanach i Suñol.

56 To date there is no critical edition or even a modern reproduction of *Los quarto libros del arte de confitería*. Extant copies are housed in Biblioteca Universitaria of Barcelona and in the Bibliothèque nationale of France.

57 Other works include *Kitab al-Filaha* [Treatise on agriculture] by Abü L-Jayr, *Kitâb al-filaha al-nabatiyya* [Book on Nabatean agriculture], and a book in verse, *Kitâb al-filaha* [Book on agriculture] by Ibn Luyûn.

58 Such extensive work has been done on New World influences in early modern Spanish cooking that I only mention a few titles here. For an overview

of the major texts that treated food that was brought to Spain, see Pérez Samper, "España y América," and Garrido Aranda. In the latter, the author records inventory from the kitchen of San Agustín de Córdoba (1679–81) that includes regular purchases of tomatoes and frijoles (208). Hernández Bermejo and León discusses the role of botanical gardens in promoting New World products in Europe. Of particular interest are those sections that deal with sixteenth-century Aranjuez and Seville (260–2). For more information on Fernandez Oviedo's role in culinary heritage, see Daneri. For long term effects of the colonizing of New World food, see Janer.

2 "Una olla de algo más vaca que carnero": Privileging Meat in the Early Modern Diet

1   All *Don Quixote* citations are from Luis Murillo's edition. All translations are my own.
2   In *Lilio de medicina*, Bernardo de Gordonio advises, "quando hablaremos de la mala complexion del estomago: mas el que tiene el estomago flaco y el estomago muy sensible, y no puede sufrir el ayuno, use caldo de carne de baca" [when we are dealing with a stomach disorder and with someone who has a weak or very sensitive stomach and cannot tolerate fasting, use beef stock] (186). Chirino acknowledges its properties for earaches. "Para el dolor del oydo echen en el gotas de cumo de carne de vaca mal asada sin sal" [For earaches, use ear drops from juice of lightly roasted beef with no added salt] (138). Finally, López de Villalobos uses beef for external healing in his instructions for a poultice for swollen joints. In his chapter "De emplastos para las junturas" [On poultices for joints], he writes, "y haced un emplastro para las junturas/ de estierco y manteca de vaca con miel" [and make a poultice for joints/ from dung and beef lard and honey] (Hernández Morejón 387).
3   The complete texts are found in the Archivo Regional de la Comunidad de Madrid [Regional archives of the Community of Madrid]: Signatura 913669/3286. See "A petición de un vecino para daños causados en su tripo por un hato de lechones" [A citizen's petition for damages incurred on his land by a herd of young pigs] and Signatura 913693/3983 "Dejar entrar reses a una viñeda; fraude en el peso de pimienta; caza indebida (1642–8)" [Allowing cattle to enter a vineyard, fraud in black pepper weight, wrongful hunting (1642–8)]. I am indebted to Natalia Maillard Alvarez for her transcriptions of these and other archival documents.
4   For more on the history of the Mesta in early modern Spain, see Martín, Valdeón, and García Sanz.

5 An *arrelde* is a four-pound weight used for weighing meat.
6 An *arroba* is a unit of weight that varied between 24–36 pounds according to the region. It was also a liquid measure that varied between 25–34 pints.
7 The maravedi [mrv] is a small monetary unit upon which other coins are measured. Its value fluctuated over the years until finally, under Isabel II in the nineteenth century, it was replaced by the centime [cent].
8 Braudel also comments that meat consumption was not limited to the rich and that Spain (and other parts of Europe) consumed an exceptional amount of meat in the early modern era compared to other parts of the world (146–52).
9 For more of the theory of capital and the role of taste in acquiring it, see Bourdieu, especially chapter 3, "The Habitus and the Space of Life Styles" (165–222).
10 For changing economic trends in Europe, see Mennell 32–3, and for those in Spain, see Bennassar (128–41) and Yun Casalilla.
11 Nola's cookbook was originally written in Catalan and was titled *Libre de coch*. It was first translated to Castilian in 1525. For more information, see chapter one (26–32).
12 Matilla Tascón reports that in 1606 beef was sold at 19 maravedies (mrvs.) through the Feast of Saint John (24 June) and mutton was sold at consistently higher prices throughout the year: 23 mrvs. (from 25 Feb. to 25 Mar.), 31 mrvs. (from 25 Mar. to 24 Apr.), 25 mrvs. (from 25 Apr. to 25 May), and 23 mrvs. (from 24 May to Saint John's Day) (111). That same year the state earned almost twice the revenue in taxes from mutton than it did from beef (21,906 reales vs 11,611 reales) (68).
13 With an increase in the sub-Saharan African population in Spain, mutton is once again appearing in the marketplace but there is still a clear preference for lamb over mutton.
14 *Carnada* and *quixote* are not terms used today to refer to cuts of meat nor are they terms that butchers in Spain recognize. However, *carnada* is probably a form of *carnaza*, a term today that refers to either the shoulder clod or the blade bolar. *Quixote* refers to the cheek meat. For an excellent resource for translating cuts of meat from Spanish to English, see *Manual de carnes bovina y ovina*. For these specific translations, see pp. 25–7, 44, 60–61.
15 Examples of leg of young mutton (today's *leg of lamb*) recipes in Martínez Montiño's cookbook include: "Gigote de una pierna de carnero" [Leg of lamb stew] (25), "Una pierna de carnero estofada" [Leg of lamb stewed] (47), "Otra pierna estofada de otra manera" [Leg of lamb stewed in another way] (48), "Otra pierna estofada de otra manera" [Leg of lamb stewed in another way] (49), "Una pierna de carnero rellena" [A leg of lamb

stuffed] (50), "Una pierna de carnero a la Francesa" [Leg of lamb French style] (51), "Otra pierna de otra manera" [Another leg of lamb in another way] (52).

16 For more information on cooking appliances, cookware, and utensils, see Marín *Relieves* (51, 54–5); for specifics within the Hispanic-Muslim tradition, see Waines (726–7); for the early modern period, see Scappi (629–62); and for information on Europe more generally, see Sarti, particularly 126–91.

17 This practice of beginning the meal with options that included the one-pot stew followed by roast selections was also the norm in France (Fábregas 11).

18 In his article "The Smellscape of *Don Quixote*," Steve Wagschal discusses the *olla podrida* and the possibility that it does not neatly fit into the contrasting patterns of food for the elite and food for peasants as it is both served at the governor's table and desired by Sancho (144n22).

19 On the origins and history of the *olla podrida*, see Gómez Laguna, "Aclaraciones" (13), González Sevilla (147), Rodríguez Marín (424–9), and L. Jacinto García (*Carlos V* 91).

20 The *mojiganga* is a minor dramatic genre that was popular in early modern Spain. It is burlesque in tone and performed at the end of a full-length play. Ted Bergman defines it as "a small dramatic piece meant to complement the larger one, something different to mark the end or bring closure to the event ... [usually] a combination of pageantry and comic relief" (5–6).

21 For another foreigner's take on the *olla podrida*, see James Howell's comment (96).

22 For more on regional varieties of *cocido*, see Calera.

23 For further information on the importance of bread in the early modern diet, see Sánchez Meco (130–1, 190–2, 272–4); for more on the bread-making industry, Hiltpold and Ringrose (144–5, 194–202, 253–77) and for more on grain production, Llopís Agelán and Hiltpold. Finally, to compare with bread in early modern England and France, see Concepción de Castro and also Purkiss's book chapter on bread as a social indicator in early modern England.

24 For more on the different types of bread and their correlation with social class, see Braudel, especially 85–139.

25 The royal decree follows:

> está ordenado que ninguna persona de los que no son panaderos, ni de los que acostumbren amasar y vender, ni son de calidad que hayan de tener esto por trato y oficio, no pudiese por sí, ni por medio de las panaderas ni otras personas, ni mediante ningún trato ni partido ni otra

cautela, vender del pan cocido, ni usar de semejante trato ni granjería; mandamos, que lo contenido en la dicha Ley, pragmática, cartas y provisiones nuestras, se cumpla. (cited in Ávila Granados 64)

[be it ordered that no one who is not a baker, neither those who regularly knead and sell, nor of the quality that those of this trade and office maintain, can themselves nor via bakers or anyone else, nor via any deal or pact or stealth, sell baked bread or take advantage of a similar deal or benefit; we order that the aforementioned of our stated law, ordinance, letters, and provisions is carried out.]

26 The earliest bread recipes in England appear in the mid-sixteenth century. For more information, see Rubel.
27 Concepción de Castro notes that in the early modern era wheat was more abundant in Spain than in many European countries to the north (47).
28 A fourth recipe is "Noclos de masa dulce" [Sweet mini rolls] (410) but as the recipe does not contain yeast or a rising agent, I have left it apart.
29 The complete quote is "echarle un poco de sal blanca, cantidad de un panecillo de los de Madrid" [add a little white salt, the amount of a Madrid bread roll] (228).

3 "Salpicón las más noches": Salads, Vegetables, and New World Contributions to Spanish Fare

1 Javier Pérez Avilés, while excavating at Cerro de las Cabezas, discovered evidence of sophisticated wine making facilities that date to 700 BCE (Khalaf). In Muslim Spain, vinegar makers went from house to house to turn household wine into vinegar (Escartín González 318–19). For more on wine production in early modern Spain, see Vassberg, *Land*; Brumont; Yun Casalilla (132, 142–4); and Huetz de Lemps.
2 An *otabo* or *octavo* is a tax applied to a specific quantity of wine, vinegar, or oil during the early modern period.
3 Sorrento is in Naples; Morón, a city, and Lavajos, a small town, are located in the province of Seville.
4 Maná [manna] is the food God provided Israelites in the desert for forty days and nights (Ex. 16:11–36) but in the seventeenth century it was "una especialidad de confiteros, más pequeña que la gragea" [a speciality of candy makers, smaller than jelly beans] (Valles Rojo, *Cocina* 423).
5 For more information on food's symbolic presence in the visual arts, see Malaguzzi.

6 In *Imperial Eyes: Travel Writing and Transculturation*, Pratt examines how
   European explorers since the eighteenth century have culturally affected
   Latin America and Africa. She pays particular attention to the gendered
   narratives of male capitalists who focused on the exploitation of natural
   resources and the advantages of Western technology to develop them and
   female social explorers whose writings focused on women's issues and the
   domestic sphere.

7 For more on the introduction of New World products to Europe, see
   Terrón, Valles Rojo (*Saberes y sabores*), Garrido Aranda, and Pérez Samper
   ("España y América"), and for their conservative reception in Europe, Coe
   (48–9). For information on food's role in the representation of the New
   World and textual authority, see Rabasa and Myers.

8 *Gazpacho andaluz* needs little explanation as its popularity as a chilled tomato soup has reached well beyond the borders of Spain. Red *piquillo* peppers, although they resemble small, cone-shaped varieties of chilies, are
   not at all spicy and are commonly served stuffed with meat or fish. The
   tortilla española is very different from the Mexican tortilla. Its three main
   ingredients are potato, onion, and egg. It is found in almost any bar in
   Spain and consumed either hot or cold. Finally, *chocolate con churros*, is a
   cup of thick hot chocolate served with several thin loops of fried dough
   that are dipped in the chocolate. They are eaten both for breakfast and as
   an afternoon snack.

9 Sahagún spent over thirty years writing this compendium that was com-
   pleted in 1575–7. In his writings, he also discusses the medicinal properties of the tomato. Bernal Díaz del Castillo and Francisco Hernández also
   write about the tomato's flavour and how it is prepared (Garrido Aranda
   202). For more on the types of tomato and the linguistic distinctions
   among different varieties, see Nuez who records seven different Nahuatl
   tomatos and their Spanish translations as well as the corresponding botanical species (30).

10 Hermolaus was a fifteenth-century Italian scholar who edited Pliny's
   Natural History (1492).

11 The House of Aguilar comes from the lineage of the González de Córdoba,
   whose most famous member was Fernando González de Córdoba, "el
   gran capitán," whom Cervantes mentions in *Don Quixote*. For more on the
   arrival of the tomato and the history of its incorporation into Spanish cuisine, see Long-Solís, "El tomate."

12 Susan Smith, co-editor of *Los coloquios del alma: Cuatro dramas alegóricos de
   Sor Marcela de San Félix, hija de Lope de Vega*, explained that while there is
   no specific date attached to this first of Sor Marcela's four allegorical plays,

she believes that it was most likely penned before 1659, the date of the second play.

13 For more detail on eighteenth-century gazpacho, see Juan de la Mata's recipe "Gazpachos de todos generos" [All types of gazpacho] (164).

14 For more on the history of the production and use of paprika, see Long-Solís, *Capsicum y cultura* and Pérez de Espinardo.

15 There is an opportunity within food studies to understand how writers, in particular those of both the early modern stage and picaresque literature, used food images both to add humour to their texts and, more specifically, to add a comic dimension to certain characters whose very names are specific foods. Few critics have explored the area of "gastro-humour," that is, how food and humour intersect in different early modern genres. For an example of this type of literary analysis, see Gordon.

16 For more on the social effects of the potato, see Salaman and Gallager.

17 Góngora also writes about the sweet potato but uses the correct term, *batata* (Amado Doblas 934–5).

18 Although sweet potato pie is more common today, we cannot eliminate the possibility of a potato pie. In his banned list Martínez Montiño also includes other savoury pies made from vegetables grown underground such as turnips or truffles.

19 Both Sahagún and Hernández write about the highly valued, aromatic ear flower. For more, see Safford.

20 Calderón de la Barca also weighs in on the debate agreeing with Juan de Cárdenas when the main character of the *mojiganga, Pésame de la viuda* [Sympathy for the widow], Maria Prado, declares that chocolate does not break the fast (vv. 59–61).

21 In a search in *Corpus español, desayunar* and its variants (*desayun**) appear hundreds of times but it is not until the nineteenth century that it is regularly used to refer to breakfast as we understand it today. See Davies.

22 For more on cultural materialism in the early modern home in Europe, see Sarti, especially 126–7, and for the rise of cultural materialism in Spain, see Sánchez Jiménez. In his article he discusses how still life paintings of fruit reflected a shift in material wealth and the appearance of luxury products. He proposes three main reasons for their appearance. First, they acted as conduits for moral reflection; second they were a result of the fluctuation of market provisions and allowed people to take notice of these objects as material wealth; and third, they were examples of *imitatio* that allowed viewers to forget harsh realities while meditating on aspects of nature's perfection. Enrique García Santo-Tomás also explores questions of food in the context of material culture in chapter 4 of his monograph, *Espacio urbano y creación literaria en el Madrid de Felipe IV*.

4 "Duelos y quebrantos los sábados": Jewish and Muslim Influences on Early Modern Eating Habits

1 For a definition of the *mojiganga*, see 243n20.
2 More recently, Rosa Navarro argues that "duelos y quebrantos" refers ironically to "griefs and complaints" and not to any specific dish.
3 The law reads as follows:

> ningunos cristianos vesinos desta dicha çibdad, no sean osados de aquí adelante en ningund tiempo, de comprar ni compren carne de las dichas carneçerías de judíos e moros. So pena que qualquier que lo comprare, por la primera ves paque de pena trezientos maravedís e por la segunda ves seysçientos maravedís e por la terçera ves, sy fuere persona honrada paque de pena mill e dosyentos maravedís e sy persona ofiçial de vaxa suerte que le darán çinquenta açotes públicamente por esta dicha çibdad. Las quales dichas penas de dineros se repartan en esta manera: el terçio para el que lo descubriere e los dos terçios para esta dicha çibdad. E que es esas mismas penas yncurran los carniçeros de las dichas carniçerías de moros e judíos sy vendieren la dicha carne a cristianos. (1480, 24 febrero L.P. fol. 83v; cited in Izquierdo Benito 203)

> [No Christian citizens of this said city dare henceforth and at no time buy or sell meat from said Jewish and Moorish butcher shops. Whoever buys it is subject to a fine of three hundred maravedis for the first offence, and six hundred maravedis for the second offence and for the third offence, if the person is honourable, he shall pay one thousand two hundred maravedis and if he is an official townsmen, that he be given fifty public lashings in this said city. That such said monetary fines be distributed in this way: a third for the complainant and two thirds for said city. And that the butchers of said Jewish and Moorish butcher shops incur these said fines if they sell said meat to Christians.]

4 For more on Jewish food as evidence in Inquisitional trials and Jewish eating habits and influences on Spanish gastronomy, see L. Jacinto García (*Un banquete*), and Gitlitz and Davidson (especially pp. 3–5), and for information on Jewish social history and what Jews ate in the Middle Ages, see Cooper.
5 For Jewish food restrictions, see Sternberg, and for Muslim ones, see Harvey.
6 In Tirso's *Bellaco sois, Gómez,* Gregorio points to the quality of the hams in Ana's town:

GREGORIO: Acompáñale un jamón
de Molina, y os prometo
que a Rute y las Algarrobillas
se las apuesta.
ANA: Os lo creo. (Act 1)

[GREGORIO: Have it with a ham from Molina, and I swear to you that
anyone would bet it is from Rute or Algarrovillas.
ANA: I believe you.]

7 In the *Kitāb al-tabīj* two other recipes, "Sinhāŷī" [Sinhaya] (207) and
"Receta del sinhāŷī regio" [Recipe for royal sinhaya] (55–6), call for partridge as one of the ingredients but in these elaborate beef-based stews,
fowl is not the focus of the dish.

8 Many critics have written on the historic value of this picaresque novel,
specifically on Aldonza's Jewish ancestry and life as a *converso* (Wolfenzon,
Arellano), the erotic (Joly, Joset, Imperiale), and the feminine subject
(Parrack).

9 *Mamotreto* refers to a thick, heavy book that is generally uneven in its organization. It has also been translated as *memorandum* or *notebook*. Delicado
uses this term to organize the sixty six different sections of his novel.

10 Although the words *culantro* and *cilantro* are used interchangeably, today
we know that *culantro* [eryngium foetidum] is an entirely different plant
from *cilantro* [coriander sativum]. It is native to tropical America and the
West Indies and thus not available in Europe until the sixteenth century.
However, lexical confusion was common enough, as evidenced by the use
of *patata* for *batata* explained in chapter 3. Delicado's insertion of *culantro*
for *cilantro* is also found in cooking manuals and dietary treatises. In several recipes, Nola calls for both *culantro seco* [coriander] and *culantro verde*
[cilantro]. See, for example, "Potaje de culantro llamado primo" [Cilantro-
coriander broth called the first], "Otro potaje de culantro llamado celian-
drate segundo" [Another coriander broth called the second celiandrate],
and "Otro potaje de culantro llamado tercio" [Another cilantro broth
called the third] (275–6). Lobera de Ávila also cites *culantro* in prescribing
a diet for the convalescent (177).

11 In his edition of *La lozana andaluza*, Claude Allaigre actually changes *textones* to *tostones* but I have left the original *textones*. See 250n25.

12 The phrase *olla reposada, no la come toda barba* is generally used to express
"too much work leaves little time for rest or comfort." But, here when

Aldonza says, "olla reposada, no la comía tal ninguna barba," she is referring to how good her grandmother's stew was and that no one ("ninguna
barba") ate it slowly (while resting). Instead everyone gobbled it down because it was so good.

13 *Boronia* has no direct translation into English. It is a precursor to the "pisto
manchego" (something akin to ratatouille). The dictionary of the Real
Academia Española [*RAE*] explains that the name comes from the Arabic,
al-būrāniyya, that comes from the name, Būrān, wife to caliph al-Ma'mūn.
Today the dish continues to be prepared and generally includes tomatoes
as well. For more on the evolution of this dish, see Marín, "Sobre Būrān y
Būrānīyyā."

14 The "cuajar" [abomasum] is one of the stomach cavities of the goat. It was
prepared much like other tripe dishes.

15 The dictionary of the *RAE* defines *oruga* as the arugula plant but it is also
known as a sauce: "salsa gustosa que se hace de esta planta, con azúcar o
miel, vinagre y pan tostado, y se distingue llamándola oruga de azúcar o
de miel" [tasty sauce made from this plant, with sugar or honey, vinegar,
and toast. Calling it sugar or honey arugula differentiates it] (*Diccionario de
la lengua*).

16 Although he published anonymously, nineteenth-century critics discovered Delicado's identity, and the biographical details – his upbringing in
Jaén (born c. 1475), adulthood in Rome until the sack of Rome in 1527, and
final years in Venice (died 1534) – that contributed to his fiction. Damiani
states that, "as a result of the Inquisitorial practices against a great number
of converts and of the Expulsion Edict of 1492, which sent the Jews of
Spain into exile, Delicado joined the massive exodus of his compatriots to
Italy and established himself in Rome, where he remained until 1528" (14).

17 An important source for understanding Muslim influences in Spanish
cooking is Teresa de Castro Martínez, in particular, "Moriscos y cristianos"
and "Iberian Peninsula."

18 The *calabaza* is one of the more popular vegetables in both the Middle
Ages and the early modern period. I have translated *calabaza* as bottle
squash giving precedence to its shape. This squash is from the species *lage-
naria siceraria*, and was brought to Spain from Africa, unlike most squashes, which originated in the Americas.

19 In addition to *La lozana andaluza*, empanadas appear in countless literary
texts: *Don Quixote, El buscón,* and *Guzmán de Alfarache* to name a few.
Another famous example can be found at the end of the first chapter of
Vélez de Guevara's *El Diablo cojuelo* [The mischievous devil] in which the

city of Madrid is described as an empanada. For more, see Enrique García Santo-Tomás, *Espacio urbano* (208–9).

20 In *Exotic Nation* Barbara Fuchs examines how Spanish and European writers consider Moorish-Christian hybridity in the architecture, costume, and horsemanship of early modern Spain.

21 The anonymous *Kitāb al-tabīj* also contains several couscous recipes with variations (223–7).

22 Ground pine resembles a miniature pine tree with a purple, hairy stem. It was primarily used as an antispasmodic and today is still used by herbalists in treating rheumatism, gout, and menstrual cramps. For more on its properties, see "Pinillo."

23 For more popular rice recipes both "dry" and "brothy," see "Nostra Taula: Cocina valenciana."

24 Adamuz is still known for its honey. In 2002 Montoro-Adamuz received a *denominación de origen* ranking from the Consejería de Agricultura y Pesca de la Junta Andaluza. The saffron-Peñafiel connection remains a mystery.

25 *Textones* is especially hard to translate but López Castanier believes they consist of a combination of sugar, honey, and seeds that is formed into a sesame meringue (149). The emphasis of *hormigos made with oil* indicates Jewish preparation (no lard). This point of clarification is also seen in the works of Nola, Martínez Montiño, and other cookbook authors.

26 For information on early sugar production in Spain, see Galloway, particularly chapter 3.

27 In Nola's cookbook, sugar appears in 91 of the 242 recipes. While most often described simply as sugar, it also appears in entries as fine sugar, a chunk of sugar, white sugar, and as sugar syrup. Sugar also appears as one of the ingredients in a fish dish (366).

28 For more information on this manuscript, see Santanach i Suñol.

29 Though not electuaries, candied walnut recipes are also found in *Llibre de totes maneres de confits* (Santanach i Suñol 282), *Llibre de Sent Soví* (*The Book of Sent Sovi* 164), and later in Baeza's *Los cuatro libros del arte de confitería* (cited in Martínez Llopis, *La dulcería* 29). Santanach notes that in the 1393 French cooking manual *Le ménagier de Paris* [The Parisian household book] a similar recipe is also found, thus demonstrating the international appeal of sweetened walnuts (282n1).

30 For more information on the diffusion of vegetables from Asia to Europe that Muslims facilitated, see Riera Melis, "Las plantas," and Watson.

31 Martínez Montiño has two different recipes for Morisco-style hen: "Gallina morisca" [Morisco hen] (63) and "Gallina a la morisca" [Morisco-style hen] (407).

5 "Lantejas los Viernes": Perceptions of Health and Christian Abstinence

1 These pulses are not to be confused with American native beans, which include the common bean, the lima bean, and the scarlet runner bean, all of whose origins can be traced to Southern Mexico and Central America. Common beans have over 500 varieties that include kidney, snap, French, haricot verts, flageolet, garden, filet, green, and strong and they took on a different, more exotic status in the early modern period. For more on the history of beans in general, see Albala. For more on the origins of beans, peas and lentils, see Vavilov (324–53).

2 In the *Association for Hispanic Classical Theater* data base word search, lentils, garbanzos, and fava beans appear significantly less that any meat or fowl product and even less than other vegetables like eggplant or lettuce.

3 In addition to those characteristics listed, Juan Cruz Cruz includes three other factors: a food's spirit that can be natural, vital, or animal; the way food is digested – in the stomach, another organ, or peripheral parts; and the importance of a "contrary" food to that of the humour in excess, e.g., excessive cold is treated with heat, etc. (*Dietética medieval*, 42–65). For more on Galen's theory of the spirit, see pp. 255–6.

4 For more on the history of dietary treatises and food's role in maintaining sound health, see Luján, especially pp. 104–9.

5 For a fuller account of the onomastic of the doctor's name, see Close (139).

6 For a reading of the Hippocratic and Galenic philosophy behind Pedro Recio's orders, see Cruz Cruz, *Dietética medieval* (39–80).

7 For more on the debate of food's role and noble blood, see Maravall (54–61).

8 Tertullian, the "father of Latin Christianity," dedicates an essay to the subject called "On Fasting," in which he discusses when and how to fast. Later, Pope Nicholas I (858–67) prohibited eating the flesh of an animal on Fridays.

9 Another reaction to the Spanish custom of eating organ meat on Saturdays is found in chapter 4 (148–9). Several travellers to Spain, for example Leo of Rosmithal, Thomé Pinheiro da Veiga, and the Marchioness of Villars, also comment on the unique abstinence practices of Spain. See Díez Borque (*La vida española* 105).

10 In Nola's *Libro de guisados* 50 fish recipes appear of a total of 242 and in Hernández de Macera's *Libro de arte de cocina*, 37 of the 177. In this latter work, dried hake, barbel, eel, Conger eel, lamprey, tuna, sea bream, and grouper are the most frequent.

11 In fact, Spain is Europe's leading importer of both lentils and garbanzos and the second leading importer of dry beans and fava beans, behind Italy.

For more on Spain's legume production and trade in a global context, see Akibode.

6 "Algún palomino de añadidura los domingos": The Theatrics of Food and Celebration

1 For a reading of the exchange of dialogue between Sancho and the inn-keeper on the road to Barcelona, see Goodwin.

2 There are really no indications whether the *pavo* here refers to *turkey* or to *peacock*. Food historians translate the bird in both ways. My instinct is that *pavo* translates as turkey almost immediately following contact with the New World. The peacock was still prized among nobility but by 1611 turkeys were widely eaten and readily available. As explained on p. 168 of this chapter, Julio Valles Rojo ranks turkeys above hens and male chickens but below female chickens and capons (*Cocina* 238).

3 Both *pichón* and *palomino* translate as *squab*. The difference is that the *pichón* is the chick of the domesticated *paloma* [pigeon], and the *palomino* is the chick of the wild *paloma*, [dove].

4 While "English pasties" are typically made with beef, in Martínez Montiño's recipe he clearly indicated that "pecho de pavo" [turkey breast] can substitute for the beef (188).

5 Mrs. is an abbreviation for *maravedís*. For more on the value of this coin, see p. 242n7.

6 One *azumbre* is 2.016 litres or approximately one half gallon.

7 This preference for poultry continues a well-established taste as is evident in the multiple references to fowl as a favoured dish of the nobility in various medieval chronicles (Castro Martínez, *La alimentación* 267).

8 Molénat also reports that in fifteenth-century Toledo, chicken was the preferred dish of high officials (317).

9 For more on banquets, spectacles, and hosting extravagant parties, see García Santo-Tomás's work on smell, taste, and sight in Golden Age Spain (*Espacio urbano*) and his book of collected essays on material culture and consumption (*Materia crítica*). Among other critics who have written on the banquet in early modern Spain, see Pérez Samper, "Fiesta y aliment-ación." For a European context, see Jeanneret and for the treatment of the banquet in literary texts, see Burke, and Nadeau, "Spanish Culinary History," and "Transformation and Transgression."

10 *Albardar* is a culinary technique that entails wrapping a piece of meat or fish with bacon or fat back so that its juices will stay more intact and it will not overbrown on the outside.

11 The *MLA International Bibliography* reveals that some thirty articles, one
    book, and one dissertation have been published on Lope de Rueda in the
    last thirty years. When the search is limited to the *pasos*, only nine articles
    and one dissertation appear.

12 All citations from the *pasos* are from the Fernando González Ollé y Vicente
    Tusón's edition; the translations are my own.

13 Others have also written on the connection between these acts. For the
    connections between hunting, gathering, food, and conquest, see Gerli's
    article on the hunt of love.

14 James Parr discusses the semantic nexus of sex and food in *El burlador de
    Sevilla.*

15 Carter discusses the multiple images of honey in literature, particularly
    those with erotic undertones (98).

16 Both Alan Paterson and C.A. Soons explore the possible social and poetic
    codes behind the banquet scene. Regarding the senses, Frederick de
    Armas discusses the banquet of sense in Cervantes's *Persiles y Sigismunda*
    and Steven Wagschal focuses on the sense of smell in *Don Quixote.*

17 All translations for *La verdad sospechosa* are from Dakin Matthews. I have
    made a slight modification to the words "thicket" (river grove) and
    "clean" (fragrant) in this first translation to maintain the location of the
    event and the importance of the olfactory sense.

18 Heliotrope is used for increasing sexual emotions; carnation for sexual de-
    sires; meliot relieves melancholy. For more on the properties of essential
    oils, see Rose, and for the history of aromatics, see Genders. For the treat-
    ment of aromatic recipes found in the *Manual de mugeres* and its relation-
    ship to *La Celestina*, see Nadeau, "What Else?"

19 An *adarme* is a unit of weight equivalent to 1.79 grams or .63 ounces.

20 For a history on the legend of the cave, see Samuel Waxman, who traces
    the legend of the cave of Toledo back to the story of the Tower of Hercules
    from the *Crónica del moro Rasís*, and Manuel García Blanco. For Ruiz de
    Alarcón's use of magic in the comedia, see Augusta Espantoso Foley and
    Mary Anne Lee Vetterling, and for the debate on magic in the *Cueva de
    Salamanca*, see David Darst.

21 Few critics have explored the area of "gastro-humour" in early modern
    texts. For more information, see 145n16.

22 Platina's *On Right Pleasure and Good Health* is an example of this type of
    literature. While Platina does not banish the pleasure of eating, taste is
    of secondary importance. In *La civil conversazione* [The civil conversation]
    (1574), Stephan Guazzo reduces the banquet to an exercise in illustrating
    refined gestures. Cristoforo de Messisbugo, who wrote *Banchette,*

compositioni di vivande et apparecchio generale [Foods and general necessities for banquets] (1549), records a list of banquets he designed and carried out. These lists include the occasion, the guests, the setting, number of dishes per course, and other details of the menu.

23 This text was a standard reference for teaching good manners for more than three centuries.

24 In their edition to the text, Sevilla Arroyo and Rey Hazas explain that "de una oreja" is a euphemism for "good wine" (991n15).

25 For more on the history of blancmange, see Contreras Más.

7 *La sobremesa*: Final Reflections on the Discourse of Food in Early Modern Spain

1 For more on a researcher's own "modes of identification," see MacClancy.

Appendix of Recipes

1 *Grasa tierna* is not a term used today but I have translated it as *delicate fat* to refer to the flavour of the fat, for example, from lamb, veal or poultry, as opposed to a strong, heavy flavour, like fat from mutton, beef, or goat.

2 *Almorí* is a barley-based flavour enhancer, very salty and usually made with vinegar and honey.

3 The *dirhem* or *dram* was historically both a coin and a weight.

4 For an explanation of *terciado*, see p. 132.

5 A *cuarta* is another monetary term that is equivalent to 4 maravedis. So *cuarta y media* would translate to 6 maravedis worth of an ingredient. Elsewhere I translated a *maravedí* as *a pinch* thus, one would need about 6 pinches of cloves.

6 *Almuesta* or today *ambuesta* or *ambueza* is the amount a person can fit when holding two open, cupped-shaped hands together.

7 *Tres blancas* is a common monetary expression. A *blanca* is a coin worth half a *maravedí*, a small monetary unit upon which other coins are measured. Here, the "three-penny" bread refers to a specific sized loaf that everyone would be familiar with.

8 The measurements for herbs and spices may have originally been based on their monetary value, in other words, the quantity was defined by how much they cost, rather than how much they measured. But, in this and other recipes, the maravedi measurement has evolved to refer to a specific quantity, something akin to a "maravedi-sized pinch."

9 The word *moxí*, comes from the Hispano-Arabic *muhsi*, which originates from the classic Arabic, *mashu*, which means an egg-based tort made in an earthenware pot with honey, cheese, and eggplant.

10 *Duke's powder* is a mix of cinnamon, clove, and sugar with an optional ingredient of ginger. For Nola's recipe, see Nola (265).

11 For more information on beef salpicon, which is a shredded beef salad, see pp. 73–4.

12 An *azumbre* is equivalent to two litres, or a little over two pints. Seven *azumbres* is equivalent to 29.5 pints.

Works Cited

Abad Alegría, Francisco. *Pimientos, guindillas y pimentón: Una sinfonía en rojo.* Gijón, Spain: Ediciones Trea, 2008.

Acosta, Juan de. *Historia natural y moral de las Indias.* Ed. José Alcina Franch. Madrid: Historia 16, 1986.

Aguilera Pleguezuelo, José. *Las cocinas árabe y judía y la cocina española.* Málaga: Arguval, 2002.

Akibode, Sitou, and Mywish Maredia. "Global and Regional Trends in Production, Trade and Consumption of Food Legume Crops." 2011. *Impact Assessment: CGIAR.* Consultative Group on International Agricultural Research. http://impact.cgiar.org/sites/default/files/images/Legumetrendsv2.pdf. Consulted on 15 Jul. 2012.

Albala, Ken. *Beans: A History.* New York: Berg, 2007.

Alcanyís, Lluís. *Regiment preservatiu e curatiu de la pestilència* Ed. Jon Arrizabalaga. Barcelona: Barcino, 2008.

Alcázar, Baltasar de. "La cena jocosa." *Círculo de poesía. Revista electronica de literatura* (May 2010). Intro. Dalí Corona. http://circulodepoesia.com/nueva/2010/05/baltasar-de-alcazar-la-cena-jocosa. Consulted on 17 Jun. 2012.

Alemán, Mateo. *El Guzmán de Alfarache.* Ed. Benito Brancaforte. Madrid: Akal, 1996.

Allard, Jeanne. "Diego Granado Maldonado." *Petits Propos Culinaires* 25 (1987): 35–41.

Altamiras, Juan de. *Nuevo arte de cocina.* Madrid: Magalia Ediciones, [2000].

Alvar-Ezquerra, Alfredo. "Comer y 'ser' en la Corte del Rey Católico: Mecanismos de diferenciación social en el cambio de siglo." *Materia crítica: Formas de ocio y de consumo en la cultura áurea.* Ed. Enrique García Santo-Tomás. Madrid: Iberoamericana, 2009. 295–320.

Amado Doblas, María Isabel. "La batata de Málaga, fruto de indias preferido por la Literatura del Siglo de Oro." *Estudios sobre América: siglos XVI–XX.* Ed. Antonio María Gutiérrez Escudero and María Luisa Cuetos. Seville: Asocación Española de Americanistas, 2005. 929–44.

Andrés, José. "Creativity in Cooking Can Solve Our Biggest Challenges." TEDxMidAtlantic. Jan. 2011. http://tedxtalks.ted.com/video/ TEDxMidAtlantic-2011-Jose-Andre;Food. Consulted on 12 Mar. 2013.

Arbelos, Carlos. *Gastronomía de las tres culturas: Recetas y relatos de los siglos XIII y XVI.* Granada: Caja de Granada, 2004.

Archivo Regional de la comunidad de Madrid. Fondo Archivo histórico municipal de Fuentidueña de Tajo. Libro. Signatura 13236 1048. "Libro de los registros y aforos de vino, vinagre, aceite, carnes, tocino, pescado y reses de cerda de cada vecino." (1610–1759). Consulted on 11 May 2011.

– Fondo Archivo histórico municipal de Loeches. Expediente judicial. Signatura 96014 26. "Expediente judicial Pedro Olive Teniente de alguacil contra Jose Milas." (1642). Consulted on 12 May 2011.

– Fondo Archivo histórico municipal de San Martín de la Vega. Auto. Signatura 913632 2551. "Del alguacil mayor al mesonero por incumplimiento de pragmática sobre la venta de comidas." (1619). Consulted on 12 May 2011.

– Fondo Archivo histórico municipal de San Martín de la Vega. Denuncia. Signatura 913693 3983. "Dejar entrar reses a una viñeda; fraude en el peso de pimienta; caza indebida." (1642–48). Consulted on 13 May 2011.

– Fondo Archivo histórico municipal de San Martín de la Vega. Mandamiento. Signatura 18230 491. "Que traiga pan a la corte como se debe." (1606). Consulted on 11 May 2011.

– Fondo Archivo histórico municipal de San Martín de la Vega. Mandamiento. Signatura 18230 496. "Que se venda el pan y el trigo cocido como es costumbre." (1606). Consulted on 11 May 2011.

– Fondo Archivo histórico municipal de San Martín de la Vega. Requisición. Signatura 913669 3286. "A petición de un vecino para daños causados en su tripo por un hato de lechones." (1606). Consulted on 4 Oct. 2007.

– Fondo Archivo histórico municipal de San Martín de la Vega. Denunciación. Signatura 18390 3109. "Auto venta de vino al por menor y de tajadas de vaca." (1668–1804). Consulted on 11 May 2011.

Arellano, Ignacio. "Una alusión tradicional en *La lozana andaluza*: El caudal de un judío (Mamotreto XVI)." *Epos: Revista de Filologia* 2 (1986): 313–16.

Armas, Frederick A. de. "A Banquet of the Senses: The Mythological Structure of Persiles y Sigismunda, III." *Bulletin of Hispanic Studies* 70.4 (1993): 403–14.

Arróniz, Othón. *La influencia italiana en el nacimiento de la comedia española.*
Madrid: Gredos, 1969.

Association for Hispanic Classical Theater. Ed. Matthew Stroud and Laura Vidler.
6 Sep 2011. http://www.wordpress.comedias.org. Consulted on 9 Aug.
2012.

Aulnoy, la condesa de. *Un viaje por España en 1679.* Intro. and trans. Luis Ruiz
Contreras. Madrid: Ediciones La Nave, 1943.

Ávila Granados, Jesús. *Una historia panadera de 640 años: Gremio de panaderos de
Barcelona, el gremio de los artesanos de pan.* Barcelona: Gremio de panaderos
de Barcelona, 2008.

Barrios, Juan de. *Libro en el cual se trata del chocolate, que provechos haga, y si sea
bebida saludable o no.* Mexico: Jerónimo Ball, 1609.

Barthes, Roland. *The Pleasure of the Text.* Trans. Richard Miller. New York: Hill
and Wang, 1975.

Bautista de la Concepción, San Juan. *Espíritu de la reforma trinitaria.* Vol. 3 in
Obras completas. Ed. Juan Pujana and Arsenio Llamazares. Madrid:
Biblioteca de autores cristianos, 1998–2002.

Beinhart, Heim. *Records of the Trials of the Spanish Inquisition in Ciudad Real.* Vol.
1, *1483–1485.* Jerusalem: The Israel National Academy of Sciences and
Humanities, 1974.

Bennassar, Bartolomé. *La España del siglo de oro.* Serie General 109. Ed. Gonzalo
Pontón, 1983. Trans. Pablo Bordonava. Barcelona: Crítica, 2001.

Bergman, Ted L.L. *The Art of Humour in the Teatro Breve and Comedias of
Calderón de la Barca.* Woodbridge: Tamesis, 2003.

Biasin, Gian-Paolo. *The Flavors of Modernity: Food and the Novel.* Princeton:
Princeton University Press, 1993.

Bolens, Lucie. *La cocina andaluza, un arte de vivir: Siglos XI–XIII.* Trans. M.
Asensio Moreno. Madrid: EDAF, 1992.

The Book of Sent Soví: Medieval Recipes from Catalonia. Ed. Joan Santanach. Trans.
Robin Vogelzang. Woodbridge: Tamesis; Barcelona: Barcino, 2008.

Bourdieu, Pierre. *Distinction: A Social Critique of the Judgement of Taste.* 1984.
Intro. Tony Bennett. Trans. Richard Nice. New York: Routledge, 2010.

Braudel, Fernand. *Civilización material y capitalismo.* Trans. Josefina Gómez
Mendoza. Barcelona: Labor, 1974.

Brumont, Francis. *Paysans de Vieille-Castille aux XVIe et XVIIe siècles.* Madrid:
Casa de Velázquez, 1993.

Burke, James. "The 'Banquet of Sense' in *La verdad sospechosa.*" *Hispanic Studies
in Honor of Alan D. Deyermond: A North American Tribute.* Ed. John S.
Miletich. Madison: University of Wisconsin Press, 1986. 51–6.

Calderón de la Barca, Pedro. "Los guisados" [mojiganga]. Ed. Evangelina Rodríguez and Antonio Tordera. Alicante: Biblioteca Virtual Miguel de Cervantes, 2000. *Biblioteca virtual Miguel de Cervantes*. http://www .cervantesvirtual.com/obra-visor-din/los-guisados-mojiganga--0/html. Consulted on 3 May 2012.

– "El pésame de la viuda" [mojiganga]. Ed. Evangelina Rodríguez and Antonio Tordera. Alicante: Biblioteca Virtual Miguel de Cervantes, 2000. *Biblioteca virtual Miguel de Cervantes*. http://www.cervantesvirtual.com/ obra-visor/el-pesame-de-la-viuda-mojiganga--0/html. Consulted on 3 May 2012.

– *La púrpura de la rosa*. Ed. Ángeles Cardona, Don Cruickshank, and Martin Cunningham. Kassel: Reichenberger, 1990.

Calendario de Córdoba. Ed. Yves Ouahnon. Barcelona: Ediciones Apostrofe, 1997.

Calera, Ana María. *La cocina regional española*. Barcelona: Mundo Actual de Ediciones, 1982.

Calila y Dimna. Ed. J.M. Cacho Blecua and María Jesús Lacarra. Madrid: Clásicos Castalia, 1984.

Calvillo de Teruel, María Rosa. *Libro de apuntaciones de guisos y dulce*. Ed. Elena Di Pinto. Madrid: Visor Libros, 2013.

Camporesi, Piero. *Bread of Dreams: Food and Fantasy in Early Modern Europe*. Trans. David Gentilcore. Cambridge, MA: Polity Press, 1980.

Caravajal, Mariana de. *Navidades de Madrid y noches entretenidas*. Ed. Antonella Prato. Milan: Franco Angeli, 1988.

Cárdenas, Juan de. *Problemas y secretos maravillosos de las Indias*. Intro. Ángeles Durán. Madrid: Alianza Editorial, 1988.

Caro Dávila, Manuel. *Discurso físico, y moral sobre la questión theológica, que pregunta: si el chocolate quebranta el ayuno*. Granada: Antonio de Torrubia, 1699.

Carter, Alexandra. "Aspectos antropológicos de la alimentación humana en la literatura." *Káñina* 8.1–2 (1984): 97–101.

Castro, Américo. "Sentido histórico-literario del jamón y del tocino." *Cervantes y los casticismos españoles*. Madrid: Alianza, 1974. 25–32.

Castro, Concepción de. *El pan de Madrid: El abasto de las ciudades española del Antiguo Régimen*. Madrid: Alianza, 1987.

Castro Martínez, Teresa de. *La alimentación en las crónicas castellanas bajomedievales*. Granada: Universidad de Granada, 1996.

– "Carne/3." *Abastecimiento y consumo alimentarios en el Reino de Granada (1482–1510)*. 2007–12. http://www.geocities.ws/CollegePark/Field/4664/ Historyserver/Tes2/carne3.htm. Consulted on 20 Oct. 2014.

- "Iberian Peninsula: Moorish Heritage in the Cuisines of Spain and Portugal." 2005–8. http://www.geocities.ws/CollegePark/Field/4664/ Historyserver/papers/IberianPeninsula.htm. Consulted on 21 Oct. 2014.
- "Moriscos y cristianos: La construcción de dos identidades alimentarias en Castilla entre el Renacimeinto y la Edad moderna." http://www .geocities.ws/CollegePark/Field/4664/Historyserver/papers/Estrasbesp .htm. Consulted on 23 Sept. 2015.

Cavarozzi, Bartolomeo. *Dinner at Emmaus*. The J. Paul Getty Museum. http:// www.getty.edu/art/collection/objects/615/attributed-to-bartolomeo- cavarozzi-the-supper-at-emmaus-italian-about-1615-1625. Consulted on 17 Jun. 2011.

Cervantes, Miguel de. *Los baños de Argel*. Electronic text by Vern G.Williamsen and J.T. Abraham. 2002. *Obras d* Proyecto Cervantes. http://cervantes.tamu. edu/V2/textos/AHCT/ba%F1osargel_05.htm. Consulted on 28 Apr. 2015.
- *Entremés de La cueva de Salamanca*. Ed. Vern Williamsen. Association for Hispanic Classical Theater, 1997. http://www.comedias.org/cervantes/ cuesal.html. Consulted on 13 Mar. 2013.
- *El ingenioso hidalgo don Quijote de la Mancha*. Ed. Luis Andrés Murillo. 2 vols. Madrid: Castalia, 1978.
- *Ocho comedias y ocho entremeses: El trato de Argel; La Numancia; Viaje del Parnaso; Poesías sueltas*. Ed. Florencio Sevilla Arroyo and Antonio Rey Hazas. Madrid: Centro de Estudios Cervantios, 1995.

Charnon-Deutsch, Lou. "El discurso de la higiene física y moral en la narrativa femenina." *La mujer de letras o la letraherida: Discursos y representaciones sobre la mujer escritora en el siglo XIX*. Ed. Pura Fernández and Marie-Linda Ortega. Madrid: Consejo Superior de Investigaciones Científicas, 2008. 177–88.

Chirino, Alonso. *Menor daño de la medicina de Alonso de Chirino*. Ed. María Teresa Herrera. Salamanca: Ediciones Universidad, 1973.

La chocolatada [The chocolate party]. Tilework. Museu del Disseny, Barcelona. *Museo de cerámica, Palacio de Pedralbes, Barcelona*. By Trinidad Sánchez- Pacheco, M. Antonia Casanovas, and Maria Dolors Giral. Zaragoza: Ibercaja, 1993.

Close, Anthony. *A Companion to Don Quixote*. Woodbridge, UK: Tamesis, 2008.

Coe, Sophie D. *America's First Cuisines*. Austin: University of Texas Press, 1994.

Coe, Sophie D., and Michael D. Coe. *The True History of Chocolate*. London: Thames and Hudson, 1996.

Colmenero de Ledesma, Antonio. *Curioso tratado de la naturaleza y calidad del chocolate, dividido en quatro puntos*. Madrid: Francisco Martínez, 1631.

Colón, Cristóbal. *Diario de a bordo*. Ed Luis Arranz. Madrid: Historia 16, 1985.

Colón, Hernando. *Historia del Almirante*. Ed Luis Arranz. Madrid: Historia 16, 1984.

Contreras, Alonso de. *Vida del capitán Alonso de Contreras, caballero del hábito de San Juan, natural de Madrid, escrita por él mismo (años 1582 a 1633)*. Biblioteca virtual Miguel de Cervantes. http://www.cervantesvirtual.com/obra/vida-del-capitn-alonso-de-contreras-caballero-del-hbito-de-san-juan-natural-de-madrid-escrita-por-l-mismo-aos-1582-a-1633-0/. Consulted on 9 May 2012.

Contreras Más. *El menjar blanc: Orígenes y evolución de un plato*. Palma de Mallorca: Miguel Font, 1996.

Cooper, John. *Eat and Be Satisfied: A Social History of Jewish Food*. Northvale, NJ: Jason Aronson, 1993.

Corbin, Alain. *Time, Desire and Horror: Towards a History of the Senses*. Trans. Jean Birrell. Cambridge, MA: Polity Press, 1995.

Corominas, Joan. *Breve diccionario etimológico de la lengua castellana*. 13th ed. Madrid: Gredos, 1973.

Cortejón, Clemente. "Duelos y quebrantos (I, Cap. 1): Comentario a una nota de la primera edición crítica del 'Don Quijote.'" 1907. Internet Archive. University of Toronto Library. http://www.archive.org/details/duelosyquebranto00cort. Consulted on 29 May 2012.

Cortés, Jerónimo. *Octava y vltima impression del Lvnario y pronostico perpetuo, general, y particular para cada reynos, y prouincias*. Barcelona: G. Margarit, 1614.

Covarrubias, Sebastián de. *Tesoro de la lengua castellana o española*. Ed. Martín de Riquer. Barcelona: Horta, 1943.

Cruz Cruz, Juan. *La cocina mediterránea en el inicio del Renacimiento*. Huesca: La Val de Onsera, 1997.

– *Dietética medieval: Apéndice con la version castellana del Regimen de salud de Arnaldo de Vilanova*. Huesca: La Val de Onsera, 1997.

Cubillo de Aragón, Álvaro. *Relación del Combite y Real Banquete, que a imitación de los Persas hizo en la Corte de España el Excmo. Sr. D. Juan Alfonso Enríquez de Cabrera al duque de Agramont: Embajador del Rey de Francia Luis XIV en ocasión de pedir la mano de la Infanta Dña. Maria Teresa de Austria y Borbón*. Madrid: Andrés García de la Iglesia, 1659.

Dal Col, Raffaello, and Juan Luis Gutiérrez Granda, trans. and ed. *Arte de cocinar: Obra del maestro Bartolomeo Scappi, cocinero privado del papa Pío V*. Gijón, Spain: Ediciones Trea, 2004.

Damiani, Bruno M. *Francisco Delicado*. New York: Twayne Publishers, 1974.

Daneri, Juan José. "Fernandez Oviedo's Pineapple and Cultural Authority in Imperial Spain." *Monographic Review/Revista Monografica* 21 (2005): 26–39.

Darst, David. "El discurso sobre la magia en *La cueva de Salamanca*, de Ruiz de Alarcón." *Duquesne Hispanic Review* 9.1 (1970): 31–44.

Davies, Mark. *Corpus del Español: 100 million words. 1200s–1900s*. 2002. http://
www.corpusdelespanol.org. Consulted on 2 Aug. 2012.

Delicado, Francisco. *La lozana andaluza*. Ed. Claude Allaigre. 6th ed. Madrid:
Cátedra, 2011.

Del Río, Ángel. *Historia de la literatura española*. New York: Holt, Rinehart, and
Winston, 1967.

Del Río Barredo, María José. *Madrid, urbs regia: La capital ceremonial de la
Monarquía Católica*. Madrid: Marcial Pons, 2000.

De Marcella, Ciceri, and Julio Rodríguez Puértolas, eds. *Cancionero*.
Salamanca: Biblioteca española del siglo XV, 1990.

Díaz, Bernal. *Historia verdadera de la conquista de la Nueva España*. Madrid:
Editorial Castalia, 1999.

Diccionario de autoridades. 1732. 3 vols. Real Academia Española. Madrid:
Gredos, 1963.

Diccionario de la lengua española. Real Academia Española. 20th ed. http://
www.rae.es. Consulted on 20 Jun. 2013.

Díez Borque, José María. *La sociedad española y los viajeros del siglo XVII*.
Madrid: Taurus, 1975.

– *La vida española en la edad de oro según los extranjeros*. Barcelona: Del Serbal,
1990.

Díez Daza, Alonso. *Libro de los provechos y dannos que provienen con la sola bevida
del agua. Y como se deva escoger la mejor. Y retificar la que no es tal, y de como se a
de bever frio en tiempo de calor sin que haga daño*. Seville: Alonso de la Barrera,
1576.

Domínguez Ortiz, Antonio. *Las clases privilegiadas en la Espana del Antiguo
Régimen*. Madrid: Ediciones Istmo, 1973.

Döring, Tobias, Markus Heide, and Susanne Muehleisen, eds. *Eating Culture:
The Poetics and Politics of Food*. Munich: Heidelberg, 2003.

Douglas, Mary. "Deciphering a Meal." *Daedalus* 101.1 (winter 1972): 61–81.

Eisenberg, Daniel. "La actitud de Cervantes hacia sus antepasados judaicos."
*Cervantes y las religiones: Actas del Coloquio International de la Asociación de
Cervantistas (Universidad Hebrea de Jerusalén, Israel, 19–21 de Diciembre de
2005)*. Ed. Ruth Fine and Santiago López Navia. Madrid: Iberoamericana,
2008. 55–78.

Eléxpuru, Inés. *La cocina de al-Andalus*. Madrid: Alianza Editorial, 1994.

Elkhort, Martin. *The Secret Life of Food: A Feast of Food and Drink History,
Folklore, and Fact*. Los Angeles: Jeremy P. Tarcher, 1991.

Erasmus, Desiderius. *De civilitate*. Trans. Brian McGregor. Ed A.H.T. Levi.
Literary and Educational Writings. Vol. 5. Toronto: University of Toronto
Press, 1978–86.

Escartín González, Eduardo. *Estudio económico sobre el "Tratado" de Ibn Abdún: El vino y los gremios en al-Andalus antes del siglo XII.* Seville: Fundación El Monte, 2006.

Espantoso Foley, Augusta. *Occult Arts and Doctrine in the Theater of Juan Ruiz de Alarcón.* Geneva: Librairie Droz, 1972.

Espinosa, Pedro, and Rodríguez M. Bernal. *Demostraciones que hizo el Duque VIII de Medina Sidonia a la presencia de S.M. el Rey Felipe IV en el bosque de Doñana.* Seville: Padilla, 1994.

Fábregas, Xavier. "Las carnes en la literatura culinaria catalana medieval." *Eurocarne* 116 (May 2003): 113–17.

✓ Ferguson, Prisilla. *Accounting for Taste: The Triumph of French Cuisine.* Chicago: University of Chicago Press, 2004.

Fernández Armesto, Felipe. *Historia de la comida: Alimentos, cocina y civilización.* Trans. Victoria Ordóñez. Barcelona: Tusquets, 2004.

Fernández Llamazares, José. *Historia de la bula de la Santa Cruzada.* Madrid: Eusebio Aguado, 1859.

Fernández de Oviedo, Gonzalo. *Sumario de la natural historia de las Indias.* 1526. Ed. José Miranda. Mexico: Fondo de Cultura Económica, 1979.

Ficino, Marcilio. *Commentary on Plato's Symposium.* Ed. and trans. Sears Reynolds Jayne. Columbia: University of Missouri Press, 1949.

– *De sufficientia, fine, forma, materia, modo, condimento, authoritate, convivii. Opera omnia.* Vol. 1. Basle: Officina Henricpetrina, 1576.

– *Meditations on the Soul: Selected Letters of Marcilio Ficino.* Rochester, VT: Inner Traditions International, 1996.

Fuchs, Barbara. *Exotic Nation: Maurophilia and the Construction of Early Modern Spain.* Philadelphia: University of Pennsylvania Press, 2009.

Fudālat al-khiwān fī ṭayyibāt al-ṭaʿām wa-al-alwān: ṣūrah min fann al-ṭabkh fī al-Andalus wa-al-Maghrib fī bidāyat ʿaṣr Banī Marīn. By Ibn Razīn al-Tujībī. Beirut: Dār al-Gharb al-Islāmī, 1984.

Gallager, Catherine. "The Potato in the Materialist Imagination." *Practicing New Historicism.* Ed. Catherine Gallager and Stephen Greenblatt. Chicago: Universtiy of Chicago Press, 2000.110–35.

Galloway, J.H. *The Sugar Cane Industry: An Historical Geography from Its Origins to 1914.* Cambridge: Cambridge University Press, 1989.

García, Carlos. *La oposición y conjunción de los dos grandes luminares de la tierra o La Antipatía de franceses y españoles.* 1617. Ed. Michel Bareau. Edmonton, Canada: Alta Press, 1979.

García, L. Jacinto. *Un banquete por Sefarad: Cocina y costumbres de los judíos españoles.* Gijón, Spain: Ediciones Trea, 2007.

– *Carlos V a la mesa: Cocina y alimentación en la España renacentista.* [Toledo]: Ediciones Bremen, 2000.

García-Ballester, Luis, and Michael R. McVaugh, eds. *Arnaldi de Villanova, Opera Medica Omnia: Regimen sanitatis ad regem aragonum.* Lérida: Pagès, 1996.

García Blanco, Manuel. "El tema de la cueva de Salamanca y el entremés cervantino de este título." *Anales cervantinos* I (1951): 71–109.

García Mercadal, José. *Viajes de extranjeros por España y Portugal.* Vol. 2. Madrid: Aguilar, 1959.

García Sánchez, Expiración. "La alimentación popular urbana en al-Andalus." *Arqueología medieval* 4 (1996): 219–36.

– "Los cultivos de Al-Andalus y su influencia en la alimentación." Granada: Escuela de estudios árabes, Consejo superior de investigaciones científicas, n.d. PDF file. 183–92. http://digital.csic.es/bitstream/10261/25468/1/ Los%20cultivos%20de%20al-Andalus%20y%20su%20influencia%20en% 20la%20alimentacion_EGarcia.pdf. Consulted on 25 Apr. 2015.

– "Especias y condimentos en la sociedad andalusí: Prácticas culinarias y aplicaciones dietéticas." *El sabor del sabor: hierbas aromaticas, condimentos y especias.* Ed. Antonio Garrido Aranda. Cordoba: Universidad de Córdoba, 2004. 71–96.

García Sánchez, Expiración, ed. and trans. *Kitāb al-agdiya: Tratado de los alimentos.* By Abu marwan Abd al-Malik b. Abi l-Ala' Zuhr. Madrid: Consejo Superior de Investigaciones Científicas, 1992.

García Santo-Tomás, Enrique. *Espacio urbano y creación literaria en el Madrid de Felipe IV.* Madrid: Iberoamericana, 2004.

– ed. *Materia Crítica: Formas de ocio y de consume en la cultura áurea.* Madrid: Iberoamericana, 2009.

Garrido Aranda, Antonio, et al. "La revolución alimentaria del siglo XVI en América y Europa." *Los sabores de España y América.* Ed. Antonio Garrida Aranda. Huesca: La Val de Onsera, 1999. 197–212.

Gautschi-Lanz, Catherine. *Le roman à table: Nourritures et repas imaginaires dans le roman français, 1850–1900.* Geneva: Slatkine, 2006.

Gázquez Ortiz, Antonio. *La mesa de la España cervantina.* Madrid: Ediciones CEP, 2009.

Genders, Roy. *Growing Herbs as Aromatics.* New Canaan, CT: Keats, 1977.

Gerli, E. Michael. "The Hunt of Love: The Literalization of a Metaphor in *Fuenteovejuna*." *Neophilologus* 63 (1979): 54–8.

Gigante, Denise. *Taste: A Literary History.* New Haven: Yale University Press, 2005.

Gitlitz, David M., and Linda Kay Davidson. *A Drizzle of Honey: The Lives and Recipes of Spain's Secret Jews.* New York: St Martin's Press, 1999.

Gómez Laguna, Santiago. "Aclaraciones sobre la olla podrida." *Cuadernos de Gastronomía* 3 (June 1993): 9–14.

– "Domingo Hernández de Maceras y su libro del arte de cocina (Salamanca, 1607)." *Cuadernos de Gastronomía* 9–10 (1994): 4–6.

– "Sobre Diego Granado y su *Arte de Cocina.*" *Cuadernos de Gastronomía* 4 (July–August 1993): 21–3.

González Dávila, Gil. *Pláticas del Padre Gil González Dávila sobre las reglas de la Compañía de Jesús.* 1614. *Biblioteca virtual Miguel de Cervantes.* 1999. http://www.cervantesvirtual.com. Consulted on 31 May 2012.

González Ollé, Fernando Tusón, and Vicente Tusón, eds. *Pasos: Lope de Rueda.* Madrid: Cátedra, 1989.

González Sevilla, María Emilia. *A la mesa con los reyes de España: Curiosidades y anécdotas de la cocina de palacio.* Madrid: Temas de hoy, 1998.

Goodwin, Robert. "'Los pajaritos del aire': Disappearing Menus and After-Dinner Speaking in *Don Quixote.*" *Educated Tastes: Food, Drink and Connoisseur Culture.* Ed. Jeremy Strong. Lincoln, NE: University of Nebraska Press, 2011. 194–214.

Goody, Jack. *Cooking, Cuisine and Class: A Study in Comparative Sociology.* Cambridge: Cambridge University Press, 1982.

Gordon, Sarah. *Culinary Comedy in Medieval French Literature.* West Lafayette, IN: Purdue University Press, 2007.

Gordonio, Bernardo de. *Obras de Bernardo de Gordonio, insigne maestro, doctor de medicina en que se contienen los siete libros de la práctica, o Lilio de la medicina: Las tablas de los ingenious de curar las enfermedades; el regimineto de las agudas; el tratado de los niños, y regimiento del ama; y los pronosticos.* Madrid: Antonio Gonçalez de Reyes. 1697.

Granado, Diego. *Libro del arte de cozina.* Ed. Xavier Benet i Pinós. Lérida: Pagès, 1991.

Granja, Agustín de la. "'Vaca y carnero, olla de caballero': Algo más sobre Cervantes y Lope." *Codici del gusto.* Ed. Maria Grazia Profeti. Milan: Franco Angeli, 1992. 215–30.

Granja Santamaría, Fernando de la. *La cocina arabigoandaluza según un manuscrito inédito.* PhD thesis. Madrid, Facultad de Filosofía y Letras, 1960.

Greco, Gina L., and Christine M. Rose, eds and trans. *The Good Wife's Guide: Le ménagier de Paris; A Medieval Household Guide.* Ithaca, NY: Cornell University Press, 2009.

Guazzo, Stephan. *La civil conversazione.* 2 vols. Modena: Panini, 1993.

Guevara, Antonio de. *Menosprecio de corte y alabanza de aldea: Arte de marear.* Ed. Asunción Rallo. Madrid: Cátedra, 1984.

Gutierrez, Nancy. *"Shall She Famish Then?" Female Food Refusal in Early Modern England.* Aldershot, England: Ashgate, 2003.

Gutiérrez de Salinas, Diego. *Discursos del pan y el vino del niño Jesús. Para que los labradores den la sazón que conviene a la tierra, y el pan nazca dentro de tres días a todo lo largo: y se entienda como se ha de dar la labor a las viñas, para que se coja la tercera parte más de uvas que se gocen ordinariamente y se conserven mas tiempo las viñas, y sea mejor el vino, y no se pierda: y otras curiosidades y avisos tocantes a la Agricultura y para que se augmente y componga la República.* Alcalá: Justo Sánchez Crespo, 1598.

Harvey, L.P. *Islamic Spain 1250–1500.* Chicago: University of Chicago Press, 1992.

Heiple, Daniel L. "Renaissance Medical Psychology in *Don Quijote.*" *Ideologies and Literature* 2.9 (1979): 65–72.

Hernández, Francisco. *Quatro libros de la naturaleza y virtudes de las plantas y animales que están recibidos en el uso de medicina en la Nueva España.* Mexico: Widow of Diego López Dávalos, 1615.

Hernández Bermejo, J. Esteban, and J. León. *Neglected Crops: 1492 from a Different Perspective. Published in Collaboration with the Botanical Garden of Córdoba (Spain) as Part of the Etnobotánica 92 Programme (Andalusia, 1992).* Rome: Food and Agriculture Organization of the United Nations, 1994.

Hernández de Maceras, Domingo. *Libro del arte de Cocina.* 1607. *La alimentación en la España del Siglo de Oro.* Ed. María de los Angeles Pérez Samper. Huesca: La Val de Onsera, 1998.

Hernández Morejón, Antonio. *Historia bibliográfica de la medicina española.* Madrid: [Viuda de Jordan e hijos], 1842.

Herrera, Gabriel Alonso de. *Obra de agricultura.* 1513. Ed. José Urbano Martínez Carreras. Biblioteca de autores españoles 235. Madrid: Ediciones Atlas, 1970.

Herrero García, Miguel. *La vida española del siglo XVII: Las bebidas.* Madrid: SELE (Sindicato Exportador del Libro Español), 1933.

Hiltpold, Parl. "The Price, Production, and Transportation of Grain in Early Modern Castile." *Agricultural History* 63.1 (winter 1989): 73–91.

"Historia: La Edad Moderna." Portal official del Excmo. Ayuntamiento de Rute. N.d. http://www.rute.org/index2.html. Consulted on 13 Oct. 2007.

Hoey, Michael. *Textual Interacion: An Introduction to Written Discourse Analysis.* New York: Routledge, 2001.

Howell, James. *Epistolæ Ho-Elianæ: Familiar Letters Domestick and Foreign, Divided into Four Books; Partly Historical, Political, Philosophical; Upon Emergent Occasions.* London: D. Midwinter [etc.], 1737.

Huetz de Lemps, Alain. "El viñedo de la 'Tierra de Medina' en los siglos XVII y XVIII." Trans. Jesús Garcíca Fernández. *Estudios geográficos* 20 (1959): 111–25.

Huici Miranda, Ambrosio, ed. and trans. *La cocina hispano-magrebí durante la época almohade: Segun un manuscrito anónimo del siglo XIII.* Gijón, Spain: Ediciones Trea, 2005.

Ibn al-Karīm, Muḥammad ibn al-Ḥasan. *A Baghdad Cookery Book: The Book of Dishes (Kitāb al-ṭabīkh)*. Trans. Charles Perry. Totnes, Devon, England: Prospect Books, 2005.

Ibn Razīn al-Tuğībī. *Relieves de las mesas, acerca de las delicias de la comida y los diferentes platos: Fuḍālat-al-Hiwān Fī Tayyibāt al-Ta'ām Wa-l-Alwān.* Ed. Manuela Marín. Gijón, Spain: Ediciones Trea, 2007.

Ibn Wafid, Ábd al-Raiman ibn Muhammad. *Tratado de Agricultura*. Málaga: Universidad de Málaga, 1997.

Ibn Zuhr, Abū Marwān Abd Al-Malik. *Kitāb al-agdiya (Tratado de los alimentos)*. Ed. Expiración García Sánchez. Madrid: Consejo Superior de Investigaciones Científicas, 1992.

Imperiale, Louis. *La Roma clandestina de Francisco Delicado y Pietro Aretino*. New York: Peter Lang, 1997.

Izquierdo Benito, Ricardo. *Abastecimiento y alimentación en Toledo en el siglo XV*. Cuenca: Universidad de Castilla-La Mancha, 2002.

Janer, Zilkia. "(In)edible Nature: New World Food and Coloniality." *Cultural Studies* 21.2/3 (March/May 2007): 385–405.

Jazi R., and F.O. Asli. "Avicenne's Pharmacopoeia." *Revue d'histoire de la pharmacie* 45.317 (1998): 9–28.

Jeanneret, Michel. *A Feast of Words: Banquets and Table Talk in the Renaissance*. 1987. Trans. Jeremy Whiteley and Enna Hughes. Chicago: University of Chicago Press, 1991.

Johnson, Carroll B. "El arte viejo de hacer teatro: Lope de Rueda, Lope de Vega y Cervantes." *Lope de Vega y los orígenes del teatro español: Actas del I Congreso Internacional sobre Lope de Vega*. Ed. Manual Criado de Val. Madrid: Edi-6, 1981. 95–102.

Joly, Monique, "A propósito del tema culinario en *La lozana andaluza*." *Journal of Hispanic Philology* 13.2 (winter 1989): 125–33.

Joset, Jacques. "Para una edición comentada de *La lozana andaluza*: el mamotreto II." *Cultura neolatina* 62.1–2 (2002): 171–80.

✓ Kaplan, Lawrence. "Beans, Peas, and Lentils." *The Cambridge World History of Food*. Vol. 1. Ed. Kenneth F. Kiple and Kriemhild Coneè Ornelas. Cambridge: Cambridge University Press, 2000. 271–81.

Khalaf, Salim George. "Phoenician Wines and Vines." *Phoenician Wine*. N.d. http://phoenicia.org/wine.html. Consulted on 5 Jan. 2010.

Kitāb al-tabīj fi l-Magrib wa-l-Andalus fi 'asr al-muwahhudin li-mu'allif mayhūl (Tratado sobre cocina en el Magrib y al-Andalus en época almohade, de autor desconocido). c. 1228–43. Republished as *La cocina hispano-magrebí durante la época almohade según un manuscrito anónimo del siglo XIII traducido por*

Ambrosio Huici Miranda. Intro. Manual Marín. Gijón, Spain: Ediciones Trea, 2005.

Klein, Julius. *The Mesta: A Study in Spanish Economic History 1273–1836*. Cambridge, MA: Harvard University Press, 1920.

Laguna, Andrés. *Pedacio Dioscorides Anazarbeo, annotado por el doctor Andrés Laguna, medico dignissmio de Julio III, pontífice máximo nuevamente ilustrado, y añadido, demonstrando las figuras de plantas, y animales en estampas finas, y dividido en dos tomos*. 1555. Madrid: Alonso Balbas, 1733.

Lee Vetterling, Mary Anne. "La magia en las comedias de Juan Ruiz de Alarcón." *Cuadernos americanos* 231 (1980): 230–47.

León Pinelo, Antonio de. *Question moral si el chocolate quebranta el ayuno eclesiastica: Tratase de otras bebidas i confecciones que vsan en varias provincias*. Madrid: Widow of Juan Gonçalez, 1636. A Coruña, Spain: Órbigo, 2010.

Levi-Provençal, Évariste, and Emilio García Gómez, eds and trans. *Sevilla a comienzos del siglo XII: El tratado de Ibn-'Abdun*. Seville: Fundación Cultural del Colegio Oficial de Aparejadores, 1998.

Lévi-Strauss, Claude. *The Raw and the Cooked: Introduction to a Science of Mythology: I*. Trans. John and Doreen Weightman. New York: Harper and Row, 1964.

Libro de Sent Sovi. Intro. Santi Santamaría, Rosa Esteva, and Joan Santanach. Trans. Manel Zabala. Barcelona: Editorial Barcino, 2007.

Listerman, Randall W. "Las aceitunas of Lope de Rueda: The Role of Mencigüela." *Romance Notes* 29.2 (winter 1988): 133–7.

Lladonosa i Giró, Josep. *La cocina medieval*. Intro. Martínez Llopís. Barcelona: Laia, 1984.

Llopís Agelán, Enrique. "Castilian Agriculture in the Seventeenth Century: Depression, or 'Readjustment and Adaptation'"? *The Castilian Crisis of the Seventeenth Century: New Perspectives on the Economic and Social History of Seventeenth-century Spain*. Ed. I.A.A Thompson and Bartolomé Yun Casalilla. New York: Cambridge University Press, 1994. 77–100.

Lobera de Avila, Luis. *El banquete de nobles caballeros*. 1530. San Sebastián: R&B Ediciones, 1996.

Lobo Lasso de la Vega, Gabriel. *Manojuelo de romances nuevos y otras obras*. Madrid: Editorial Saeta, 1942.

Long-Solís, Janet. *Capsicum y cultura: La historia del chilli*. Mexico, D.F.: Fondo de cultura económica, 1986.

– "El tomate: De hierba Silvestre de las Américas a denominador común en las cocinas mediterráneas." *Cultura alimentaria de España y América*. Ed. Antonio Garrido Aranda. La Huesca: Val de Onsera, 1995. 215–35.

Lope de Rueda. *Pasos*. Ed. Fernando González Ollé and Vicente Tusón. Madrid: Cátedra, 1989.

Lope de Vega, Félix. "Amor, pleito y desafío." Ed. David Hildner. Association for Hispanic Classical Theater.1997. http://www.comedias.org/lope/amplde.html . Consulted on 19 Jun. 2012.

– *La Arcadia*. Ed. Edwon Morby. Madrid: Clásicos Castalia, 1975.

– *La corona mayor*. Alicante: Biblioteca Virtual Miguel de Cervantes, 1999. *Biblioteca virtual Miguel de Cervantes*. http://www.cervantesvirtual.com/obra/la-mayor-corona--0. Consulted on 15 Oct. 2014.

– *Los locos de Valencia*. Alicante : Biblioteca Virtual Miguel de Cervantes, 2012. *Biblioteca virtual Miguel de Cervantes*. http://www.cervantesvirtual.com/obra/los-locos-de-valencia. Consulted on 28 Apr. 2015.

López Castanier, Miguel, and Cesáreo Fernández Duro. *La cocina del Quijote, con todas las recetas*. [Spain]: Rey Lear, 2004.

López de Gómara, Francisco. *Historia general de las Indias*. Vol. 1. Barcelona: Orbis, 1985.

Luján, Nestor. *Historia de la gastronomía*. Barcelona: Folio, 1997.

Luján, Nestor, and Juan Perucho. *El libro de la cocina española: Gastronomía e historia*. Barcelona: Danae, 1970.

/ MacClancy, Jeremy. "Food, Identity, Identification." *Researching Food Habits*: *Methods and Problems*. Ed. Helen Macbeth and Jeremy MacClancy. Oxford: Berghahn, 2004. 63–74.

✓ Malaguzzi, Sylvia. *Food and Feasting in Art*. Trans. Brian Phillips. Los Angeles: J. Paul Getty Museum, 2006.

Manual de carnes bovina y ovina: Handbook of Uruguayan Meat. Montevideo, Uruguay: INAC. Instituto Nacional de Carnes, 2011. Pdf. http://www.plattevalleyfoodgroup.com/downloads/uruguay.pdf. Consulted on 31 Mar. 2015.

Manual de mugeres en el qual se contienen muchas y diversas reçeutas muy buenas Ed. Alicia Martínez Crespo. Salamanca: Ediciones Universidad Salamanca, 1995.

Manual de mugeres en el qual se contienen muchas y diversas reçeutas muy buenas. *Manual of Women in which is contained many and diverse very good recipes*. Medieval and Material Culture. http://www.larsdatter.com/manual.htm. Consulted on 1 Sept. 2012.

Maravall, José Antonio. *Poder, honor y elites en el siglo XVII*. Madrid: Siglo Veintiuno, 1979.

Marín, Manuela. "From Al-Andalus to Spain: Arab Traces in Spanish Cooking." *Food and History* 2 (2004): 35–52.

– ed. *Relieves de la mesa acerca de las delicias de la comida y los diferentes platos: Fuḍālat al-Hiwān Fi Tayyibat al-Ta'am Wa-l-Alwan*. By Ibn Razin al Tugibi. 2nd half of 13th century. Gijón, Spain: Ediciones Trea, 2007.

– "Sobre Būrān y *Būrānīyyā*." *Al-Qantara* 2 (1981): 193–207.

Markham, Gervase. *The English Housewife: Containing the Inward and Outward Virtures which Ought to Be in a Complete Woman; as Her Skill in Physic, Cookery, Banqueting-stuff, Distillation, Perfumes, Wool, Hemp, Flax, Dairies, Brewing, Baking, and All Other Things Belonging to a Household.* Ed. Michael R. Best. Kingston, ON: McGill-Queen's University Press, 1986.

Marradón, Bartolomé. *Diálogo del uso del tabaco, los daños que causa, etc. y del chocolate y otras bebidas.* Seville: Gabriel Ramos Vejarano, 1618.

Martín, José Luis, J. Valdeón, and Ángel García Sanz. "La lucha por los pastos." *Cuadernos Historia 16.* 66 (1996): 5–17.

Martinelli, Candida. *An Anonymous Al-Andalus Cookbook from the 13th Century.* Candida Martinelli's Italophile Site. http://italophiles.com/al_andalus .htm. Consulted on 23 Jul. 2011.

Martínez Llopis, Manuel. *La dulcería Española: Recetarios histórico y popular.* Madrid: Alianza Editorial, 1999.

– *Historia de la gastronomía española.* Huesca: La Val de Onsera, 1995.

Martínez Montiño, Francisco. *Arte de Cocina, pastelería, vizcochería y conservería.* 1611. Valencia: Librerías París-Valencia, 1997.

Mata, Juan de la. *Arte de repostería.* 1747. Valladolid: Editorial Maxtor, 2003.

Matilla Tascón, Antonio. *Abastecimiento de carne a Madrid (1477–1678).* Madrid: Instituto de Estudios Madrileños, 1994.

Matthews, Dakin, trans. *La verdad sospechosa* [The truth can't be trusted]. Juan Ruiz de Alarcón. Ed. Vern Williamsen. Association for Hispanic Classical Theater, 1998. http://www.comedias.org/play_texts/translat/trutru1.html. Consulted on 10 Jun. 2013.

Mattiolo, Pietro Andrea. *De plantis epitome utliissima.* Frankfurt am Main: [J. Feyerabend], 1586.

McMahon, Elise-Noël. "*Gargantua, Pantagruel,* and Renaissance Cooking Tracts: Texts for Consumption." *Neophilologus* 76 (1992): 186–97.

Meads, Chris. *Banquets Set Forth: Banqueting in English Renaissance Drama.* Manchester: Manchester University Press, 2001.

Mennell, Stephen. *All Manners of Food: Eating and Taste in England and France from the Middle Ages to the Present.* Urbana: University of Illinois Press, 1996.

Messisbugo, Cristoforo de. *Banchette, compositioni di vivande et apparecchio generale.* Ferrara: Giovanni de Buglhat et Antonio Hucher Compagni, 1549.

Micón, Francisco *Alivio de los sedientos, en el qual se trata de la necesidad que tenemos de bever frio y refrescado con nieve, y las condiciones que para esto son menester, y quales cuerpos lo pueden libremente soportar.* Barcelona: Diego Galván, 1576.

Miguel-Prendes, Sol. 2003. "Chivalric Identity in Enrique de Villena's *Arte Ciscoria.*" *La Corónica* 32.1 (2003): 307–42.

Mintz, Sidney. *Sweetness and Power: The Place of Sugar in Modern History*. New York: Viking Press, 1985.

Mira de Amescua, Antonio. *La mesonera del cielo y hermitaño galan*. Ed. Vern Williamsen. Association for Hispanic Classical Theater, 1991. http://www .comedias.org/mira/mescie.html. Consulted on 15 May 2012.

Modern Language Association International Bibliography. EBSCO. 2014. http:// eds.b.ebscohost.com.proxy.iwu.edu/ehost/search/advanced?sid=ceef988a-8b0e-4155-aad1-5203e7fb5acc%40sessionmgr115&vid=0&hid=126. Consulted on 15 Jun. 2014.

Molénat, J.P. "Menus des pauvres, menus des confrères a Tolède dans la deuxième moitié du XVe siècle." *Manger et boire au moyen âge*. Nice: Centre d'études medievales de Nice, 1984. 313–18.

Monardes, Nicolás. *La historia medicinal de las cosas que traen de nuestras islas occidentales*. Madrid: Ministerio de Sanidad y Consumo, 1989.

✓ Montanari, Massimo. *The Culture of Food*. Trans. Carl Ipsen. Oxford: Blackwell, 1994.

Morel-Fatio, Alfred Paul Victor, ed. *Ambrosio de Salazar et l'etude de l'espagnol en France sous Louis XIII*. Vol. 1. Paris: A. Picard et fils, 1901. *HathiTrust Digital Library*. http://babel.hathitrust.org/cgi/pt?id=ucl.$b735850;view=1up; seq=7. Consulted on 23 Sept. 2015.

Moreno Gómez, Jesus. "Los duelos y quebrantos en la solidaridad popular." *Isla de Arriarán* 25 (June 2005): 279–92.

Moreto, Augustín. *La fuerza al natural*. Alicante: Biblioteca virtual Miguel de Cervantes, 2013. http://www.cervantesvirtual.com/obra/comedia-famosa-la-fuerza-del-natural/. Consulted on 24 Apr. 2015.

Murcott, Anne, Warren Belasco, and Peter Jackson, eds. *The Handbook of Food Research*. New York: Bloomsbury, 2013.

Murillo, Bartolomé. *La cocina de los ángeles*. 1646. RMN-Grand Palais, Musée du Louvre, Paris.

Myers, Kathleen A. "New World Phenomena in Oviedo's Illustrations." *Early Images of the Americas: Transfer and Invention*. Ed. J.M. Williams, et al. Tuscon: University of Arizona Press, 1993. 183–213.

Nadeau, Carolyn. "Spanish Culinary History in Cervantes' 'Bodas de Camacho.'" *Revista Canadiense de Estudios Hispánicos* 29.2 (winter 2005): 347–61.

– "Transformation and Transgression at the Banquet Scene in *La Celestina*." *Objects of Culture in Imperial Spain*. Ed. Frederick de Armas and Mary Barnard. Toronto: University of Toronto Press, 2013. 205–27.

– "What Else Happened in the Early Modern Kitchen? Reading Celestina's Kitchen through the *Manual de mugeres*." *Comida y bebida en la lengua española, cultura y literaturas hispánicas.* Ed. Andjelka Pejovic, Vladimir Karanovic, and Mirjana Sekulic. Kragujevac, Serbia: FILUM, 2012: 289–303.

Navarro, Rosa. ¿Qué comía Alonso Quijano los sábados? *Comida y bebida en la lengua española, cultura y literaturas hispánicas.* Ed. Andjelka Pejovic, Vladimir Karanovic, and Mirjana Sekulic. Kragujevac, Serbia: FILUM, 2012. 261–71.

Nola, de. *Libro de guisados.* In *La cocina mediterránea en el inicio del Renacimiento.* Ed. Juan Cruz Cruz. Huesca: La Val de Onsera, 1997. 227–375.

Norton, Marcy. *Sacred Gifts, Profane Pleasures: A History of Tobacco and Chocolate in the Atlantic World.* Ithaca, NY: Cornell University Press, 2008.

"Nostra Taula: Cocina valenciana." ComarcaRural, 2001. http://www. comarcarural.com/valencia/recetario/arroces_secos/paelladesepiaiflori-col.htm. Consulted on 5 Feb. 2012.

Nuez, Fernando. *El cultivo del tomate.* Madrid: Ediciones Mundi-Prensa, 1995.

Oudin, César, trans. *L'Ingénieux Hidalgo Don Quichotte de la Manche: Nouvelles exemplaires.* By Miguel de Cervantes. Ed. Jean Cassou. Paris: Gallimard, 1949.

Parr, James. "Erotismo y alimentación en *El Burlador de Sevilla*: El mundo al revés." *Edad de oro* 9 (1990): 231–9.

Parrack, John C. "Identity, Illusion, and the Emergence of the Feminine Subject in *La Lozana andaluza*." *Women in the Discourse of Early Modern Spain.* Ed. Joan F. Cammarata. Gainesville, FL: University Press of Florida, 2003. 35–53.

Paterson, Alan K. "Reversal and Multiple Role-Playing in Alarcón's *La verdad sospechosa*." *Bulletin of Hispanic Studies* 61 (1984): 361–8.

Pepys, Samuel. *The Diary of Samuel Pepys.* Vol. 9. Ed. Robert Latham and William Matthews. Berkeley: University of California Press, 1970.

Pérez de Espinardo, Jesús. *El libro del pimentón.* Murcia: Turbinto, 2000.

Pérez Samper, María de los Angeles. *La alimentación en la España del Siglo de Oro: Domingo Hernández de Maceras "Libro del arte de Cocina."* Huesca: La Val de Onsera, 1998.

– "España y América: El encuentro de dos sistemas alimentarios." *Las raíces de la memoria: América Latina, ayer y hoy, quinto encuentro debate.* Barcelona: Universitat de Barcelona, 1996. 171–88.

– "Fiesta y alimentación en la España moderna: El banquete como imagen festiva de abundancia y refinamiento." *Espacio, Tiempo y Forma, Serie IV, Historia Moderna* 10 (1997): 53–98.

Peterson, T. Sarah. *Acquired Tastes: The French Origins of Modern Cooking.* Ithaca, NY: Cornell University Press, 1994.

Peyrebonne, Nathalie. "El paratexto de los libros de cocina." *Paratextos en la literatura española. Siglos XV–XVIII.* Ed. María Soledad Arredondo, Pierre Civil, and Michel Moner. Madrid: Casa de Veláquez, 2009.

Pinheiro da Veiga, Thomé. *Fastiginia: O fastos geniales*. Trans. Narciso Alonso Cortés. Valladolid: Colegio de Santiago, 1916. HathiTrust Digital Library. http://babel.hathitrust.org/cgi/pt?id=njp.32101073400978;view=1up; seq=5. Consulted on 14 Mar. 2013.

"Pinillo." *Plantas medicinales: Infojardin*. 2012. http://www.infojardin.net/fichas/plantas-medicinales/ajuga-chamaepitys.htm. Consulted on 3 Feb. 2012.

Platina. *On Right Pleasure and Good Health*. Ed. and trans. Mary Ella Milham. Tempe, AZ: Medieval and Renaissance Texts and Studies, 1998.

Plouvier, L. "L'introduction du sucre en pharmacie." *Revue d'histoire de la pharmacie* 47.322 (1999): 199–216.

Pratt, Mary Louise. *Imperial Eyes: Travel Writing and Transculturation*. New York: Routledge, 1992.

Purkiss, Diane. "Crammed with Distressful Bread? Bakers and the Poor in Early Modern England." *Renaissance Food from Rabelais to Shakespeare: Culinary Readings and Culinary Histories*. Ed. Joan Fitzpatrick. Farnham, Surrey: Ashgate, 2010. 11–23.

Quevedo, Francisco de. *Francisco de Quevedo: Poesía original complete*. Ed. J.M. Blecua. Barcelona: Planeta, 1981.

– *La vida del buscón*. Ed. Carolyn A. Nadeau. Newark, DE: Cervantes and Co, 2007.

Rabasa, José. *Inventing America: Spanish Historiography and the Formation of Eurocentricism*. Norman: University of Oklahoma Press, 1993.

Restrepo Manrique, Cecilia. "Reseña del libro '*Arte de Cocina; pastelería; vizcochería y conservería*': Compuesta por Francisco Martínez Montiño, Cocinero Mayor del Rey Nuestro Señor. Barcelona: Tusquets, 1982. http://www.historiacocina.com/paises/articulos/montino.htm. Consulted on 10 Jan. 2009.

Riera Melis, Antoni. "Jerarquía social y desigualdad alimentaria en el Mediterráneo noroccidental durante la Baja Edad Media: La cocina y la mesa de los estamentos populares." *La alimentación mediterránea: Historia, cultura, nutrición*. Ed. Xavier Medina. Barcelona: Institut Català de la Mediterrània, 1996. 81–107.

– "'Panem nostrum. Quotidianum da nobis hodie': Los sistemas alimenticios de los estamentos populares en el mediterráneo noroccidental en la baja edad media." *La vida cotidiana en la edad media: Nájera, Del 4 al 8 de agosto 1997*. Logroño: Instituto de estudios riojanos, 1998. 25–46. *Biblioteca Gonzalo de Berceo*. 2007. PDF. 15 Jul. 2012.

– "Las plantas que llegaron de Levante: Acerca del legado alimentario islámico en la Cataluña medieval." *Anuario de estudios medievales* 31.2 (2001):

797–841. http://estudiosmedievales.revistas.csic.es/index.php/
estudiosmedievales/article/view/269/274. Consulted on 23 Jul. 2011.

Ringrose, David R. *Madrid and the Spanish Economy, 1560–1850*. Berkeley:
University of California Press, 1983. *The Library of Iberian Resources Online*.
http://libro.uca.edu/ringrose/mad7.htm. Consulted on 30 May 2012.

Rodinson, Maxime, A.J. Arberry, and Charles Perry. *Medieval Arab Cookery*.
Totnes, Devon, England: Prospect Books, 2001.

Rodríguez Marín, Francisco. "El yantar de Alonso Quijano el Bueno." *Estudios
cervantistas*. Madrid: Ediciones Atlas, 1947. 421–39.

Rojas, Agustín de. *El vieje entretenido*. Vol. 1, 1603. Ed. Jacques Joset. Madrid:
Espasa-Calpe, 1977.

Rose, Jeanne. *The Herbal Body Book*. New York: Putnam, 1976.

Rosenberger, Bernard. "Diversité des manières de consommer les céréales
dans le Mahgreb precolonial." *La alimentación en las culturas islámicas*. Ed.
Manuela Marín and David Waines. Madrid: Agenica Española de
Cooperación Internacional, 1994. 309–54.

– "Usos del azúcar en tres libros de cocina hispánicos (siglos XIII–XV)." *El
sabor del sabor: Hierbas aromaticas, condimentos y especias*. Ed. Antonio Garrido
Aranda. Cordoba: Universidad de Córdoba, 2004. 97–120.

Rubel, William. "Sir Hugh Plat's Manuscript: An English Bread circa 1560."
The Magic of Fire: Traditional Foodways with William Rubel. http://www
.williamrubel.com/. Consulted on 1 Jun. 2012.

Rubio Gago, Manuel E. "El consumo de pan tradicional en León y su dimen-
sión social." *Revista de Folklore* 213 (May–June 1998): 75–83. http://www
.funjdiaz.net/folklore/indice.cfm. Consulted on 31 May 2012.

Rucquoi, A. "Alimentation des riches, alimentation des pauvres dans une ville
castillane ai XVe siècle." *Manger et boire au moyen âge*. Nice: Centre d'études
medievales de Nice, 1984. 297–312.

Ruiz de Alarcón, Juan. *La cueva de Salamanca*. Ed. Vern Williamsen. Association
for Hispanic Classical Theater, 1998. http://www.comedias.org/alarcon/
cuevsa.html. Consulted on 12 Jul. 2012.

– *Las paredes oyen*. Ed. Vern Williamsen. Association for Hispanic Classical
Theater, 1998. http://www.comedias.org/alarcon/pareoy.html. Consulted
on 12 Jul. 2012.

– *El semejante a sí mismo*. Ed. Vern G. Williamsen. Association for Hispanic
Classical Theater, 1998. http://www.comedias.org/alarcon/semesi.html.
Consulted on 12 Jul. 2012.

– *La verdad sospechosa*. Association for Hispanic Classical Theater. http://
www.comedias.org/alarcon/versos.pdf. Consulted on 10 Jun. 2013.

Safford, William Edwin. "The Sacred Ear-Flower of the Aztecs: Xochinagaztli."
   The Annual Report of the Board of Regents of the Smithsonian Institution.
   61st Congress, 3rd session, report 1217. Washington, D.C., 1910. 427–31.
Sahagún, Bernardino de. *Historia general de las cosas de Nueva España*. Vol. 2. Intro.
   Alfredo López Austin and Josefina García Quintana. Madrid: Alianza, 1988.
Salaman, Redcliffe N. *The History and Social Influence of the Potato*. Cambridge:
   Cambridge University Press, 1970.
Sánchez Jiménez, Antonio. "Bodegones poéticos: Pintura, fruta y hortalizas
   como bienes de consumo moral y literario en Lope de Vega y Luis de
   Góngora." *Materia crítica: Formas de ocio y de consumo en la cultura áurea*. Ed.
   Enrique García Santo-Tomás. Madrid: Iberoamericana, 2009. 191–210.
Sánchez Meco, Gregorio. *El arte de la cocina en tiempos de Felipe II*. El Escorial:
   Consejalía de cultura, 1998.
San Félix, Sor Marcela de. "Muerte del Apetito." *Obra Completa: Coloquios
   espirituales, loas y otros poemas*. Ed. Electa Arenal and Georgina Sabat de
   Rivers. Barcelona: Promociones y Publicaciones Universitarias, 1988.
   IntraText CT, *Èulogos*, 2007. http://www.intratext.com/IXT/ESL0014/_
   PN.HTM. Consulted on 15 Jun. 2014.
Santanach i Suñol, Joan, ed. *Llibre de totes maneres de confits*. Els Nostres
   Clàssics B 22. Barcelona: Barcino, 2003.
Sarti, Raffaella. *Europe at Home: Family and Material Culture, 1500–1800*. New
   Haven: Yale University Press, 2002.
Scappi, Bartolomeo. *Opera [Dell'arte del cucinare]*. Bologna: Arnaldo Forni
   Editore, 1981.
– *The Opera of Bartolomeo Scappi (1570): L'arte et prudenza d'un maestro cuoco*.
   Trans. Terence Scully. Toronto: University of Toronto Press, 2008.
Scully, Terence, ed. and trans. *The Vivendier*. Totnes, Devon, England: Prospect
   Books, 1997.
Shergold, N.D. *A History of the Spanish Stage: From Medieval Times until the End
   of the Seventeenth Century*. Oxford: Clarendon Press, 1967.
Simón Palmer, María del Carmen. *Bibliografía de la gastronomía y la alimentación
   en España*. Gijón, Spain: Ediciones Trea, 2003.
– *La cocina de palacio 1561–1931*. Madrid: Editorial Castalia, 1997.
– *Libros antiguos de cultura alimentaria (siglo XV–1900)*. [Cordoba]: Excma.
   Diputación Provincial de Córdoba, c. 1994.
Smith, Susan M. and Georgina Sabat de Rivers, eds. *Los coloquios del alma:
   Cuatro dramas alegóricos de Sor Marcela de San Félix, hija de Lope de Vega*.
   Newark: Juan de la Cuesta, 2006.
Solís, Antonio de. *Euridice y Orfeo*. In *Comedia de Antonio de Solís*. Vol. 1. Ed.
   Manuela Sánchez Reguerira. Madrid: Consejo Superior de Investigaciones
   Científicas, 1984. 147–222.

Soons, C.A. "*La verdad sospechosa* in its Epoch." *Romanische Forschungen* 74 (1962): 399–402.

Sorapán de Rieros, Juan. *Medicina española contenida en proverbios vulgares de nuestra lengua*. 1616. Madrid: Cosano, 1949.

Sternberg, Robert. *The Sephardic Kitchen: The Healthful Food and Rich Culture of the Mediterranean Jews*. New York: HarperCollins, c. 1996.

Stoler, Ann Laura, and Karen Strassler. "Castings for the Colonial: Memory Work in 'New Order' Java." *Society for Comparative Study of Society and History* 42.1 (Jan. 2000): 4–48.

Tannahill, Reay. *Food in History*. New York: Three Rivers Press, 1988.

Terrón, Eloy. *España, encrucijada de culturas alimentarias: Su papel en la difusión de los cultivos americanos*. Madrid: Ministerio de Agricultura, Pesca y Alimentación, 1992.

Thirsk, Joan. *Food in Early Modern England: Phases, Fads, Fashions 1500–1760*. London: Hambledon Continuum, 2006.

This, Hervé. "Let's Have an Egg." *Eggs in Cookery: Proceedings of the Oxford Symposium of Food and Cookery 2006*. Ed. Richard Hoskins. Totnes, Devon, England: Prospect Books, 2007. 250–8.

Tirso de Molina (Gabriel Téllez). *El amor médico*. Ed. Vern Williamsen. Association for Hispanic Classical Theater, 1997. http://www.comedias.org/tirso/Amomed.html. Consulted on 25 Apr. 2012.

– *Bellaco Sois, Gómez*. Ed. Vern Williamsen. Association for Hispanic Classical Theater, 2000. http://www.comedias.org/tirso/bellso.html. Consulted on 11 Mar. 2013.

– *El colmenero divino*. Ed. Vern Williamsen. Association for Hispanic Classical Theater, 1996. http://www.comedias.org/tirso/coldiv.html. Consulted on 15 Oct. 2014.

– *La elección por la virtud*. Ed. Vern Williamsen. Association for Hispanic Classical Theater, 1998. http://www.comedias.org/tirso/elecvi.html. Consulted on 11 Mar. 2013.

– *Santo y sastre*. Ed. Vern Williamsen. Association for Hispanic Classical Theater, 1998. http://www.comedias.org/tirso/sansas.html. Consulted on 19 Jun. 2012.

Tobin, Ronald. *Tarte à la crème: Comedy and Gastronomy in Molière's Theater*. Columbus: Ohio State University Press, 1990.

Torres de Mendoza, Luis. *Colección de documentos inéditos relativos al descubrimiento, conquista y organización de las antiguas posesiones españolas de América y Oceania: Sacados de los Archivos del Reino, y muy especialmente del de Indias*. Madrid: M. Bernaldo de Quirós, 1868.

Uchamany, Eva Alexandra. *La vida entre el judaísmo y el cristianismo en la Nueva España 1580–1606*. Mexico: Archivo General de la Nación, 1992.

Val, Joaquín del, ed. *Libro del Arte de cocina por Diego Granado*. 1599. Madrid: Sociedad de Bibliófilos españoles, 1971.

Valles Rojo, Julio. *Cocina y alimentación en los siglos XVI y XVII*. [Valladolid]: Junta de Castilla y León, 2007.

– *Don Quijote y Sancho no pudieron ser gastronomos: Algunos pasajes del Quijote relacionados con la comida*. Valladolid [?], Spain: Iberaval, 2005.

– *Saberes y sabores del legado colombiano: Gastronomía y alimentación en España y América. S XVI–XXI*. Valladolid: Ayuntamiento de Valladolid, 2006.

Vassberg, David E. *Land and Society in Golden Age Castile*. Cambridge: Cambridge University Press, 1984.

– *The Village and the Outside World in Golden Age Castile: Mobility and Migration in Everyday Rural Life*. Cambridge: Cambridge University Press, 1996.

Vavilov, Nickolay Ivanovich. *Origin and Geography of Cultivated Plants*. Ed V.R. Dorofeyev. Trans. Doris Löve. Cambridge: Cambridge University Press, 1992.

Vélez de Guevara, Luis. *El diablo cojuelo*. Madrid: Clásicos castellanos, 1918.

La vida de Lazarillo de Tormes y de sus fortunas y adversidades. Ed. Alberto Blecua. Madrid: Castalia, 1982.

Villena, Enrique de. *Arte cisoria*. Ed. Russell V. Brown. Barcelona: Humanitas, 1984.

– *Obras completas*. Ed. Pedro M. Cátedra. Madrid: Turner, 1994–2002.

Vital, Laurent. *Relación del primer viaje de Carlos V a España*. Trans. Bernabé Herrero. Madrid: Artes gráficas, 1958.

Vives, Juan Luis. "Diálogo séptimo: La comida de la escuela." *Linguae Latinae Exercitatio Ejercicios de lengua latina*. Valencia: Ajuntament de Valencia, 1994. 18–25. Biblioteca Valenciana Digital. http://bivaldi.gva.es/va/corpus/unidad.cmd?idCorpus=1&idUnidad=10046&posicion=1. Consulted on 25 Apr. 2015.

Wagschal, Steven. "The Smellscape of *Don Quixote*: A Cognitive Approach." *Cervantes* 32.1 (spring 2012): 125–62.

Waines, David. "The Culinary Culture of Al-Andalus." *The Legacy of Muslim Spain*. Ed. Salma Khadra Jayyusi. New York: Brill, 1994. 725–38.

Watson, Andrew M. *Agricultural Innovation in the Early Islamic World: The Diffusion of Crops and Farming Techniques, 700–1100*. Cambridge: Cambridge University Press, 1983.

Waxman, Samuel M. "Chapters on Magic in Spanish Literature." *Revue Hispanique* 38 (1916): 325–463.

Wolfenzon, Carolyn. "La lozana andaluza: Judaísmo, sífilis, exilio y creación." *Hispanic Research Journal* 8.2 (April 2007): 107–22.

WorldCat Advanced Search. OCLC Online Computer Library Center. http://firstsearch.oclc.org.proxy.iwu.edu/WebZ/FSPrefs?entityjsdetect=:javascript

=true:screensize=large:sessionid=fsapp5-35179-i9ccalh8-vi71us:entitypage-num=1:0. Consulted on 25 Oct. 2014.

Wuthnow, Robert, James Davison Hunter, Albert Bergesen, and Edith Kurzweil, *Cultural Analysis: The Work of Peter L. Berger, Mary Douglas, Michel Foucault, and Jürgen Habermas*. Boston: Routledge and Kegan, 1984.

Yates, Francis A. *Giordano Bruno and the Hermetic Tradition* Chicago: University of Chicago Press, 1964.

Yun Casalilla, Bartolomé. *Sobre la transición al capitalismo en Castilla: Economía y sociedad en Tierra de Campos (1500–1830)*. Valladolid: Junta de Castilla y León, 1987.

Index of Recipes

General Index

TORONTO IBERIC

1 Anthony J. Cascardi, *Cervantes, Literature, and the Discourse of Politics*
2 Jessica A. Boon, *The Mystical Science of the Soul: Medieval Cognition in Bernardino de Laredo's Recollection Method*
3 Susan Byrne, *Law and History in Cervantes'* Don Quixote
4 Mary E. Barnard and Frederick A. de Armas (eds), *Objects of Culture in the Literature of Imperial Spain*
5 Nil Santiáñez, *Topographies of Fascism: Habitus, Space, and Writing in Twentieth-Century Spain*
6 Nelson Orringer, *Lorca in Tune with Falla: Literary and Musical Interludes*
7 Ana M. Gómez-Bravo, *Textual Agency: Writing Culture and Social Networks in Fifteenth-Century Spain*
8 Javier Irigoyen-García, *The Spanish Arcadia: Sheep Herding, Pastoral Discourse, and Ethnicity in Early Modern Spain*
9 Stephanie Sieburth, *Survival Songs: Conchita Piquer's* Coplas *and Franco's Regime of Terror*
10 Christine Arkinstall, *Spanish Female Writers and the Freethinking Press, 1879–1926*
11 Margaret Boyle, *Unruly Women: Performance, Penitence, and Punishment in Early Modern Spain*